Modern Concepts of
Acute and
Chronic Hepatitis

Modern Concepts of
Acute and
Chronic Hepatitis

Edited by
GARY GITNICK, M. D.

University of California at Los Angeles
School of Medicine
Los Angeles, California

PLENUM MEDICAL BOOK COMPANY
NEW YORK AND LONDON

Library of Congress Cataloging in Publication Data

Modern concepts of acute and chronic hepatitis / edited by Gary Gitnick.
    p.   cm.
  Includes bibliographies and index.

  ISBN-13: 978-1-4615-9521-2   e-ISBN-13: 978-1-4615-9519-9
  DOI: 10.1007/978-1-4615-9519-9

  1. Hepatitis. I. Gitnick, Gary L.
  [DNLM: 1. Hepatitis. WI 700 M691]
RC848.H42M63   1989
616.3′623 — dc19
DNLM/DLC   88-22557
for Library of Congress   CIP

© 1989 Plenum Publishing Corporation
Softcover reprint of the hardcover 1st edition 1989

233 Spring Street, New York, N.Y. 10013

Plenum Medical Book Company is an imprint of Plenum Publishing Corporation

This book is dedicated to my family—

my wife Cherna;
our children Neil, Kim, Jill, and Tracy;
and our parents Ann, Sonia, and Jack.

Contributors

Ferruccio Bonino • Division of Gastroenterology, San Giovanni Battista Molinette Hospital, 10126 Turin, Italy

John Bartels • Division of Allergy, Immunology, and Infectious Diseases, University of Medicine and Dentistry of New Jersey, New Brunswick, New Jersey 08903-0019

Albert J. Czaja • Division of Gastroenterology, Mayo Clinic and Mayo Medical School, Rochester, Minnesota 55905

Gary L. Davis • Division of Gastroenterology, Hepatology, and Nutrition, University of Florida College of Medicine, Gainesville, Florida 32610

V. J. Desmet • Laboratory of Cytochemistry and Histochemistry, University Hospital St. Raphael, Catholic University, Leuven, B-3000 Leuven, Belgium

Stephen M. Feinstone • Laboratory of Infectious Diseases, National Institute of Allergy and Infectious Diseases, National Institutes of Health, Bethesda, Maryland 20892

Michael A. Gerber • Department of Pathology, Tulane University School of Medicine, New Orleans, Louisiana 70112

Gary Gitnick • Department of Medicine, University of California at Los Angeles School of Medicine, Los Angeles, California 90024

David J. Gocke • Division of Allergy, Immunology, and Infectious Diseases, University of Medicine and Dentistry of New Jersey, New Brunswick, New Jersey 08903-0019

George F. Grady • Massachusetts Center for Disease Control, Department of Public Health, and Department of Medicine, Tufts University School of Medicine, Boston, Massachusetts 02130

Ian D. Gust • Macfarlane Burnet Centre for Medical Research, Fairfield Hospital, Melbourne, Australia 3078

Raymond S. Koff • Department of Medicine, Framingham Union Hospital, Framingham, Massachusetts 01701; and Division of Medicine, Boston University School of Medicine, Boston, Massachusetts 02118

Ronald L. Koretz • Division of Gastroenterology, Olive View Medical Center, Sylmar, California 91342; and Department of Medicine, University of California School of Medicine, Los Angeles, California 90024

Saul Krugman • Department of Pediatrics, New York University Medical Center, New York, New York 10016

Christopher D. Lind • Division of Gastroenterology, Hepatology, and Nutrition, University of Florida College of Medicine, Gainesville, Florida 32610

Jurgen Ludwig • Departments of Medicine and Pathology, Mayo Clinic and Foundation, Rochester, Minnesota 55905

Ian R. Mackay • Clinical Research Unit of the Walter and Eliza Hall Institute of Medical Research and the Royal Melbourne University, Victoria 3050, Australia

Jack Peicher • Department of Gastroenterology, University of Southern California, Los Angeles, California 90033

Robert P. Perrillo • Gastroenterology Section, Veterans Administration Medical Center; and Division of Gastroenterology, Washington University School of Medicine, St. Louis, Missouri 63106

Hans Popper • The Lillian and Henry M. Stratton–Hans Popper Department of Pathology, Mount Sinai School of Medicine of the City University of New York, New York 10029

Jorge Rakela • Departments of Medicine and Pathology, Mayo Clinic and Foundation, Rochester, Minnesota 55905

Fredric G. Regenstein • Gastroenterology Section, Veterans Administration Medical Center; and Division of Gastroenterology, Washington University School of Medicine, St. Louis, Missouri 63106

Mario Rizzetto • Division of Gastroenterology, San Giovanni Battista Molinette Hospital, 10126 Turin, Italy

Eugene R. Schiff • Division of Hepatology, University of Miami School of Medicine, and Hepatology Section, Veterans Administration Medical Center, Miami, Florida 33125

Roger D. Soloway • Department of Medicine, University of Texas Medical Branch, Galveston, Texas 77550-2778

Andrew Stolz • Department of Medicine, UCLA School of Medicine, Los Angeles, California 90024; and Wadsworth Veterans Administration Center, Los Angeles, California 90073

Swan N. Thung • The Lillian and Henry M. Stratton–Hans Popper Department of Pathology, Mount Sinai School of Medicine of the City University of New York, New York 10029

Victor M. Villarejos • International Center for Medical Research and Training, Louisiana State University, San Jose, Costa Rica

Barbara G. Werner • Massachusetts Center for Disease Control, Department of Public Health, and Department of Medicine, Tufts University School of Medicine, Boston, Massachusetts 02130

Preface

The literature of medicine continues to expand at a remarkable pace. The number of papers and monographs published has increased dramatically in the past five years. Nowhere has this increase been as dramatic as in the field of acute and chronic hepatitis. Why then should there be still another book?

Despite the sheer volume of words published, it is still difficult to find in any one volume a compilation of all of the most significant work. Most monographs have considered either chronic or acute hepatitis, not both. Few works have addressed both the clinician and the basic scientist. This book addresses both of these audiences and considers both of these diseases. It was designed to provide an authoritative but concise assessment of our changing concepts of acute and chronic hepatitis. It covers what is currently known and, based on the most convincing research, believed about these diseases. To fulfill this ambitious goal, only authors with international reputations in their fields of expertise were invited to contribute.

In the evolution of our current thoughts on the pathogenesis and management of acute and chronic hepatitis, our ideas have changed several times. This book presents the facts as they are known today and, in areas where all the facts are not established, presents the well-founded opinions of those considered to be authorities. The authors present established and usually confirmed data and do not deal extensively with areas of speculation or unconfirmed material.

Accordingly, the reader of this text will not find an extensive discussion of the utilization of interferon in the management of acute or chronic hepatitis simply because the available data remain too uncertain to offer reliable guidelines. On the other hand, the book does describe new and as yet incompletely developed topics such as the use of the hepatitis B virus DNA assay and the development of an unconfirmed assay for non-A, non-B hepatitis. The former subject is covered here because a number of groups have contributed sufficient findings to justify its discussion within the limits of the available data. The latter is presented because although the data have not been confirmed, the material, while controversial, is of such far-reaching interest that the authors and editor felt justified in including it.

This text attempts then to reach a balance between that which is currently accepted and thought to be established and that which is new and of reasonable importance.

Mrs. Susan Dashe was responsible for the administrative organization of this text. She worked diligently to bring together the chapters in a timely manner and to assist the editor in the overall development of the book. I am grateful to her for her superb efforts and her dedication to the development of this text.

                                                                            Gary Gitnick, M.D.
Los Angeles

Contents

I. Acute Hepatitis

III. Chronic Active Hepatitis

Modern Concepts of
Acute and
Chronic Hepatitis

I

Acute Hepatitis

History of Acute Viral Hepatitis

SAUL KRUGMAN

INTRODUCTION

The disease that is called viral hepatitis today has an ancient history. Reports of epidemic jaundice were described in Greece during the fifth century BC, and many outbreaks were described during the nineteenth and twentieth centuries. A review of the medical literature by Blumberg[1] in 1923 revealed that there were 11 outbreaks from 1812 to 1886, 51 from 1886 to 1920, and more than 200 in New York State alone from 1920 to 1922.

Epidemics of so-called "campaign jaundice" were prevalent during various wars. For example, more than 70,000 cases occurred among Union troops during the Civil War, and many hundreds of thousands of cases occurred among American, British, and French troops during World War II. In retrospect, it is likely that these outbreaks were caused by hepatitis A virus (HAV).

The first recognized outbreak of hepatitis B occurred in Bremen, Germany, in 1883.[2] During a smallpox immunization program at that time, many thousands of persons were inoculated with vaccine prepared from glycerinated lymph of human origin. Of 1289 vaccinated shipyard workers, 191 (15%) developed jaundice several weeks to 8 months postinoculation. By contrast, jaundice was not observed in several hundred uninoculated employees. It is likely that the source of the human lymph was a hepatitis B carrier.

During the first half of the twentieth century, outbreaks of "long incubation period" hepatitis were observed in many countries of the world among several groups: (1) patients who attended venereal disease, diabetic, and tuberculosis clinics; (2) persons who received blood transfusions; (3) persons who were inoculated with mumps or measles convalescent serum; and (4) military person-

---

SAUL KRUGMAN • Department of Pediatrics, New York University Medical Center, New York, New York 10016.

nel who received yellow fever vaccine during World War II.[3−6] These infections were caused by the use of hepatitis B-contaminated needles, syringes, blood, and blood products. The yellow fever vaccine at that time contained human serum that was obtained from an unrecognized hepatitis B carrier.

Initially, knowledge of the pathogenesis of the disease was based on clinical and pathologic observations. The concept proposed by Virchow[7] in 1865 was accepted for many years. He proposed that so-called "catarrhal jaundice" was caused by a plug of mucus in the ampulla of Vater. However, the presence of diffuse hepatic necrosis was demonstrated by Eppinger[8] in 1922 and by Rich[9] in 1930. These findings indicated that an infectious agent was the cause of the disease.

During the late 1930s and early 1940s, studies in human volunteers by various investigators in Europe and in the United States provided convincing evidence of a viral etiology.[10−13] Their findings indicated that two viral agents were responsible for the epidemics of jaundice in military personnel during World War II. At that time, MacCallum[14] proposed the terminology of hepatitis A virus (HAV) and hepatitis B virus (HBV). The evidence for two types of viral hepatitis was based on differences in the incubation period and on presumed differences in the mode of transmission.

Human volunteer studies during the 1940s revealed that feces or serum obtained during the acute phase of infectious hepatitis (hepatitis A) induced the disease after an incubation period of 15–33 days. By contrast, acute-phase serum obtained from patients with homologous serum jaundice (hepatitis B) induced the disease after a longer incubation period (50–160 days). Both Havens et al.[15] and Neefe et al.[13] failed to transmit hepatitis B by oral inoculation of infectious serum that produced the disease regularly when administered parenterally. On the basis of these findings, it was assumed that percutaneous inoculation was the only mode of transmission of HBV.

The observations of the epidemiology, natural history, and prevention of hepatitis A and hepatitis B during the 1940s were confirmed and extended during the course of a study by Murray[16] and by our Willowbrook hepatitis studies begun during the mid-1950s. The development of serum enzyme assays in 1955 provided sensitive markers of hepatitis infection with or without jaundice. The ability to detect anicteric hepatitis enabled us to clarify further the epidemiology of the disease.[17]

During the 1960s, we identified two types of viral hepatitis; each type had distinctive epidemiologic, clinical, and immunologic features.[18] One type, designated MS-1, resembled hepatitis A, and the other, designated MS-2, resembled hepatitis B. The MS-2 strain of hepatitis B was infectious orally as well as parenterally. Therefore, contrary to the prevailing concept at that time, the findings indicated that hepatitis B could be transmitted from person to person by intimate physical contact. These new epidemiologic findings were confirmed during the late 1960s, when the discovery of Australia antigen by Blumberg *et al.*[19] and its association with hepatitis B[20] led to the development of specific tests for identification of hepatitis B infections. The Willowbrook studies confirmed the existence of homologous immunity following hepatitis A and hepatitis B infections. However, one hepatitis agent did not confer immunity against the other virus.

The period between the mid-1960s and the mid-1980s proved to be a golden era in the history of hepatitis A and hepatitis B research. Other types of hepatitis that were identified included hepatitis D, non-A, non-B (NANB), and epidemic NANB hepatitis.

HEPATITIS A

In 1973, Feinstone *et al.*[21] detected HAV particles in stools from patients who were infected with the MS-1 strain of the virus. The identification of hepatitis A antigen in stool specimens and in the liver of marmoset monkeys provided a source of hepatitis A antigen (HAAg). By the mid-1970s, highly sensitive immunoassays were developed for the detection of HAV and its antibody (anti-HAV). The development of IgM-specific anti-HAV serologic tests enabled physicians to distinguish recent HAV infection from a past infection.

The first successful cultivation of HAV was reported by Provost and Hilleman[22] in 1979. This important contribution was confirmed by other investigators; it provided the technology needed for the development of a hepatitis A vaccine.

The RNA genome of HAV, a picornavirus, was molecularly cloned and partially sequenced during the 1980s. These clones can be used as sensitive probes for the detection of viral RNA in clinical samples and cell cultures. These new developments make it possible to prepare genetically engineered hepatitis A vaccines.

HEPATITIS B

The sequence of events that led to the identification of HBV began in 1965, when Blumberg and colleagues identified an antigen in serum obtained from an Australian aborigine. The subsequent association of the Australia antigen with hepatitis B was confirmed by various investigators. Extensive studies during the 1960s and 1970s revealed the distribution of this antigen in various population groups and in patients whose diseases appeared to be unrelated to hepatitis B. Seroepidemiologic surveys found Australia antigen to be present in the blood of 0.1–0.3% of healthy donors, in 10–20% of persons living in various African and Asian countries, in 10–15% of patients with leukemia or Hodgkin's disease, in 20–30% of institutionalized patients with Downs' syndrome, and in about 20% of patients with viral hepatitis.

The convincing data to support the conclusion that Australia antigen was a hepatitis B antigen were reported by Prince[20] and by Giles *et al.*[23] Thus, it was obvious that the prevalence of the Austrialia antigen in African and Asian persons and in patients with leukemia and Downs' syndrome indicated that these high-risk groups were likely to contract chronic hepatitis B infection.

Electron microscopic studies by Dane *et al.*[24] in 1970 demonstrated the presence of a 42-nm particle in the blood of patients with hepatitis B. The surface component of this particle was shown to be immunologically distinct from the core component. The accumulated evidence indicated that the Dane particle was HBV; its surface component was designated as hepatitis B surface antigen (HB_sAg). The core component contained endogenous DNA and hepatitis core antigen (HB_cAg). A third antigen related to infectivity, hepatitis B e antigen (HB_eAg), was subsequently described by Magnius and Espmark[25] in 1972.

The development and use of sensitive specific markers of hepatitis B infection enabled many investigators to clarify the natural history of hepatitis B infection. During the 1970s, it was observed that chronic hepatitis B infection was a possible cause of cirrhosis of the liver[26,27] and primary hepatocellular carcinoma.

The development of tests to measure hepatitis B antibody provided the technology to identify units of blood that contained anti-HB_s. These antibody-positive units were used for the preparation of hepatitis B immunoglobulin (HBIG). Our preliminary studies indicated that HBIG was effective for the prevention of modification of hepatitis B.[28]

During the course of our studies on the natural history of hepatitis B, in 1970 we developed, by serendipity, a crude inactivated hepatitis B vaccine. This development was the result of an investigation designed to determine the effect of heat (boiling for 1 min) on the infectivity of a 1 : 10 dilution of MS-2 serum in distilled water.[29] A previous study had revealed the presence of HBV and HB_sAg in MS-2 serum. The 1-min boil destroyed the infectivity of HBV, but the heat-inactivated MS-2 serum proved antigenic. Later, it was shown that the inactivated MS-2 serum was immunogenic and partially protective; it possessed the characteristics of an inactivated hepatitis B vaccine.[28] By 1975, various investigators had developed plasma-derived subunit hepatitis B vaccines.[29,30] The successful cloning of HB_sAg by DNA recombinant technology led to the development and licensure of a yeast recombinant hepatitis B vaccine by 1987.

HEPATITIS D VIRUS

Rizzetto[31] detected by immunofluorescence an antigen in liver cell nuclei and in the serum of HBsAg carriers who had chronic liver disease. This unique antigen (HDAg) was distinct from HB_cAg. Studies in chimpanzees have revealed that it is a transmissible agent associated with but distinct from HBV. It is a 35-nm particle containing an RNA core and HBsAg as its surface component. Replication of this agent is initiated and maintained by the helper function provided by HBV infection. Delta infection of a chronic hepatitis B carrier may increase the risk of a complicating fulminant hepatitis B infection.

NON-A, NON-B HEPATITIS

Before the 1970s, hepatitis B was the most commonly recognized cause of posttransfusion hepatitis. In spite of the institution of routine screening of blood for HB_sAg and the recruitment of an all-volunteer blood donor population, the problem of posttransfusion hepatitis was not solved. It soon became apparent that NANB agents were present in the blood of certain donors.[32] Today, certain NANB hepatitis viruses are the causative agents of more than 90% of cases of posttransfusion hepatitis in the United States. It has been estimated that 0.5–8% of U.S. blood donors are asymptomatic carriers of these viruses. Unfortunately, to date, these agents have not been characterized. No specific tests are available for the identification of NANB hepatitis carriers.

EPIDEMIC NON-A, NON-B HEPATITIS

Seroepidemiologic studies of waterborne epidemics of hepatitis in India, Asia, and South America demonstrated no evidence of HAV or HBV infection. This epidemic form of NANB hepatitis has features different from hepatitis A: (1) longer incubation period (mean, 40 days), (2) older age distribution (mean, 27 years), (3) high mortality in pregnant women, and (4) high fetal wastage.[33,34]

CONCLUSION

Progress in viral hepatitis research during the past two decades has been phenomenal. The explosion of new knowledge has improved our understanding of the natural history of HAV, HBV, HDV, and NANB hepatitis infection. The appropriate use of safe and effective plasma-derived and recombinant hepatitis B vaccines should protect millions of infants, children, and adults worldwide.

Meantime, viral hepatitis continues to be a major public health problem, and it is a significant physical, emotional, and economic burden to humankind throughout most of the world.

REFERENCES

1. Blumberg G: Infectious jaundice in the United States. *JAMA* **81**:353–358, 1923.
2. Lurman A: Eine icterusepidemie. *Berl Klin Wochenschr* **22**:20–23, 1855.
3. Flaum A, Malmros, H, Persson E: Eine nosocomiale icterus epidemic. *Acta Med Scand (Suppl)* **16**:544–553, 1926.
4. Findlay GM, MacCallum FO: Note on acute hepatitis and yellow fever immunization. *Trans R Soc Trop Med Hyg* **51**:297–308, 1937.
5. Beeson PB: Jaundice occurring one to four months after transfusion of blood or plasma. Report of seven cases. *JAMA* **121**:1332–1334, 1943.
6. Beeson PB, Chesney G, McFarlan AM: Hepatitis after injection of mumps convalescent plasma. 1. Use of plasma in mumps epidemic. *Lancet* **1**:814–815, 1944.
7. Virchow R: Uber das Vorkommen aund den Nachweiss des Hepatogenen, insbesondere des Katarrhalischen Icterius. *Virchows Arch Pathol Anat Physiol* **32**:117–125, 1865.
8. Eppinger H: Die pathogenese des icterus. *Verh Dtsch Gesell int Med* **34**:15, 1922.
9. Rich AR: The pathogenesis of the forms of jaundice. *Bull Johns Hopkins Hosp* **47**:338–377, 1930.
10. Voegt H: Zur aetiologie der hepatitis epidemica. *MMW* **89**:76–79, 1942.
11. Havens WP Jr, Ward R, Drill VA, et al: Experimental production of hepatitis by feeding icterogenic materials. *Proc Soc Exp Biol Med* **57**:206–208, 1944.
12. Neefe JR, Stokes J Jr, Gellis SS: Homologous serum hepatitis and infectious (epidemic) hepatitis. *Am J Med Sci* **210**:561–575, 1945.
13. Neefe JR, Gellis SS, Stokes J Jr: Homologous serum hepatitis and infectious (epidemic) hepatitis: Studies in volunteers bearing on immunological and other characteristics of the etiological agents. *Am J Med* **1**:3–22, 1946.
14. MacCallum FO: Homologous serum jaundice. *Lancet* **2**:691–692, 1947.
15. Havens WP Jr: The period of infectivity of patients with homologous serum jaundice and routes of infection in this disease. *J Exp Med* **83**:441–447, 1946.
16. Murray R: Viral hepatitis. *Bull NY Acad Med* **31**:341–358, 1955.
17. Krugman S, Giles JP: Viral hepatitis, type B (MS-2 strain): Further observations on natural ' history and prevention. *N Engl J Med* **288**: 755–760, 1973.
18. Krugman S, Giles JP, Hammond J: Infectious hepatitis: Evidence for two distinctive clinical, epidemiological and immunological types of infection. *JAMA* **200**:365–373, 1967.
19. Blumberg BS, Alter HJ, Visnich S: A "new" antigen in leukemia sera. *JAMA* **191**:541–546, 1967.
20. Prince AM: An antigen detected in the blood during the incubation period of serum hepatitis. *Proc Natl Acad Sci USA* **60**:814–821, 1968.
21. Feinstone SM, Kapikian AZ, Purcell RH: Hepatitis A: Detection by immune electron microscopy of a viruslike antigen associated with acute illness. *Science* **182**:1026–1028, 1973.
22. Provost P, Hilleman MR: Propagation of human hepatitis A virus in cell culture *in vitro. Proc Soc Exp Biol Med* **160**:213–221, 1979.
23. Giles JP, McCollum RW, Berndson LWJ, Krugman S: Viral hepatitis: Relationship of Australia/SH antigen to the Willowbrook MS-2 strain. *N Engl J Med* **281**:119–122, 1969.

24. Dane DS, Cameron CH, Briggs NM: Virus-like particles in serum of patients with Australia antigen-associated hepatitis. *Lancet* **1**:695–698, 1970.

25. Magnius LO, Espmark JA; Specificities in Australia antigen-positive sera distinct from the Le Bouvier determinants. *J Immunol* **109**:1017–1021, 1972.

26. Gitnick, GL, Schoenfield LJ, Sutnick AL, et al: Australia antigen in chronic active liver disease with cirrhosis. *Lancet* **2**:285–288, 1969.

27. Wright R, McCollum RW, Klatskin G: Australia antigen in acute and chronic liver disease. *Lancet* **2**:7–121, 1969.

28. Krugman S, Giles JP, Hammond J: Viral hepatitis type B: Prevention with specific hepatitis B immune serum globulin. *JAMA* **218**:1665–1670, 1971.

29. Hilleman MR, Buynak EB, Roehm RR, et al: Purified and inactivated human hepatitis B vaccine. A progress report. *Am J Med Sci* **270**: 401–404, 1975.

30. Purcell RH, Gerin JL: Hepatitis B subunit vaccine: A preliminary report of safety and efficacy in chimpanzees. *Am J Med Sci* **270**:395–399, 1975.

31. Rizzeto M, Canese MG, Arico S: Immunofluorescence detection of a new antigen–antibody system (anti) associated to hepatitis B in liver and in serum of HBsAg carriers. *Gut* **18**:997–1003, 1977.

32. Prince AM, Brotman B, Grady GF, et al: Long-incubation posttransfusion hepatitis without serologic evidence of exposure to hepatitis B virus. *Lancet* **2**:241–246, 1974.

33. Khuroo MS: Study of an epidemic of non-A, non-B hepatitis: Possibility of another human hepatitis virus distinct from posttransfusion non-A, non-B type. *Am J Med* **68**:818–824, 1980.

34. Wong DC, Purcell RH, Sreenivasan, et al: Epidemic and endemic hepatitis in India: Evidence for a non-A, non-B hepatitis virus aetiology. *Lancet* **2**:876–879, 1980.

The Clinical Features of Acute Viral Hepatitis

RAYMOND S. KOFF

INTRODUCTION

Acute viral hepatitis attributable to infection by the hepatitis A virus (HAV), the hepatitis B virus (HBV), the hepatitis D (delta) virus, and any of the three or more non-A, non-B hepatitis viruses is associated with a broad spectrum of clinical features. This spectrum largely reflects the severity of illness and varies enormously from inapparent asymptomatic infection at one extreme, through symptomatic anicteric and icteric hepatitis, to confluent hepatic necrosis and fatal fulminant hepatitis at the other. It would be misleading to suggest that all clinical features are associated with disease severity; a set of extrahepatic syndromes, which appear to have no direct relationship to the severity of illness, is also encountered during the course of a variable proportion of viral hepatitis cases. These are either manifestations of extrahepatic tissue damage directly induced by the agents of viral hepatitis (an example of which may be the association of aplastic anemia with non-A, non-B viral hepatitis[1]) or immunologically mediated tissue injury. The serum sickness-like syndrome seen in hepatitis B is the classic example of the latter. It should be emphasized that while certain clinical features suggest infection with a specific type of viral hepatitis, absolute differentiation of etiologic agents in individual cases cannot be undertaken on this basis alone.

Most patients who are recognized to have acute viral hepatitis exhibit a

RAYMOND S. KOFF • Department of Medicine, Framingham Union Hospital, Framingham, Massachusetts 01701; and Division of Medicine, Boston University School of Medicine, Boston, Massachusetts 02118.

typical constellation of features. While most of these features are well known to the practitioner, when they appear as singular manifestations, which they occasionally do, unaccompanied by other characteristic symptoms, diagnostic accuracy may suffer. In addition to this issue, atypical clinical patterns, such as cholestatic and relapsing hepatitis, are seen in a small number of affected patients and present other diagnostic concerns. Other clinical variants, such as prolonged hepatitis and the syndrome of fulminant hepatitis, are discussed elsewhere in this volume.

INAPPARENT ASYMPTOMATIC HEPATITIS

Recognition of this form of acute viral hepatitis is infrequent. It produces no symptoms. It is detected only by the demonstration of laboratory abnormalities in persons who are monitored because of exposure to hepatitis or in whom fortuitous screening shows evidence of mild hepatocellular injury or serologic evidence of acute hepatitis infection. Inapparent asymptomatic hepatitis has been identified in all etiologic forms of human viral hepatitis: hepatitis A, hepatitis B, hepatitis D, and infections caused by non-A, non-B viral hepatitis agents. These instances of inapparent asymptomatic hepatitis virus infection appear to be particularly common in infants and young children, in transfusion-associated hepatitis (largely non-A, non-B infections), and in populations in which susceptibility to persistent HBV infection may be increased. The contrast between asymptomatic and symptomatic hepatitis in different age groups has been particularly well established in outbreaks of hepatitis A. In most cases of hepatitis A in children aged 2 years or younger, the disease is asymptomatic or unrecognized as viral hepatitis.[2] By contrast, symptomatic hepatitis has been reported in 75–97% of adults with hepatitis A; 40–70% of these cases were associated with jaundice.[3]

Although most of these inapparent asymptomatic infections are associated with mild and transient serum aminotransferase elevations, in some patients with hepatitis A, B, or D (always associated with HBV infection) serologic evidence of acute infection without laboratory features of hepatitis may be identified. Undoubtedly, when serologic markers of non-A, non-B hepatitis virus infections become available, these agents will also be shown occasionally to produce infections without evidence of hepatocellular injury.

It should be emphasized that at this time some serum aminotransferase elevations may be inappropriately attributed to sporadic non-A, non-B viral hepatitis. Drug ingestion or systemic disorders may be responsible for the laboratory abnormalities identified in some of these patients. Misclassification as non-A, non-B viral hepatitis reflects diagnostic confusion. The frequency with which this error occurs is unknown and will remain uncertain until specific serologic markers of infection by these non-A, non-B hepatitis agents become available. In the interim, the diagnosis of sporadic non-A, non-B hepatitis should not be considered definitive, and careful review of the drug history and identification of other coexisting diseases are essential.

SYMPTOMATIC HEPATITIS

Symptomatic acute viral hepatitis may be anicteric or icteric. Infrequently, jaundice may be recognized in an asymptomatic person in whom serologic or other evidence of acute hepatitis is present on laboratory testing. In general, the clinical features of anicteric hepatitis are similar to those of icteric hepatitis, but the intensity and duration of symptoms may be reduced and abbreviated in those with anicteric disease. Transient unexplained fever, symptoms of an upper respiratory infection, and symptoms of gastroenteritis, either alone or in combination, may be the sole clinical manifestations of anicteric viral hepatitis. The characteristic malaise, fatigue, and anorexia of icteric hepatitis may be so diminishing in severity that the affected patient fails to seek medical attention.

The symptoms of acute hepatitis are nearly identical in all etiologic forms of viral hepatitis, although some sets of features are more suggestive of specific etiologic agents. For example, in most adult patients with acute hepatitis A, the clinical onset of illness appears to be rather abrupt and patients may often identify a specific day on which they first developed symptoms and became ill. By contrast, in hepatitis B, hepatitis D, and non-A, non-B hepatitis virus infections, the onset of symptoms is usually more insidious and the transition from health to illness cannot be pinpointed as readily as in hepatitis A. Fever and headache are more commonly described in hepatitis A than in the other etiologic forms. Despite these observations, only serologic studies are reliable enough to distinguish between the etiologic agents.

Prodromal Features

During the acute phase of illness, a variety of symptoms may be identified before the recognition of jaundice. In a small proportion of patients, no symptoms occur before the onset of jaundice. When it does occur, the prodromal phase is variable in duration but tends to be shorter in hepatitis A than in hepatitis B, hepatitis D, or non-A, non-B viral hepatitis. In hepatitis A, the average duration of preicteric symptoms is a few days to about 1 week in most cases. In about 3–10% of cases, the preicteric phase may exceed 1 week, and in some cases it may last as long as 2 weeks. In hepatitis B, the preicteric phase may be considerably prolonged and in some cases has been as long as 2 months. Preicteric phases of less than 1 week are seen in only 25% of hepatitis B cases. Prodromal features of hepatitis D and non-A, non-B viral hepatitis are often so transient that a true prodrome may fail to be recognized before the onset of jaundice. However, documentation of a prodrome closely resembling that of hepatitis B, with a serum sickness-like syndrome, has been reported in non-A, non-B viral hepatitis.[4] In sporadic non-A, non-B viral hepatitis a preicteric phase of more than 2 weeks duration was seen in 95% of cases.[5]

Prodromal features include a variety of constitutional, gastrointestinal (GI), and respiratory symptoms and a set of extrahepatic serum sickness-like syndromes involving the skin, joints, kidneys, and small blood vessels. The main features of the clinical disease include lassitude, fatigue, anorexia, nausea and vomiting, abdominal discomfort (usually in the right upper quadrant), fever (rarely exceeding 39°C), chilliness (without shaking chills), headache, flulike symptoms, nasal discharge, sore throat, and cough. Anorexia may be most striking in the afternoon and evening; lunch and dinner are often poorly tolerated. Abnormalities in gustatory and olfactory acuity have been identified in affected patients. Loss of taste for food may be accompanied by loss of taste for cigarettes. This finding is not specific for acute viral hepatitis (it may be noted in drug-induced hepatitis, alcoholic hepatitis, and hepatic congestion due to heart failure), and it has become less relevant, since the number of cigarette smokers has diminished. Although vomiting is a common feature of the acute illness, it is rarely severe or prolonged in patients with typical acute viral hepatitis. Pernicious vomiting, leading to dehydration and electrolyte abnormalities, suggests an atypical, more serious, variant of viral hepatitis. In uncomplicated cases, a weight loss of < 5 kg may occur during the prodrome and acute phase of illness.

Myalgias and photophobia are described and diffuse arthralgias may be seen in as many as one third of patients. However, a history of arthralgias can be elicited in only about 10% of patients with hepatitis A.[6,7] Whether arthralgias represent a constitutional symptom or a *forme fruste* of the serum sickness-like syndrome remains uncertain, although the latter seems unlikely because the full-blown serum sickness syndrome appears to be extremely rare in hepatitis A.

Frank arthritis, angioedema, urticaria, and maculopapular eruptions are the major extrahepatic immunologically mediated manifestations observed during the prodrome of viral hepatitis. Frank arthritis is most closely associated with hepatitis B. During the prodrome of the illness, 1–10% of patients with hepatitis B may have evidence of an acute migratory polyarthritis. A similar syndrome is rarely found in non-A, non-B viral hepatitis[4] and has yet to be reported with certainty in hepatitis A as a prodromal symptom. However, in relapsing hepatitis A virus infection, isolated instances of arthritis and vasculitis associated with cryoglobulinemia were recently described.[8] The arthritis of hepatitis B is typically a symmetric polyarthritis affecting the distal joints (e.g., the proximal interphalangeal joints), but larger axial and appendicular joints also have been involved. A superficial resemblance to acute rheumatoid arthritis has been noted, but the viral hepatitis-associated disease usually subsides with the development of jaundice, and residual joint disease is not seen. Skin rashes have been reported in as many as one third of patients with viral hepatitis[9] and have been described in all etiologic forms (its occurrence in hepatitis D is uncertain, since rashes in this setting may be attributable to hepatitis B). Angioedema and urticarial eruptions may develop during the prodrome of hepatitis B and may be associated with arthritic symptoms. The most common rash, regardless of etiologic form, is a transient macular erythema. A papular eruption is also seen in some patients, and a papulovesicular eruption localized to the trunk and anterior surfaces of the upper extremities, with or without pruritus, has been described in transfusion-associated and sporadic non-A, non-B viral hepatitis.[9] In a small number of these patients, skin biopsies failed to demonstrate evidence of deposition of immunoglobulin or complement components in tissue samples. The mechanisms responsible for these lesions remains to be established.

A rare skin lesion in the United States, but not uncommonly observed in Japan and Italy, termed the Gianotti–Crosti syndrome or papular acrodermatitis of childhood, has been associated with hepatitis B, hepatitis A, and other non-hepatitis infectious agents.[10–12] In affected infants and children with anicteric hepatitis B, the syndrome is characterized by the occurrence of nonpruritic symmetric flat papules on the face, extremities, and buttocks, associated with lymphadenopathy. The cutaneous lesions may persist for several weeks.

Necrotizing vasculitis, with or without glomerulonephritis, has been associated with HBV infections. While in most reported cases the vasculitis and renal abnormalities have been correlated with persistent HBV infection, there is anecdotal evidence that vasculitis and glomerulonephritis may rarely become manifest during the acute phase of infection. Acute Raynaud's phenomenon with digital vasospasm and infarction of the fingers has been reported during the incubation period of hepatitis B.[13] Vasculitis has rarely been identified as a consequence of relapsing HAV infection.[8]

Myocarditis was reported in a patient with fulminant hepatitis B in whom HB$_s$Ag was identified in endothelial cells of intramyocardial blood vessels but not in extracardiac vessels or renal glomeruli.[14] These observations suggest a selective targeting of extrahepatic tissues in some patients.

In the absence of fulminant hepatitis, neurologic involvement may occur during the prodrome or acute icteric phase of acute viral hepatitis. In isolated cases, the Guillain–Barré syndrome has been recognized during the preicteric phase of hepatitis B[15] and following the onset of jaundice in hepatitis A.[16] Mononeuritis (cranial or peripheral nerve) has been reported in both hepatitis A and hepatitis B during the preicteric and icteric phases of illness.[17]

With the exception of those few patients with extrahepatic manifestations, in whom joint, cutaneous, or neurologic signs may be elicited, physical examination of the patient in the prodrome of typical icteric viral hepatitis may be unrewarding or may reveal minimal hepatomegaly only.

Icteric and Convalescent Phases

Just before the recognition of jaundice, nearly all patients recognize a darkening of the urine to a brownish color. Once jaundice is manifest, nausea and vomiting become less prominent; anorexia, malaise, and weakness may increase briefly before their disappearance. Other constitutional symptoms also tend to resolve following the onset of jaundice. In about one half of patients with typical icteric acute viral hepatitis, pruritus is noted concomitantly with the onset of jaundice or a few days later when jaundice has reached its peak or has begun to recede. With the onset of jaundice, stool color lightens, which may be recognized by as many as 40% of patients during the first week of jaundice.

Jaundice gradually disappears, usually within 2–6 weeks after its onset. In children and in patients with hepatitis A, jaundice tends to be short lived and persists for no longer than 2 weeks in about 85% of cases. In a handful of patients with hepatitis A, prolonged jaundice associated with pruritus may persist for as long as 8 months (cholestatic viral hepatitis). In other etiologic forms of viral hepatitis, particularly hepatitis B and bloodborne non-A, non-B viral hepatitis, the duration of jaundice may be considerably longer than in typical hepatitis A, but the cholestatic variant appears to be exceedingly rare.

In a small number of patients, most of whom have non-A, non-B viral hepatitis, clinical evidence of aplastic anemia may be recognized during the icteric or convalescent phase of illness.[18] While the precise mechanism responsible for this devastating complication is uncertain, a direct attack of the hepatitis agent on the bone marrow has been postulated.

Physical examination may demonstrate slight tenderness over the liver on direct palpation or on light punch percussion over the right upper quadrant. Exquisite tenderness is rarely found; if present, it suggests other diagnoses. The liver is usually enlarged and may measure 12–14 cm in the vertical span. The edge of the liver is usually rounded, but nodularity is not found. In about 10–15% of patients, the spleen tip may be detected,[3] and in a similar proportion posterior cervical lymphadenopathy has been described. Careful examination of the skin will show small spider angiomata in about 5–50% of patients. These findings are transient, rapidly disappearing during the convalescent phase. Ascites and peripheral edema are not present in typical cases; such evidence of sodium and fluid accumulation suggests the presence of a severe variant of viral hepatitis or another disorder. Alterations of mental status are not observed in typical acute hepatitis. Mental slowing, drowsiness, insomnia, and asterixis suggest severe disease, i.e., fulminant hepatic failure.

CLINICAL VARIANTS

Cholestatic Hepatitis

The rare clinical syndrome of cholestatic hepatitis is characterized by pro-longed jaundice, with total serum bilirubin levels in excess of 10 mg/dl, associated with pruritus, fever, diarrhea, and weight loss.[19] Despite these symptoms, most patients feel reasonably well and in time will recover completely without sequelae. Ultrasonographic studies of affected patients show no dilation of the extrahepatic biliary tree. It is worth noting, however, that the gallbladder wall may be transiently thickened, with a double-wall appearance and the presence of sludge within the gallbladder lumen in patients with typical (noncholestatic) acute viral hepatitis.[20] These abnormalities resolve during the convalescent phase. The clinical course of cholestatic hepatitis lasts at least 12 weeks. Serologic studies indicate that hepatitis A is responsible for most instances of cholestatic hepatitis; the role of other agents remains speculative.

Relapsing Hepatitis

Secondary rises in serum aminotransferases associated with recurrent symptoms of hepatitis have been identified in patients with serologically documented hepatitis A.[21] Such relapses have occurred 2–8 weeks after the initial onset of symptoms. In general, the peak aminotransferase level is lower in the secondary rise than in the initial episode. Secondary peak bilirubin levels may be higher or lower than at the initial bout. Despite the prolonged illness associated with relapsing hepatitis, the illness has resolved in most instances.

CONCLUSION

In general, acute viral hepatitis produces a spectrum of clinical illness that varies broadly, regardless of the responsible agent. While some clinical features suggest infection with a specific hepatitis virus, the experienced clinician understands that diagnostic accuracy in individual cases is dependent on serologic testing rather than on clinical acumen. Similarly, when the manifestations of hepatitis occur as singular events, or when extrahepatic features are the most salient symptoms and signs, in the absence of the typical constellation of findings, a high index of suspicion will be required for accurate diagnosis. Recognition of cholestatic and relapsing hepatitis require awareness of these atypical variants in the assessment of the patient in whom an unanticipated course has developed.

REFERENCES

1. Carquel A, Vigano P, Davoli C, et al: Sporadic acute non-A, non-B hepatitis complicated by aplastic anemia. *Am J Gastroenterol* **78**:245–247, 1983.
2. Hadler SC, Webster HM, Erben JJ, et al: Hepatitis A in day-care centers. A community-wide assessment. *N Engl J Med* **302**:1222–1227, 1980.
3. Lednar WM, Lemon SM, Kirkpatrick JW, et al: Frequency of illness associated with epidemic hepatitis A virus infections in adults. *Am J Epidemiol* **122**:226–233, 1985.
4. Perrillo RP, Pohl DA, Roodman ST, et al: Acute non-A, non-B hepatitis with serum sickness-like syndrome and aplastic anemia. *JAMA* **245**:494–496, 1981.
5. Shammaa MH: Acute viral hepatitis in Lebanon: Evidence for an HAV-like non-A, non-B hepatitis. *Liver* **4**:39–44, 1984.
6. Routenberg JA, Dienstag JL, Harrison WO, et al: Foodborne outbreak of hepatitis A: Clinical and laboratory features of acute and protracted illness. *Am J Med Sci* **278**:123–137, 1979.
7. Bamber M, Thomas HC, Bannister B, et al: Acute type A, B, and non-A, non-B hepatitis in a hospital population in London: Clinical and epidemiological features. *Gut* **24**:561–564, 1983.
8. Inman, RD, Hodge M, Johnston MEA, et al: Arthritis, vasculitis, and cryoglobulinemia associated with relapsing hepatitis A virus infection. *Ann Intern Med* **105**:700–703, 1986.
9. Liehr H, Seelig R, Seelig HP: Cutaneous papulo-vesicular eruptions in non-A, non-B hepatitis. *Hepatogastroenterology* **32**:11–14, 1985.
10. Schneider JA, Poley JR, Orcutt MA, et al: Papular acrodermatitis (Gianotti–Crosti syndrome) in a child with anicteric hepatitis B, virus subtype adw. *J Pediatr* **101**:219–222, 1982.
11. Sagi EF, Linder N, Shouval D: Papular acrodermatitis of childhood associated with hepatitis A virus infection. *Pediatr Dermatol* **3**:31–33, 1985.
12. Draelos ZK, Hansen RC, James WD: Gianotti–Crosti syndrome associated with infections other than hepatitis B. *JAMA* **256**:2386–2388, 1986.
13. Cosgriff TM, Arnold WJ: Digital vasospasm and infarction associated with hepatitis B antigenemia. *JAMA* **235**:1362–1363, 1976.
14. Ursell PC, Habib A, Sharma P, et al: Hepatitis B virus and myocarditis. *Hum Pathol* **15**:481–484, 1984.
15. Ng PL, Powell, LW, Campbell CB: Guillain–Barré syndrome during the pre-icteric phase of acute type B viral hepatitis. *Aust NZ J Med* **5**:367–369, 1975.
16. Bosch, VV, Dowling, PC, Cook SD: Hepatitis A virus immunoglobulin M antibody in acute neurological disease. *Ann Neurol* **14**:685–687, 1983.
17. Pelletier G, Elghozi D, Trepo C, et al: Mononeuritis in acute viral hepatitis. *Digestion* **32**:53–56, 1985.
18. Zeldis JB, Dienstag JL, Gale RP: Aplastic anemia and non-A, non-B hepatitis. *Am J Med* **74**:64–68, 1983.
19. Gordon SC, Reddy KR, Schiff L, et al: Prolonged intrahepatic cholestasis secondary to acute hepatitis A. *Ann Intern Med* **101**:635–637, 1984.
20. Maudgal DP, Wansbrough-Jones MH, Joseph AHA: Gallbladder abnormalities in acute infectious hepatitis. A prospective study. *Dig Dis Sci* **29**:257–260, 1984.
21. Jacobson IM, Nath BJ, Dienstag JL: Relapsing viral hepatitis type A. *J Med Virol* **16**:163–169, 1985.

Histopathology and Ultrastructural Features of Acute Hepatitis

SWAN N. THUNG, MICHAEL A. GERBER, and HANS POPPER

INTRODUCTION

Acute and chronic hepatitides represent liver diseases, which pose major public health problems. Since the discovery of hepatitis B surface antigen by Blumberg and colleagues more than 20 years ago,[1] research in viral hepatitis has made rapid progress. Using modern knowledge of viral hepatitis as background, including hepatitis in animal models, this chapter describes its histopathology and immunopathology, employing current views on pathogenesis.

MORPHOLOGY OF CELLULAR ALTERATIONS IN HEPATITIS

Hepatocellular Degeneration, Necrosis, and Regeneration

Hepatocellular degeneration[2] is defined as an alteration unfavorable to the cell, organ, or organism. Light microscopic indications of diffuse hepatocellular degeneration in properly fixed and processed specimens are variations in size, shape, and staining quality of the cytoplasm and nuclei of hepatocytes. These

SWAN N. THUNG and HANS POPPER • The Lillian and Henry M. Stratton–Hans Popper Department of Pathology, Mount Sinai School of Medicine of the City University of New York, New York 10029.   MICHAEL A. GERBER • Department of Pathology, Tulane University School of Medicine, New Orleans, Louisiana 70112.

features correlate electron microscopically with organelle changes and account for the functional deficiency of the viable hepatocytes. This deficient function is reflected in elevation of serum aminotransferase activities and clinically in easy fatigability. Circumscribed hepatocellular degeneration is seen as cytoplasmic alterations, such as swelling or irregular clumping. In its extreme form, the swelling of the cytoplasm is called ballooning or hydropic degeneration (Fig. 1). The cells are enlarged and have pale rarified cytoplasm. They appear empty, with clumps of cytoplasmic remnants around the nucleus. The plasma membrane of the affected cells is indistinct and the nuclei may show karyolysis. Electron microscopic examination shows that ballooning is associated with dilation of the cisternae of the endoplasmic reticulum with detachment of ribosomes and loss of glycogen from the cytoplasm.[3] These cells may undergo a rapid lytic process and disappear (drop out). Remnants of these cells attract lymphocytes and macrophages and less often other types of inflammatory cells. The entire lesion is described as focal necrosis (Fig. 2). Clumping or condensation of the cytoplasm represents another type of hepatocellular degeneration associated with loss of the basophilic nucleic acids, the eosinophilic degeneration.[4] The hepatocytes shrink, develop an angular or rhomboid shape, and appear darker and more eosinophilic than the neighboring hepatocytes. These cells eventually round up and are extruded from the liver cell plates into the perisinusoidal or Disse spaces to become eosinophilic bodies (Fig. 3). Ultrastructurally, these degenerating cells shrink and have electron-dense cytoplasm. Although eosinophilic bodies are less common than ballooned cells, they are more conspicuous because they live longer than the ballooned cells. Focal necrosis and eosinophilic bodies can occur in any lesion with hepatocellular necrosis but are most conspicuous in acute viral hepa-

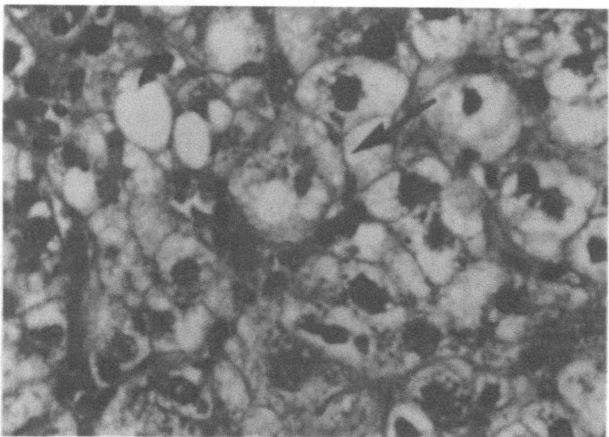

FIGURE 1. Ballooning or hydropic degeneration of hepatocyte (arrow). The cell is enlarged and has pale rarified cytoplasm and karyolysis of the nucleus. (H&E.)

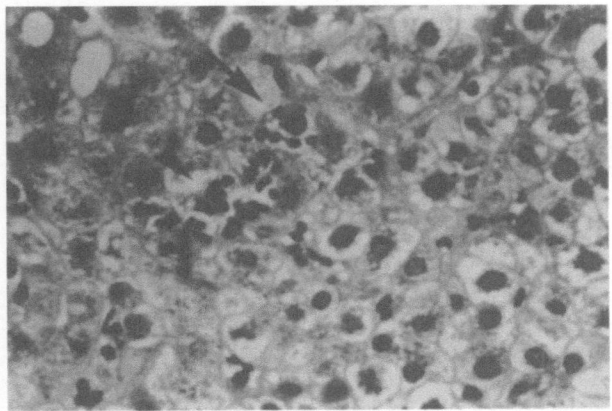

FIGURE 2. Remnants of necrotic hepatocyte attract lymphocytes and macrophages (focal necrosis, arrowhead). An eosinophilic body surrounded by lymphocytes is also present (arrow). (H&E.)

titis (Fig. 2). Liver cell death by apoptosis represents rapid budding of the cytoplasm to form numerous globules and nuclear fragmentation.[5] Small sinusoidal eosinophilic bodies, the size of erythrocytes or much smaller, are seen in apoptosis (Fig. 4). In contrast to necrosis, apoptosis is not associated with an inflammatory reaction and is thought to be the result of programmed cell death.

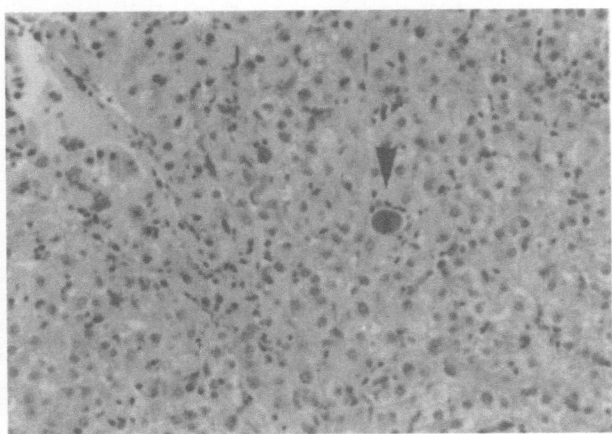

FIGURE 3. A hepatocyte undergoing eosinophilic degeneration and roundup; it is extruded into the perisinusoidal space to become an eosinophilic body (arrow). (H&E.)

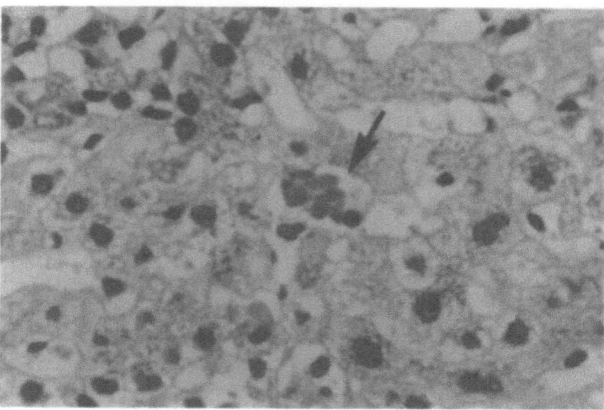

FIGURE 4. Multiple small eosinophilic bodies are seen in sinusoidal space in apoptosis (arrow). (H&E.)

Fat accumulation is rare in viral hepatitis.[6] In large droplet steatosis, single fat globules displace the nuclei to one side (Fig. 5). It is usually of longer duration than small- and medium-size droplet steatosis. The cell membrane appears prominent as in plant cells. In small- to medium-size droplet steatosis, many fat globules are seen in each hepatocyte without displacement of the nucleus. While large-droplet steatosis has surprisingly little functional impact, the small- droplet steatosis may be significant functionally, if many hepatocytes are involved.

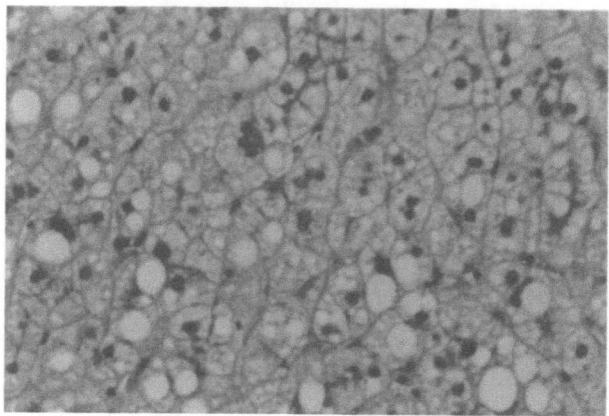

FIGURE 5. Fat accumulation in hepatocytes. Small-, medium-, and large-droplet steatosis is seen. (H&E.)

The extent of necrosis in different patients with hepatitis varies considerably. Necrosis may involve scattered single hepatocytes throughout the lobules (spotty necrosis), seen in classic acute viral hepatitis. Necrosis of contiguous hepatocytes may occur and may involve perivenous zone 3 (centrolobular) and sometimes zone 2 (midzonal) of Rappaport's acinus.[7] The areas of necrosis may connect perivenous-to-perivenous or perivenous-to-periportal zones (bridging necrosis)[8]; they may affect adjacent lobules or acini (multilobular necrosis)[9] and may involve many adjacent acini in a substantial part of the liver (massive necrosis). In the most severe cases (fulminant hepatitis with acute hepatic failure), no hepatocytes are discernible. Portal tracts and central veins are approximated and the reticulin network, which is empty due to dropout of hepatocytes, collapses (Fig. 6).

Regeneration of hepatocytes develops early in acute hepatitis, almost coincident with the degenerative changes, and is reflected in mitoses and multiple nuclei. Multinuclear enlarged (giant) hepatocytes result from fusion rather than from incomplete division of hepatocytes. They occur in many forms of neonatal and infantile hepatitis and rarely in adult hepatitis. These giant cells seem to survive for up to half a year. In various disorders, particularly those associated with submassive or massive hepatic necrosis, regenerating hepatocytes in periportal areas are arranged in cords. If they develop distinct lumen, they may resemble bile ductules (ductular hepatocytes).[10] These ductular hepatocytes share characteristics of both hepatocytes and bile duct cells (metaplasia). They are surrounded by a basement membrane and contain carcinoembryonic antigen similar to duct cells; they also produce α_1-antitrypsin and contain intermediate filaments such as cytokeratins typical for hepatocytes and large mitochondria, resembling hepatocytes.

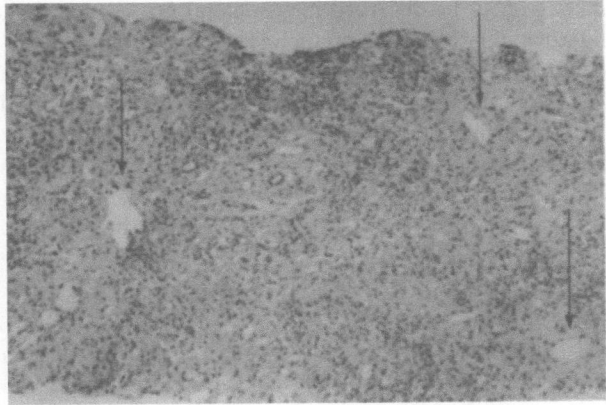

FIGURE 6. Liver biopsy specimen showing massive necrosis. All hepatocytes have disappeared, and the terminal hepatic venules (arrows) are approximated. (H&E.)

In normal liver after the age of 5 years, hepatocytes are arranged in single cell plates, with the nuclei in the center of the cells. Regeneration may lead to formation of two or more cell-thick plates, recognized by the perisinusoidal position of the nuclei. This kind of regeneration occurs in response to acute liver injury or may form hepatocellular nodules, in the absence of recognizable acute injury, such as in nodular regenerative hyperplasia or in cirrhosis.

Cholestasis, Bile Ductular Proliferation, and Bile Duct Changes

Morphologically, cholestasis[11] is defined as an accumulation of brown-greenish bile pigment in hepatocytes, in bile canaliculi, or in Kupffer cells. It is not a significant feature in acute viral hepatitis B. In hepatitis A and in the enteric form of non-A, non-B hepatitis, however, it is frequent. Cholestasis is often multifactorial, its mechanism is not established, and different sites of initiation are postulated. The clinical, biochemical, as well as morphologic findings in this condition may simulate those of mechanical biliary obstruction of larger intra-hepatic and extrahepatic bile ducts. The hepatocytes are swollen and have a rarified cytoplasm with bile-stained fine strands (feathery degeneration). This may proceed to focal necrosis. Bile plugs are present in dilated canaliculi. Prolonged cholestasis is recognized by the presence of bile in activated Kupffer cells. Acute cholestasis is usually in the perivenous area. There may be periportal proliferation of bile ductules surrounded by neutrophils.[12] Around proliferated bile ductules neutrophils accumulate, but do not indicate bacterial infection. In dehydrated patients, the proliferating bile ductules may contain dense bile plugs.[12] They are not necessarily accompanied by other forms of cholestasis and not always by elevation of serum alkaline phosphatase activities.

Bile duct alterations are frequent in hepatitis but are usually mild. Evidence of bile duct damage may be observed in parenteral non-A, non-B hepatitis and consists of slight irregularity of the epithelia which are rounded and surrounded by acute and chronic inflammatory cells.[13,14] In contrast to primary biliary cirrhosis, the basement membrane of the damaged bile ducts in viral hepatitis is intact. Moreover, the bile duct changes in viral hepatitis differ from those in orthotopic liver transplant rejection and in sclerosing cholangitis. In the latter, the bile duct epithelium is atrophic and is surrounded by periductal fibrosis; in the advanced stage, the bile ducts are replaced by bile duct scars.

Sinusoidal Cell Activation and Lobular Inflammation

Sinusoidal cell activation represents an excess number of sinusoidal cells caused by activation and proliferation of Kupffer cells, which are usually peri-odic acid Schiff positive and diastase resistant (DPAS positive).[15,16] There are also other inflammatory cells, such as lymphocytes, monocytes, polymorphonuclear leukocytes, and plasma cells in and around sinusoids. This type of sinusoidal cell activation, not associated with hepatocellular alterations, is seen in the early stages of primary biliary cirrhosis, in nonhepatotropic viral infections (e.g., adenovirus, Epstein–Barr virus, coxsackievirus), in lymphomas, and in some forms of non-A, non-B hepatitis (Fig. 7). In other forms of hepatitis, sinusoidal cell activation and diffuse inflammation are usually associated with hepatocellular damage and focal necrosis. In acute viral hepatitis, the wall of the terminal hepatic (central) venules is infiltrated by lymphocytes or macrophages, or both (endophlebitis).

Kupffer cells, together with endothelial cells, have phagocytic and endocytotic capacities, hence may act as scavenger cells.[17] They may also function as antigen-presenting cells and secrete inflammatory modulators, such as eicosanoids or cytokines, as do nonresident monocytes and lymphocytes. The secretory products are chemotactic, mitogenic, protein synthesis-stimulating, and other regulatory factors.[18,19] Eicosanoids also increase capillary permeability and vasoconstriction. Cytotoxic T lymphocytes may lyse infected hepatocytes that display viral antigens together with HLA class I or II antigens on their plasma membranes.[20]

Portal Inflammation

In both acute and chronic hepatitis, an inflammatory reaction, composed mainly of lymphocytes and monocytes, is present in the portal areas. A few plasma cells and eosinophilic and neutrophilic leukocytes may be observed. The

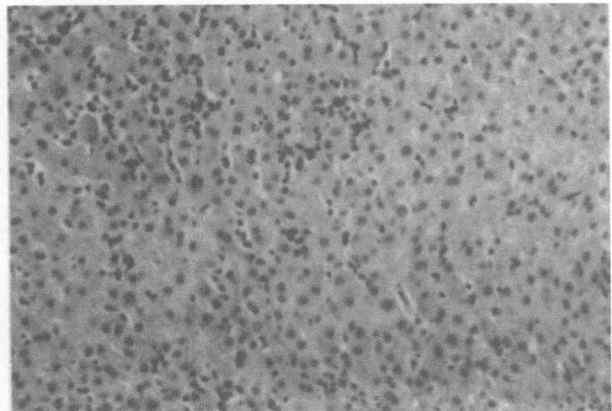

FIGURE 7. Hypercellularity of the hepatic lobule due to sinusoidal cell activation and inflammation in acute viral hepatitis. (H&E.)

inflammatory response may be confined to the portal tracts, which may be enlarged (as recognized by the discrepancy between the size of the portal tract and its portal vein and bile duct), or it may extend into the periportal area and disrupt the limiting plate. Limiting plate refers to the first layer of hepatocytes around a portal tract. When the extension of the inflammatory exudate into the periportal zone is accompanied by destruction of periportal hepatocytes, the process is called piecemeal necrosis[21,22] (Fig. 8). Characteristically, piecemeal necrosis is seen in chronic active hepatitis and may lead to trapping of single or groups of hepatocytes in the periportal connective tissue. They then assume an acinar arrangement. Piecemeal necrosis must be distinguished from spillover of portal inflammatory exudate without necrosis of periportal hepatocytes. The portal lymphoid accumulation can be large and dense and may contain germinal centers, as often seen in parenteral hepatitis non-A, non-B or δ hepatitis.[23]

Fibrosis

Portal and periportal fibrosis[24–26] often follows portal and periportal inflammation and perhaps reflects healing, particularly if the excess collagen fibers concentrically surround portal tracts and periportal zones. By contrast, active fibrosis results in stellate-shaped portal tracts, because connective tissue septa radiate into the parenchyma. These fibrotic septa contain arterioles and particularly proliferating bile ductules surrounded by inflammatory cells. Stellate portal fibrosis may also become arrested as in septal hepatitis. In areas of older fibrosis, elastic fibers increase in addition to the collagen fibers. When fibrotic septa link

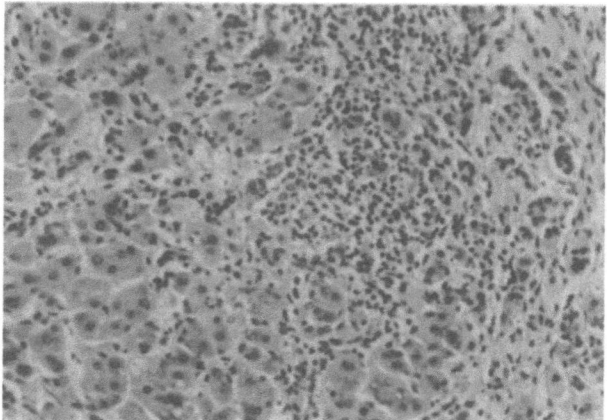

FIGURE 8. Extension of the inflammatory exudate into the periportal zone, accompanied by necrosis of periportal hepatocytes in chronic active hepatitis. (H&E.)

the perivenous to the periportal zones, they disturb the hepatic microcirculation by creating anastomoses between afferent portal vein and hepatic artery branches, as well as efferent hepatic vein tributaries, allowing blood to bypass the parenchyma.

EVOLUTION OF ACUTE VIRAL HEPATITIS

Characteristic Histologic Features

Acute viral hepatitis (AVH) is a diffuse necroinflammatory lesion of the liver of less than 6 months duration almost always accompanied by biochemical abnormalities and clinical symptoms.[27,28] It results primarily, but not exclusively, from infection by hepatotropic viruses A (HAV), B (HBV), parenteral and enteric non-A, non-B (NANB), and D (HDV). With some exceptions, the histologic changes produced by HAV, HBV, and NANB are similar. None of the individual phenomena described earlier is diagnostic of AVH; therefore, the diagnosis is based on a combination of features. The classic form of AVH is acute hepatitis with spotty necrosis. The fully developed stage is characterized by panlobular disarray, increased cellularity, and pleiomorphism of hepatocytes. This appearance is caused by a combination of changes consisting of hepatocellular degeneration and necrosis, hepatocellular regeneration, sinusoidal cell activation, and inflammation. The two types of degenerative changes, i.e., eosinophilic degeneration with formation of eosinophilic bodies, and ballooning degeneration leading to focal necrosis, are diffuse throughout the acinar parenchyma. Regeneration is reflected in mitoses and multinuclear hepatocytes. The various and simultaneous processes of hepatocellular degeneration and regeneration produce marked variations of size, shape, and staining qualities of hepatocytes. The parenchymal changes in AVH are always accompanied by a mesenchymal reaction in that the sinusoidal lining cells become larger and more numerous. Inflammatory reaction, composed predominantly of monocytes and lymphocytes, is diffuse throughout acini and portal tracts. Endophlebitis of the terminal hepatic venules is observed. Since the life span of DPAS-reactive macrophages is relatively long, they may be seen as "tombstones" even after subsidence of hepatitis. Cholestasis, intracellular and canalicular, is usually mild.

Although little is known about the pathology of the early stage of AVH in humans, the changes have been described in detail in chimpanzees on the basis of serial biopsies, but they are milder than in humans. For instance, chimpanzee hepatitis A shows severe periportal necroinflammation and an intact perivenous zone.[29] Hepatocellular necrosis is minimal, while sinusoidal cell activation and inflammation are present. This early lesion coincides with the first rise in aminotransferase activities. In the subsiding or late stage, hepatocellular degeneration and inflammation regress.

Different Forms of Acute Viral Hepatitis

Acute Hepatitis with Confluent Necrosis

In less than 3% of patients with acute hepatitis, the necrosis is more extensive than spotty necrosis, leading to bridging or multilobular necrosis.[8,9] All other features of classic acute hepatitis are also seen. Although there is extensive loss of hepatocytes, the reticulin network is preserved initially. Later, it collapses and forms passive septa or bridges. Formation of fibrotic septa from active fibroplasia need not follow. The parenchyma shows regenerative changes of hepatocytes. Occasionally, more often in older persons, hepatocellular regeneration may be impaired. Although the clinical features of patients with confluent necrosis is usually more severe, histopathologic examination of a biopsy specimen is the only means by which bridging or multilobular necrosis can be recognized. Why some cases heal, leaving either a scarred or substantially normal liver, while others progress to massive necrosis or cirrhosis is not clear. The prognostic implications of bridging necrosis for chronicity of liver disease remain controversial.

Acute Hepatitis with Massive Necrosis

In general, in 0.1–1% of cases with AVH massive hepatic necrosis develops. In the most severe cases, the patients present clinically as fulminant hepatitis with acute hepatic failure.[30] The serum aminotransferase activities, which are usually high in acute hepatitis, may decline in massive necrosis, because there are much fewer hepatocytes left to leak the enzymes. Elastic fibers, which can be demonstrated even in small amounts by Victoria blue stain, increase subsequently. Therefore, the amount of elastic fibers indicates the age of massive hepatic necrosis.[31] In patients who survive, regeneration of parenchymal cells is prominent. This is evidenced by the formation of twin plates, mitoses and multiple nuclei of hepatocytes, and proliferation of ductular hepatocytes as well as real ductules around portal tracts. Survival depends largely on hepatocellular regeneration, reflected by a rise of serum α-fetoprotein.[32] In older patients, however, regeneration may be impaired, associated with a poorer prognosis. Massive hepatic necrosis may result from infection with HBV, HBV and HDV (co- or superinfection), both forms of NANB, less commonly HAV, herpes virus, adenovirus, and cytomegalovirus. In nonhepatotropic viral infections, massive necrosis is frequently observed in patients with defective immune mechanisms. Fulminant hepatitis D in the Amazon basin and Central Africa is characterized by hepatocytes with many small vacuoles in the cytoplasm (so-called morula cells), and granular eosinophilic necrosis, but these changes have not been described in hepatitis D in the United States.[33]

Evidence for Transition to Chronicity

Reliable morphologic criteria to predict transition of AVH to chronicity have not been established, except perhaps for the presence of HBsAg-laden ground-glass hepatocytes,[34] which may be detected during the transition of acute to chronic hepatitis B. However, ground-glass hepatocytes in acute hepatitis may also be seen in acute hepatitis A, hepatitis D, or NANB superimposed on a chronic HBV carrier or reactivation of hepatitis B in an asymptomatic carrier. Other changes suspicious of a possible chronic course include bridging hepatic necrosis, extensive periportal fibrosis, true piecemeal necrosis, bile duct alterations, and heavy infiltration of portal tracts by inflammatory cells, particularly plasma cells, or lymphoid follicles.

Differentiation and Immunopathology of Acute Viral Hepatitis, Types A, B, and Non-A, Non-B

The parenchymal, mesenchymal, and portal alterations described earlier represent the main features observed in acute hepatitis, regardless of the etiologic agent implicated. Some features, however, are recognized as unusual and may reflect specific histologic patterns of viral hepatitis A, hepatitis B, or NANB.

In acute viral hepatitis A, parenchymal changes are more prominent in periportal zones than in perivenous areas, particularly in children. Generally, parenchymal alterations are less severe than in hepatitis B. Proliferation of Kupffer cells is mild, but mononuclear inflammatory cell infiltration is more severe than in hepatitis B and would thus suggest a tendency to chronicity, which in fact is virtually absent in this disease. The portal and periportal distribution of the necroinflammatory lesions in HAV infection is observed in chimpanzees and marmosets, as well as in humans.[35-37] Centrilobular cholestasis is frequently prominent, and the disease is more severe in adults. HAV antigen can be demonstrated in the liver for several weeks by immunohistochemical methods. The viral antigen is expressed as fine granules in the cytoplasm of hepatocytes and Kupffer cells scattered throughout the lobules, although necroinflammation is usually prominent in periportal areas. Immune mechanisms, probably cell-mediated cytotoxicity, appear to play a role in the pathogenesis of hepatic injury[38] but have not been elucidated; a direct viral cytopathic effect has also been proposed.

In acute viral hepatitis B, necroinflammatory lesions are predominantly perivenous. Endophlebitis is frequent. The sinusoidal cells are markedly activated, but lymphocytes predominate. They are often closely attached to the cell membranes of normal or altered hepatocytes and sometimes appear to lie within them (Fig. 2). Acidophilic bodies are usually in close contact with lymphocytes. These findings are consistent with the hypothesis that HBV-induced hepatocellular injury is mediated by the host immune response to virus-encoded or virus-induced target antigens (perhaps HBcAg or HBeAg) that are expressed on the hepatocellular surface during viral replication.[39] There is increasing evidence that HLA-restricted cytotoxic T lymphocytes directed against a molecular complex of viral and histocompatibility antigens on the hepatocellular surface represent the effector cells.[40]

HBV-associated liver diseases have been studied in great detail in humans and chimpanzees by a variety of immunohistochemical procedures.[41] These tests have been done on frozen sections and in routinely processed liver specimens using antibodies to hepatitis B core, e, and surface antigens (HBcAg, HBeAg, and HBsAg). Few or no viral components are detected in acute and fulminant hepatitis B, although HBcAg and HBsAg may be demonstrable during the late incubation period and in early acute hepatitis B, particularly in chimpanzees. HDV infection is always associated with HBV and may occur as co- or superinfection. HDAg can be reliably and readily demonstrated in nuclei and less frequently in cytoplasm of hepatocytes. It is suspected that in contrast to HBV, HDV has a direct cytopathic effect on hepatocytes.

Light microscopic changes of moderate differential diagnostic value in hepatitis NANB have been demonstrated in chimpanzees and also in humans. Fat accumulation, which is considered unusual in acute viral hepatitis except in children, is common in acute hepatitis NANB. It is usually mild and microvesicular and is particularly common after exposure to blood and its products (concentrates). Bile duct alterations as described above are frequent, but are usually mild. Two types of lobular lesions are noted in parenteral hepatitis NANB[23]: (1) many acidophilic bodies with only limited inflammatory reaction, and (2) conspicuous sinusoidal cell reaction, particularly lymphocytes lining up, streak like in the sinusoids, similar to the changes in infectious mononucleosis and toxoplasmosis. Compared with hepatitis B, lymphocytes are not prominent. When present, they reside in the sinusoids and rarely abut hepatocytes. Heavy lymphoid cell accumulation may be observed in portal triads, often forming lymphoid follicles. Giant cell transformation is observed in some adults with chronic hepatitis NANB.

In the enteric form of NANB hepatitis, first recognized in epidemics with high mortality of pregnant women, but lacking chronicity, cholestasis with pseudogland formation of hepatocytes is more common,[40] and macrophages and even neutrophils predominate over lymphocytes.[42] Immunohistochemical studies in NANB hepatitis have not been useful. The viral antigens seem to be weak immunogens. Several different ultrastructural alterations have been reported in the hepatocytes of chimpanzees or patients with parenteral NANB hepatitis[43,44]: (1) intranuclear particles, 15–27 nm in diameter; (2) circular and tubular fused membranes in the cytoplasm; and (3) tubular profiles in dilated cisternae of endoplasmic reticulum. In contrast to the immunohistochemical studies, the ultrastructural changes in hepatocytes appear to be helpful in the diagnosis of NANB hepatitis. In chimpanzees, lymphocytotoxicity was considered important in liver injury[45] in contrast with the usual assumption that NANB viruses are cytopathic.

Role of the Liver Biopsy in Differential Diagnosis

Acute hepatitis can easily be diagnosed from a compatible clinical history and physical examination supported by characteristic biochemical serum tests. Therefore, liver biopsy is indicated only when the etiology of acute hepatitis is not clear or in prolonged, unresolving, or relapsing hepatitis. The differential diagnosis of acute hepatitis encompasses not only hepatitis A, B, D, and the NANBs, but also hepatitis caused by not primarily hepatotropic viruses, several bacterial infections, autoimmune processes, drugs, alcohol, acute biliary obstruction, orthotopic liver transplant rejection, and various metabolic and nonspecific forms of hepatic injury.[28]

Mechanical Biliary Obstruction

Portal and periportal changes closely mimicking those of large bile duct obstruction may be seen in some forms of AVH, particularly in hepatitis with bridging necrosis and in cholestatic viral hepatitis. The diagnosis is usually established by observing the characteristic necroinflammatory changes in the lobules, which in AVH are not directly associated with cholestasis.

Drug-Induced Hepatitis

Drug-induced hepatitis may closely resemble viral hepatitis clinically, biochemically, and morphologically. Certain features, however, such as cytotoxic hepatocyte alterations with little inflammatory response, fatty change, granuloma formation, infiltration by eosinophils, bile duct damage, and induction cells, suggest a drug-related cause. Simultaneous presence of these different features is suspicious of the effects of drugs with multiple injurious metabolites.

Nonspecific Reactive Hepatitis

This entity is particularly difficult to differentiate from the late and residual stages of acute hepatitis when macrophages predominate over lymphocytes. In nonspecific reactive hepatitis, the necroinflammatory changes are less pronounced and are neither uniform nor diffuse.

Chronic Hepatitis

The differentiation of acute from chronic hepatitis is discussed in Chapter 18. Acute hepatitis with confluent necrosis and collapse may be mistaken for cirrhosis, histologically. However, areas of necrosis or collapse contain no or very little collagen and elastic fibers, in contrast to fibrous septa in cirrhosis.

Acute Hepatitis Due to Nonhepatotropic Viruses

Many viruses other than the hepatitis viruses may affect the liver. The extensive use of immunosuppressive treatment has increased the number of such cases. The hepatic changes consist of proliferation of sinusoidal lining cells, which may be prominent with the formation of retothelial nodules. Focal eosinophilic necrosis of hepatocytes is a common finding, and eosinophilic bodies are often seen. Necrosis of liver cells may be extensive, especially early in life and in patients with defective immune response. Nuclear or cytoplasmic viral inclusions may establish the diagnosis.

Acute Orthotopic Liver Transplant Rejection

Damage to vessels (endothelialitis) is characteristic in transplant rejection and involves terminal hepatic venules, as well as portal veins.[46] Lesions of small bile ducts with vacuolation and necrosis of the epithelium are also more pronounced than in AVH, whereas more or less extensive hepatocellular necrosis accompanies early lesions.

ACKNOWLEDGMENTS. This work was supported in part by grant DK 30854 from the National Institutes of Health. We are grateful to Mrs. Marva Barbee for secretarial help.

REFERENCES

1. Blumberg BS, Alter HJ, Visnich S.: A "new" antigen in leukemia sera. *JAMA* **191**:541–546, 1965.
2. Popper H: Hepatocellular degeneration and death, in Arias IM, Popper H, Schachter D, Shafritz DA (eds): *The Liver. Biology and Pathology.* New York, Raven, 1982, pp. 771–784.
3. Schaffner F: The structural basis of altered hepatic function in viral hepatitis. *Am J Med* **49**:658–668, 1970.
4. Ishak KG: Light microscopic morphology of viral hepatitis. *Am J Clin Pathol* **65**:787–827, 1976.
5. Wyllie AH, Kerr JFR, Curie AR: Cell death: The significance of apoptosis. *Int Rev Cytol* **68**:251–306, 1980.

6. Leevy CM: Fatty liver: A study of 270 patients with biopsy proven fatty liver and a review of the literature. *Medicine (Baltimore)* **41**:249–278, 1982.
7. Rappaport AM: Anatomic considerations, in Schiff L (ed): *Diseases of the Liver*. Philadelphia, JB Lippincott, 1975, pp. 1–57.
8. Boyer JL, Klatskin G: Pattern of necrosis of acute viral hepatitis. Prognostic value of bridging (subacute hepatic) necrosis. *N Engl J Med* **283**:1063–1071, 1970.
9. Schmid M, Cueni B: Portal lesions in viral hepatitis with submassive hepatic necrosis. *Hum Pathol* **3**:209–214, 1972.
10. Gerber MA, Thung SN, Shen SC, et al: Phenotypic characterization of hepatic proliferation: Antigen expression by proliferating epithelial cells in fetal liver, massive hepatic necrosis and nodular transformation of the liver. *Am J Pathol* **110**:70–74, 1983.
11. Popper H, Schaffner E: Cholestasis, in Berk JE (ed): *Bockus Gastroenterology*. Vol. 5. Philadelphia, WB Saunders, 1985, pp. 2697–2731.
12. Lefkowitch HJ: Bile ductular cholestasis: An ominous histopathologic sign related to sepsis and "cholangitis lenta." *Hum Pathol* **13**:19–24, 1982.
13. Christoffersen P, Poulsen H, Scheuer PJ: Abnormal bile duct epithelium in CAH and cirrhosis. *Hum Pathol* **3**:227–235, 1972.
14. Bamber M, Murray AK, Weller IVD, et al: Clinical and histological features of a group of patients with sporadic non-A, non-B hepatitis. *J Clin Pathol* **34**:1175–1180, 1981.
15. Review by an International Group: Morphologic criteria in viral hepatitis. *Lancet* **1**:333–337, 1971.
16. Popper H, Paronetto F, Barka T: PAS positive structures of nonglycogenic character in normal and abnormal liver. *Arch Pathol Lab Med* **70**:300–313, 1960.
17. Kirn A, Gut J-P, Bingen A, et al: Murine hepatitis induced by frog virus 3: A model for studying the effect of sinusoidal cell damage on the liver. *Hepatology* **3**:105–111, 1983.
18. Keppler D, Frapp S, Hagman W, et al: The relation of leukotrienes to liver injury. *Hepatology* **5**:883–891, 1985.
19. Popper H, Keppler D: Networks of interacting mechanisms of hepatocellular degeneration and death, in Popper H, Schaffner F (eds): *Progress in Liver Diseases*. Vol. VIII. Orlando, Fla, Grune & Stratton, 1986, pp. 209–235.
20. McMichael AJ: HLA restriction of human cytotoxic T cells. *Springer Semin Immunopathol* **3**:3–22, 1980.
21. DeGroote J, Gedigk P, Popper H, et al: A classification of chronic hepatitis. *Lancet* **2**:626–628, 1968.
22. Popper H: Changing concepts of the evolution of chronic hepatitis and the role of piecemeal necrosis. *Hepatology* **3**:758–762, 1983.
23. Dienes HP, Popper H, Arnold W, et al: Histologic observations in human hepatitis non-A, non-B. *Hepatology* **2**:562–571, 1982.
24. Popper H, Udenfriend S: Hepatic fibrosis: Correlation of biochemical and morphologic investigations. *Am J Med* **49**:707–721, 1970.
25. Popper H: Pathologic aspects of cirrhosis. A review. *Am J Pathol* **87**:228–258, 1977.
26. Anthony PP, Ishak KG, Nayak NC, et al: The morphology of cirrhosis. *J Clin Pathol* **31**:395–414, 1978.
27. Leevy CM, Popper H, Sherlock S (Criteria Committee): Diseases of the liver and biliary tract: Standardization of nomenclature, diagnostic criteria, and diagnostic methodology. *Fogarty International Center Proceedings No. 22*. DHEW Publication No. (NIH) 76-725. Washington, DC, U.S. Government Printing Office, 1976.
28. Gerber MA, Thung SN: Viral hepatitis: Pathology, in Berk JE (ed): *Bockus Gastroenterology*. Vol. 5. Philadelphia, WB Saunders, 1985, pp. 2825–2855.

29. Dienstag JL, Popper H, Purcell RH: The pathology of viral hepatitis types A and B in chimpanzees. A comparison. *Am J Pathol* **85:**131–148, 1976.
30. Lucke B: Pathology of fetal epidemic hepatitis. *Am J Pathol* **20:**471–593, 1944.
31. Thung SN, Gerber MA: The formation of elastic fibers in livers with massive hepatic necrosis. *Arch Pathol Lab Med* **106:**468–469, 1982.
32. Bloomer JR, Waldman TA, McIntire KR, et al: Relationship of serum alpha-fetoprotein to severity and duration of illness in patients with viral hepatitis. *Gastroenterology* **68:**342–350, 1975.
33. Buitrago B, Popper H, Hadler SC: Specific histologic features of Santa Marta hepatitis: A severe form of hepatitis delta virus infection in northern South America. *Hepatology* **6:**1285–1291, 1986.
34. Houthoff HJ, Niermeijer P, Gips CH, et al: Hepatic morphologic findings and viral antigens in acute hepatitis B. *Virchows Arch Pathol Anat* **389:**153–166, 1980.
35. Popper H, Dienstag JL, Feinstone SM, et al: Pathology of viral hepatitis in chimpanzees. *Virchows Arch Pathol Anat* **387:**91–106, 1980.
36. Krawczynski KK, Bradley DW, Murphy BL, et al: Pathogenetic aspects of hepatitis A virus infection in enterally inoculated marmosets. *Am J Clin Pathol* **76:**698–706, 1981.
37. Abe H, Beninger PR, Ikejiri N, et al: Light microscopic findings of liver biopsy specimens from patients with hepatitis type A and comparison with type B. *Gastroenterology* **82:**938–947, 1982.
38. Vallbracht A, Gabriel P, Maier K, et al: Cell-mediated cytotoxicity in hepatitis A virus infection. *Hepatology* **6:**1308–1314, 1986.
39. Van der Oord JJ, de Vos R, Desmet VJ: In situ distribution of major histocompatibility complex products and viral antigens in chronic hepatitis B virus infection: Evidence that HBc-containing hepatocytes may express HLA-DR antigens. *Hepatology* **6:**981–989, 1986.
40. Gerber MA: Immunopathology of chronic hepatitis, in *Pathogenesis of Liver Diseases. IAP Monograph No. 28.* Baltimore, Williams & Wilkins, 1987, pp. 54–63.
41. Gerber, MA, Thung SN: The diagnostic value of immunohistochemical demonstration of hepatitis viral antigens in the liver. *Hum Pathol* **18:**771–774, 1987.
42. Khuroo MS, Saleem M, Teli MR, et al: Failure to detect chronic liver disease after epidemic non-A, non-B hepatitis. *Lancet* **2:**260–261, 1980.
43. Shimizu YK, Feinstone SM, Purcell RH, et al: Non-A, non-B hepatitis: Ultrastructural evidence for two agents in experimentally infected chimpanzees. *Science* **205:**197–200, 1979.
44. De Vos R, Vanstapel MJ, Desmyter J, et al: Are nuclear particles specific for non-A, non-B hepatitis? *Hepatology* **3:**532–544, 1983.
45. Sugitani M: Identification of lymphocyte subsets in chimpanzee livers with non-A, non-B acute hepatitis—Using serial needle biopsies. *Acta Hepatol Jpn* **27:**309–316, 1986.
46. Snover DC, Sibley RK, Freese DK, et al: Orthotopic liver transplantation: A pathological study of 63 serial liver biopsies from 17 patients with special reference to the diagnostic features and natural history of rejection. *Hepatology* **4:**1212–1222, 1984.

Viral Hepatitis
Extrahepatic Manifestations

JOHN BARTELS and DAVID J. GOCKE

INTRODUCTION

Viral hepatitis has long been reported to be associated with manifestations of extrahepatic tissue injury, but it is only with the development of specific markers for the hepatitis A and hepatitis B viruses during the past two decades that clear links between infection with hepatitis viruses and extrahepatic manifestations have been well defined. In general, it appears that the cause of tissue injury in all these extrahepatic manifestations is the deposition of immune complexes composed of viral antigen, antibody, and complement in affected tissues. Convincing evidence of the role of such immune complexes in extrahepatic tissue injury has been provided in recent years by elegant electron microscopic and immunofluorescent techniques that have set the standard for further study in the field. The best-documented extrahepatic syndromes associated with viral hepatitis are the serum sickness-like prodrome of acute viral hepatitis, the glomerulonephritis seen mainly in children, and some cases of systemic vasculitis accompanying hepatitis B. Other syndromes for which some evidence of association is available include essential cryoglobulinemia, myocarditis, and certain neurologic disorders, including Guillain–Barré syndrome. The available evidence for each of these syndromes is reviewed below.

JOHN BARTELS and DAVID J. GOCKE • Division of Allergy, Immunology, and Infectious Diseases, University of Medicine and Dentistry of New Jersey, New Brunswick, New Jersey 08903-0019.

SERUM SICKNESS PRODROME OF ACUTE VIRAL HEPATITIS

A transient serum sickness-like syndrome characterized by a skin rash and joint pains occurring during the incubation period (the prodrome) of acute viral hepatitis is the most common extrahepatic manifestation of hepatitis virus infection. The syndrome usually consists of mild arthralgias accompanied by a pruritic skin rash that may be maculopapular, urticarial, or petechial. Occasionally, the joint involvement is severe enough to cause frank arthritis with heat, swelling, and diminished motion, which may prompt a workup for other causes of acute arthritis. In some cases, muscle pain and weakness is a prominent complaint, but actual myositis is rare. These symptoms usually precede the onset of jaundice and other symptoms of hepatitis by a few days or as long as 2–3 weeks. Since they are transient, usually lasting only 2–3 days, and often mild, they may never come to medical attention unless specifically elicited by the physician. However, the physician needs to be aware of these manifestations of viral hepatitis so as to consider the viral hepatitis prodrome in the differential diagnosis of the patient with a skin rash and joint pain.

Niermeijer and Gips[1] in Germany carried out a prospective study of the natural history of acute hepatitis B in 38 patients of whom 30% had extrahepatic complaints consisting of urticaria, rashes, myalgia, and arthropathy. These symptoms occurred anywhere from 8 weeks before to 1½ weeks after the peak SGPT elevation. The average time of appearance of these prodromal symptoms was about 2 weeks before the peak of the hepatic injury.

Stewart and colleagues[2] studied 489 cases of viral hepatitis occurring over a 3-year period in West London; 20% of the cases were found to have HB_sAg in the serum. Joint symptoms were present in 118 of 324 adults (36%) and increased in frequency with age. Interestingly, there was no difference in the incidence of joint symptoms (about 30%) between the HB_sAg-positive and -negative patients. In 38% of those patients with HB_s antigenemia, joint pain lasted longer than 2 weeks, while only 15% of those in whom HB_sAg was not detected had this duration of symptoms. The association between age and arthralgia was strongest in those in whom HB_s antigenemia was not detectable. HB_s antigenemia was not detected in 80% of these patients, but the problem with the study is that other HBV markers and hepatitis A antibody tests were not performed. Thus, it remains unclear precisely how many of these patients had A, B, and non-A, non-B hepatitis, respectively. It seems safe to say, however, that many probably had non-B hepatitis, which disputes the concept that extrahepatic manifestations are associated only with hepatitis B. In a study of a foodborne outbreak of hepatitis A among Navy recruits, in whom the diagnosis of hepatitis A was made with modern radioimmunoassay (RIA) techniques, 14% of 130 affected persons had a skin rash, and 10% had arthralgias.[3] Thus, the evidence seems fairly clear that the serum sickness syndrome can be seen with all three types of viral hepatitis.

In patients with the serum sickness-like prodrome, circulating immune complexes composed of HB_sAg, anti-HB_s, and complement have been detected in both the serum and synovial fluid. These circulating immune complexes can often be demonstrated by cryoprecipitation. Studies by Wands et al.[4] showed that the immunoglobulin composition of these circulating complexes is extremely critical in determining whether or not extrahepatic tissue injury occurs. These workers found that complexes containing the complement-fixing IgG_1 and IgG_3 subtypes are isolated exclusively from patients exhibiting joint and skin involvement. They also showed that the presence of these complement-fixing complexes correlated closely with decreases in serum C3 and C4 levels and with the presence of skin and joint symptoms during the prodromal phase and that the complexes cleared with disappearance of these symptoms and the onset of jaundice. Dienstag et al.[5] provided additional insight into the pathogenesis of the skin lesions in such patients. Light and electron microscopic studies of biopsies of urticarial skin lesions from two patients with the serum sickness prodrome of hepatitis B demonstrated a necrotizing venulitis. In addition, immunofluorescent techniques showed that HB_sAg, IgM, and C3 were deposited in the involved cutaneous vessel walls but not in simultaneously obtained uninvolved skin. In one patient, typical HBV-like structures resembling Dane particles and the 20-nm spherical forms of HB_sAg were observed within an intraendothelial vacuole of a cell lining a vessel wall from an urticarial skin lesion. This localization of the very large particulate form of HB_sAg within endothelial cells of venules contrasts with the localization of the smaller HB_eAg complexes in the glomerular basement membrane and subepithelial regions in the glomerular basement membrane and subepithelial regions of renal glomeruli, as described in children with membranous nephritis.

A variety of skin lesions have been reported to be part of the prodromal complex. In addition to urticaria, these range from erythematous maculopapular lesions, purpura, scarletinaform rash, subcutaneous nodules, and petechiae. These skin manifestations are usually present only transiently during the incubation phase of hepatitis and often are not seen by a physician. Biopsies have been done on them infrequently. However, Weiss et al.[6] described a patient who had both erythematous maculopapular lesions and purpuric lesions associated with HB_s antigenemia and hypocomplementemia. On biopsy, the maculopapular lesion showed mild perivascular mononuclear cell infiltration around small and medium-size vessels in the upper and middle dermis, but immunofluorescent staining for immunoglobulin, complement, and HB_sAg deposits was negative. Biopsy of the purpuric lesion, however, showed more marked perivascular infiltrates in the dermis, with fibrinoid necrosis in the vessel walls. In addition, immunofluorescent studies displayed deposits of IgM and C3 at the sites of vascular injury, although HB_sAg could not be detected. Weiss *et al.* report that the maculopapular rash in their patients subsequently became purpuric. They suggest that these rashes represent various stages of development and that the ability to demonstrate HB_sAg in the sites of tissue injury by immunofluorescence may be a temporal phenomenon. This is certainly consistent with the experience in HBV-related polyarteritis and in experimental models of serum sickness, in which the ability to demonstrate the responsible antigen is transient because of destruction of the antigenic determinants by proteolytic enzymes released by the inflammatory response.

Papular acrodermatitis of childhood should also be mentioned here. As originally described by Gianotti in children,[7] this syndrome is characterized by a papular eruption on the face and limbs lasting 15–20 days and always accompanied by acute hepatitis B. The skin eruption precedes signs of liver injury usually by 20 days or more, and the hepatitis is generally anicteric. In most cases, HB_sAg is present at the onset of the skin eruption. Claudy *et al.*[8] recently described this same syndrome in three adult patients. Papular acrodermatitis should probably be regarded as part of the spectrum of cutaneous manifestations during the prodrome of acute hepatitis B.

GLOMERULONEPHRITIS

Hepatitis B as an immune complex-mediated cause of glomerulonephritis was first reported in 1971 by Coombes *et al.*[9] in a 53-year-old man. Since that time, a great deal of work, mostly in children, has firmly established this entity as one of the best-studied extrahepatic manifestations of viral hepatitis. Brzosko *et al.*[10] originally called attention to the association between hepatitis B and childhood glomerulonephritis of varying histologic types. Immune complexes containing HB_sAg and anti-HB_s were found in the glomeruli of 56% of kidney biopsy specimens in which immunoglobulins and complement were identified. This group extended their findings in a report on renal biopsy specimens of 98 children with either nephrotic syndrome or gromerulonephritis, or both.[11] It was found that 24 of these children had glomerular deposits of HBV antigens, 21 of whom had a histologic diagnosis of membranous glomerulonephropathy. Only 2 of the other 74 had membranous type lesions. Of the total of 23 with membranous glomerulopathy, 21 had either HB_sAg, HB_cAg, or both in glomerular deposits. HB_eAg was not looked for. This association was further developed by Takekoshi *et al.*,[12] who studied 163 Japanese children with renal disease. Of these, all of 11 with a histologic diagnosis of membranous glomerulonephritis had HB_s antigenemia, whereas HB_sAg was detected in the sera of only 7 of the other 152 patients with other histologic diagnoses. Neither the Japanese group nor Levy *et al.*[13] were able to find HB_sAg deposits in the glomeruli of HB_s antigenemic children with glomerulonephritis, as Brzosko *et al.* had reported. Complicating this apparent discrepancy was the use of different methods by each group; the Polish group used sensitive indirect immunofluorescent antibody-staining techniques, while the other workers used a less sensitive direct immunofluorescent method. A possible explanation of these differences comes from more recent work exploring the role of other hepatitis B virus antigen–antibody complexes in glomerulonephritis. In 1979, Takekoshi *et al.*[14] described two patients with HB_s antigenemia and membranous glomerulonephritis with typical electron-dense deposits in the basement membrane and subepithelial space in whom deposits of HB_eAg were demonstrated along the glomerulocapillary walls. Immunoglobulin and complement were present, but not HB_sAg. The estimated molecular weight of HB_eAg when associated with IgG is about 300,000, which correlates well with chronic bovine serum albumin (BSA)–immune-complex glomerulonephritis in animals in which a membranous type glomerulonephritis develops because of the deposition of relatively low-molecular-weight immune complexes (in the range of $3–5 \times 10^5 \ M_r$) in the subepithelial space of the glomeruli. By contrast, it is estimated that HB_sAg and HB_cAg produce large immune complexes with antibody with molecular weights in the range of 4×10^6 and 9×10^6, respectively.

This same Japanese group presented more evidence implicating HB_eAg–antibody complexes in the pathogenesis of hepatitis-associated glomerulopathies in 1981.[15] Six children who were chronic HBV carriers with membranous glomerulonephritis were studied. Four had active renal disease and two inactive disease. Sections of kidney biopsy material were stained with fluorescein-labeled human anti-HB_e, anti-HB_s, and anti-HB_c. No HBV antigens were detected in the glomeruli of the two children with inactive disease, but HB_eAg was found in all four with active disease. HB_sAg was found in the glomeruli of only one of these four children. It is interesting to note that the two with inactive disease had HB_sAg and anti-HB_e in the serum. The finding of HB_sAg in the glomeruli of only one child with glomerulonephritis and HB_eAg in all is interesting in that it may explain discrepancies between investigators who have found HB_sAg in the kidneys in hepatitis-associated glomerulonephritis and those who have not. Perhaps the large HB_sAg–Ab complexes are "innocent bystanders" that deposit in kidneys already damaged by smaller HB_eAg–Ab immune complexes.

Two recent case reports add support to the notion that HB_eAg–Ab immune complexes are important in inciting glomerulonephritis. Cadrobbi *et al.*[16] describe a 3-year-old boy with chronic active hepatitis B who was initially HB_sAg/HB_eAg-positive, but who then converted to HB_eAg-negative and anti-HB_e-positive. Later, he developed membranous glomerulonephritis coincident with the reappearance of HB_eAg with anti-HB_e in the serum. On steroid treatment, the patient again became HB_eAg-negative/anti-HB_e-positive and had resolution of proteinuria. Eventually, the child went on to develop anti-HB_s with disappearance of HB_sAg. In this case, glomerulonephritis developed in a setting in which HB_eAg–Ab immune complexes were likely to form. It is of interest that this patient was the only one of 13 initially HB_eAg-positive patients who had spontaneous recurrence of HB_eAg after conversion to anti-HB_e. Another report from the Japanese group that originally implicated HB_eAg–Ab immune complexes describes a 15-year-old boy with chronic glomerulonephritis whose serum was HB_sAg- and HB_eAg-positive.[17] He was treated with interferon with disappearance of HB_eAg and simultaneous resolution of proteinuria. HB_sAg remained positive in this case despite clinical remission.

Finally, an interesting study by Thomas et al.[18] suggests that the pathogenesis of HBV-related glomerulopathies may be related to the consumption of complement. Patients with chronic active hepatitis B, and one with membranous nephritis and polyarteritis nodosa, were found to have increased metabolic clearance of the third component of complement (C3) as compared with those with acute hepatitis B. Complement-mediated damage may be the final mechanism for causation of nephritis induced by a variety of immune complexes. Perhaps when markers for other hepatitis agents are available, studies will show that deposition of immune complexes containing antigens of these viruses are a cause of other cases of glomerulonephritis.

POLYARTERITIS AND OTHER FORMS OF VASCULITIS

The association of some cases of polyarteritis with HBV infection is now well recognized.[19–21] Approximately 20–40% of patients with polyarteritis have persistent HBV infection, which appears to be the underlying etiologic factor for their vasculitis. Usually the onset of signs and symptoms of vasculitis occurs several months to years after the initial HBV infection and consists of the usual multisystem manifestations of polyarteritis, i.e., fever, peripheral neuropathy, arthralgia, hypertension, renal damage, and signs of major vascular occlusions. In some cases, there is no preceding history of recognized hepatitis. The presence of persistent HBV infection is manifest as an ongoing HB_s antigenemia, commonly accompanied by evidence of mild asymptomatic hepatic injury. Usually, the serum concentrations of the hepatic enzymes are in the range 100–400 IU/100 ml, and jaundice is absent. Occasionally, the patient may exhibit significant biochemical and histologic evidence of chronic active hepatitis. Biopsy of affected organs displays the fibrinoid necrosis and perivascular infiltration in the walls of small arteries and arterioles characteristic of polyarteritis. Angiographic studies are frequently helpful in demonstrating aneurysms or vasculitic lesions in the abdominal viscera and elsewhere. Patients with HBV-related polyarteritis have circulating immune complexes composed of HB_sAg and anti-HB_s in the serum. When fresh vasculitic lesions are examined during the early stages of the disease, deposits of HB_sAg, IgG, and C3 can be demonstrated by immunofluorescent techniques in the sites of vascular damage.[19] The case for the association of classic polyarteritis nodosa and other forms of vasculitis with hepatitis B has recently been strengthened by application of immunologic techniques similar to those employed in the study of HBV-associated glomerulonephritis. In one remarkable report, Michalak[22] from Warsaw described seven well-studied cases of classic polyarteritis that came to autopsy. The material for this study consisted of necropsy specimens from unselected patients who had been clinically diagnosed as having polyarteritis nodosa: one was female and six were male, ranging in age from 27 to 59 years. HB_sAg and HB_cAg were detected in the cytoplasm and nuclei of hepatocytes in all seven cases, indicating the presence of ongoing infection with HBV. Histologic changes in the liver varied from minimal to chronic aggressive hepatitis. In all cases, deposits of HB_sAg, immunoglobulins, globulin, and C1q were detected in vascular lesions by use of immunofluorescent techniques. The idea that these deposits represented HB_sAg–anti-HB_s immune complexes was supported by the successful elution of HB_sAg from the deposits by treatment with buffers known to dissociate antigen–antibody complexes, but not by treatment with phosphate-buffered saline. Immune-complex glomerulonephritis was also found in six of the cases. In five of the seven patients, serum samples had been assayed for HB_sAg antemortem, and all five were positive. HB_s antigenemia persisted for 2–12 months and was associated with persistent elevations of SGOT and SGPT in four of the patients. One patient had a history of an acute episode of jaundice clinically characterized as acute hepatitis. The HB_sAg-containing immune complexes were present more abundantly in early exudative and fibrinoid vascular lesions, whereas lesser amounts were seen in lesions undergoing involution, and the complexes were totally absent in healed lesions. In addition, HB_sAg were detected by the Shikata stain in the cytoplasm of the hepatocytes in all cases. Double staining with fluorescein-labeled anti-HB_s and rhodamine B-labeled reagents for identification of immunoglobulins and complement showed the vascular deposits of HB_sAg to be an integral part of the immunoglobulin and complement deposits. In the small arteries, homogeneous HB_sAg deposits were localized diffusely throughout the intima in areas of narrowing or occlusion of the lumen, chiefly at points of branching. In larger arteries, HB_sAg deposits were distributed along the elastic membrane, subendothelially and in the hyperplastic intima. As a rule, the HB_sAg deposits were accompanied by deposits of IgG, IgM, globulin, C1q, and fibrin. Also, deposition of HB_sAg, Ig, and complement could be seen in the germinal centers of the spleen and lymph nodes, sites typical for the trapping of immune complexes. The continuous production of large amounts of HB_sAg in patients infected with HBV, its release from hepatocytes into the circulation, the continued anti-HB_s production, and HB_sAg immune-complex formation all conform to similar events in chronic viral infections that produce immune-complex disease in animals. In addition, the demonstration of HB$_s$Ag-immune complexes in recent exudative and fibrinoid vascular lesions provides substantial evidence for a primary pathogenetic role of those complexes.

An interesting report by Drueke et al.[23] from France provides some sense of perspective on the frequency of polyarteritis nodosa in patients with persistent HBV infection. In a study of 266 persistent HB$_s$Ag carriers undergoing long-term hemodialysis, three were observed to have classic polyarteritis nodosa. In 384 other hemodialysis patients without HB$_s$ antigenemia, no cases of vasculitis were observed. In the three HB$_s$Ag-associated cases of polyarteritis nodosa, the HB$_e$Ag was found in two patients, and C3 was low in one. Circulating immune complexes were demonstrated in all three patients. HB$_s$Ag and anti-HB$_s$ were identified in PEG precipitates by RIA and immune electron microscopic techniques in all three. Direct immunofluorescence on a muscle biopsy specimen from one patient was positive for HB$_s$Ag, but not for IgG, IgM, C3, or C1q. In one case, circulating immune complexes could not be demonstrated after initiation of corticosteroid therapy, and in another case, the immune complexes disappeared intermittently. In the latter case, transient disappearance of circulating immune complexes appeared to be related to a decrease in disease activity.

A report from England sheds some light on the frequency of this relationship between polyarteritis and HBV infection. In a study of 17 cases of biopsy-proved polyarteritis, Travers et al.[24] found evidence of HBV infection (persistent HB$_s$ antigenemia) in four cases (23%). Unfortunately, other HBV markers were not examined, nor was any immunologic workup carried out. Hepatic enzyme abnormalities were seen in all four of the HB$_s$Ag-associated cases, but similar enzyme abnormalities were seen in approximately one half of the other patients. In agreement with previous reports, there was nothing to distinguish the HB$_s$Ag-associated cases from non-HBV cases with regard to clinical signs and symptoms, organ involvement, or course of the disease.

In a comprehensive study of 80 patients with various forms of vasculitis, Gover et al.[25] in Denver found that four had concurrent HBV infection; polyarteritis nodosa was present in two, and a cutaneous vasculitis was the diagnosis in the other two. The two cases of cutaneous vasculitis presented clinically as Schönlein–Henoch purpura. In one of these patients, skin biopsy specimens demonstrated granular deposits of IgM, C3, C4, and HB$_s$Ag and electron-dense deposits of aggregated 20-nm particles resembling HB$_s$Ag in postcapillary venules. Other evidence for circulating HB$_s$Ag immune complexes included an increased serum C1q-binding activity, decreased serum complement, and a cryoprecipitate containing both HB$_s$Ag and an IgM-type of anti-HB$_s$. Negative-staining electron microscopy of the cryoprecipitate obtained from the serum demonstrated aggregated 20-nm particles resembling intact HB$_s$Ag.

Recently, several additional reports of individual cases of polyarteritis nodosa associated with HBV infection appeared. One of these was an interesting report by Kinderman[26] of histologically proved polyarteritis in which steroid therapy was associated with clinical and histologic improvement and disappearance of HB_s antigenemia. About 1 year later, the patient became acutely ill again and was found to have HB_sAg immune complexes in the serum and in vessel walls prior to death. This case illustrates again the transient nature of the HB_sAg immune complexes and emphasizes the need to look during early acute phases in order to demonstrate HB_sAg in complexes. It also suggests the possibility that some HB_sAg-negative cases of polyarteritis nodosa may represent cases in which HB_s antigenemia may have been missed because the patients were seen late in their course. Another case, reported by Bruckstein and Zimmon,[27] presented with acute abdominal pain and underwent exploratory laparotomy before the diagnosis became evident. Govindan et al.[28] reported a case of HBV-related polyarteritis presenting as temporal arteritis. On biopsy of a tender, painful temporal nodule, fibrinoid necrosis and inflammatory infiltration of the media were found. This coincided with the presence of HB_sAg and HB_eAg in the serum. In the context of temporal arteritis, Fainaru et al.[29] reported from Israel on 47 patients with biopsy-proved temporal arteritis in whom they remark that more than one half the patients had laboratory evidence of liver damage. The possible association of these cases with hepatitis virus infection was not commented on and needs further exploration. Other cases of HBV-related polyarteritis nodosa were reported by Barbado et al.[30] and Dally et al.[31] Finally, on the subject of vasculitis, a good overview of polyarteritis nodosa and related disorders was published by Travers.[32]

With respect to the management and course of patients with biopsy-proved polyarteritis, there have been two interesting reports.[33,34] In one report, the fatality rate was similar for HB_sAg-positive and HB_sAg-negative patients with polyarteritis (42% and 44%, respectively); in the other, HBV-related disease seemed to be more severe. Death usually resulted from vasculitic problems. Among the survivors, the disease in the HB_sAg-positive group appeared to be easier to control and to require less intensive immunosuppressive therapy. Nonetheless, the number of patients in all these studies was limited, and polyarteritis must be regarded as a potentially fatal condition, whether or not it is associated with HBV.

Although apparently unrelated to HBV infection, some other recent observations on polyarteritis are relevant in this context. Elkon et al.[35] described four patients in whom polyarteritis developed within 2 years of onset of hairy cell leukemia. The one patient tested had circulating immune complexes, but more extensive immunologic studies were not done. Although all four patients had received transfusions, HB_sAg was said to be absent in all. Could these cases have been induced by non-A, non-B hepatitis virus(es)? Or does some other tumor-associated agent or antigen cause a persistent antigenic load? Or is there a defect in clearance of antigen–antibody complexes in patients with hairy cell leukemia? Elkon *et al.* comment in their discussion that one of these patients had strikingly prolonged clearance of heat-damaged red blood cells.

Finally, the phenomenon of polyarteritis in children must be reexamined in light of the new findings on HBV-related immune-complex disease, especially the frequency with which HBV may cause childhood nephropathy. Ettlinger *et al.*[36] reviewed the Mayo Clinic experience with childhood polyarteritis, pointing out the similarities between the highly fatal infantile form of polyarteritis and some cases of Kawasaki's disease (or mucocutaneous lymph node syndrome). Patients with these diseases have not been systematically studied for HBV markers or other immunologic features, and Kawasaki's disease is certainly more common in areas where HBV disease is more prevalent, such as Japan and Hawaii.[37]

CRYOGLOBULINEMIA

Essential mixed cryoglobulinemia (EMC) is an immune-complex disease characterized by arthralgias, purpura, weakness, vasculitis, and a diffuse glomerulonephritis. Mild arthralgias or nondeforming arthritis involving multiple joints and purpuric lesions, especially on the lower extremities, may persist for many years. These symptoms may be accompanied by Sjögren's syndrome, thyroiditis, or Raynaud's phenomenon. Approximately 50% of patients exhibit glomerulonephritis and systemic vasculitis that may appear suddenly during the course of the disease and are often rapidly progressive and fatal. The characteristic laboratory finding is the presence of cold-insoluble proteins (cryoglobulins). These cryoglobulins are usually composed of IgG, IgM, and even IgA (i.e., mixed); the term "essential" is applied when the syndrome cannot be associated with infection, connective tissue disease, or a lymphoreticular neoplasm. Complement levels may also be depressed, and vasculitis is seen on biopsy of involved tissues.

Levo *et al.*[38] called attention to the fact that a group of patients seen in New York with the EMC syndrome had evidence of previous HBV infection. They found that 14 of 19 patients with EMC had HB_sAg or anti-HB_s in the cryoprecipitate. Electron microscopic examination in four of these cryoprecipitates exhibited particles similar to those associated with HBV. It should also be noted that Levo *et al.* found liver involvement in 86% of their patients with EMC. Realdi *et al.*[39] also found a high frequency of HB_sAg and anti-HB_s in the serum of patients with EMC.

In recent years, additional reports on the putative association of EMC with HBV infection have appeared. Bombardieri *et al.*[40] in Italy found liver involvement in 21 of 30 patients with EMC. The patients had no clinical symptoms of liver disease but did have hepatosplenomegaly, mild elevations of hepatic enzymes, abnormal BSP retention, and low albumin levels. Histologically, chronic persistent hepatitis, chronic active hepatitis, and cirrhosis were all seen. Forty-four percent of the Italian EMC patients had either HB_sAg or anti-HB_s in either the serum or in the cyroprecipitates, or in both. Unfortunately, data on HBV markers in a comparable control group are not provided. Galli et al.[41] from Milan reported on 35 cases of EMC. Thirteen of these patients (37%) had either occult or clinically apparent liver disease. None had evidence of secondary factors, such as chronic infection, connective tissue, or lymphoproliferative disease. Of these 13, HB_sAg was found in the serum of two, anti-HB_s in the serum of eight, and anti-HB_c in the serum of 10. Examination of cryoprecipitates from these patients showed HB_sAg in the cryoprecipitates of two (those that were HB_s antigenemic), and anti-HB_s was found in two other cryoprecipitates. Of the 22 patients without liver disease, 12 showed evidence of previous exposure to HBV in the form of anti-HB_s or anti-HB_c in the serum. None of these patients was positive, either in the serum or the cryoprecipitate, for HB_sAg, but six had anti-HB_s in the cryoprecipitate. Galli et al. conclude that their findings are at variance with the hypothesis of Levo et al. that HBV is involved in the pathogenesis of EMC. Again, no data on the frequency of HBV markers in comparable control populations were provided.

The association of EMC and infection has also been questioned by Dienstag and Wands and colleagues[42] in Boston. These investigators examined the records of patients with EMC seen at the Massachusetts General Hospital (MGH) between January 1976 and May 1979. During this period, 12 patients with a diagnosis of EMC were found. They had arthralgias, purpura, and weakness with or without renal disease and had no evidence of neoplasia, infection, or other connective tissue syndrome. As a control group, 22 subjects with mixed cryoglobulinemia secondary to some other recognized disease process were studied. The patients were tested for hepatitis markers in both serum and cryoprecipitates, and the cryoprecipitates were examined by electron microscopy for HBV particles. None of the patients with EMC had detectable HB_sAg or anti-HB_s in the serum, whereas 5 of the 22 patients with secondary cryoglobulinemia were positive for either HB_sAg or anti-HB_s. HB_sAg and HBV particles could not be detected in 10 patients with EMC in whom fresh cryoprecipitates could be obtained for study, although one cryoprecipitate contained anti-HB_s. Of 12 patients with secondary cryoglobulinemia in whom cryoprecipitates were examined, four were positive for HB_sAg or anti-HB_s. Dienstag and Wand and coworkers conclude that EMC was not related to HBV infection in their patients. The Boston authors point out that at MGH many of the patients with EMC described by Levo and colleagues could have been classified as patients with chronic hepatitis and secondary immune complex-mediated extrahepatic features. Perhaps the point is that a clinical syndrome that passes for EMC may often be associated with chronic liver disease, especially if the disease is related to HBV infection.

SYNDROMES POSSIBLY ASSOCIATED WITH VIRAL HEPATITIS

Myocarditis

Several early studies associated both serum and infectious hepatitis with electrocardiographic (ECG) and gross pathologic cardiac abnormalities.[43-45] In a study by Bell[44] in 1971, the gross and microscopic autopsy findings in 30 patients with fetal hepatitis were described. Thirteen of these patients were classified as serum hepatitis and the remainder as infectious hepatitis. One half the patients were found to have ECG abnormalities, generally minor. Seven of the 30 had clinically evident pulmonary edema during the course of their illness. Nine patients were found to have interstitial lymphocytic infiltrates in the myocardium. No particular correlation was noted with the stage of hepatitis at which myocarditis appeared, but it is noteworthy that all apparently presented initially as hepatitis. Unfortunately, these observations were made before the availability of markers for hepatitis viruses, so the role of specific hepatitis viruses remains unclear. This difficulty is highlighted by a case report of a patient with viral hepatitis and myocarditis who was clearly documented to have had coxsackie B3 virus disease by serologic methods.[45] This virus is a known cause of myocarditis and, in this case, the hepatitis was the unusual manifestation. Two other recent studies seem to make the association between hepatitis B and myocarditis clearer. Mahapaton and Ellis[46] report two cases in which patients with serologically documented acute hepatitis B presented with symptoms of myocarditis. Serology for other known causes of viral myocarditis was negative.

An even stronger case for the association between hepatitis B and myocarditis was made in the description of a case of fulminant fetal hepatitis B by Ursell et al.[47] At autopsy, these workers found interstitial inflammatory infiltrates similar to those described by Bell. They were also able to demonstrate HB_sAg in cardiac tissue, mostly in arterioles, but not in kidney, liver, or lung. Despite these findings, this patient did not manifest clinical myocarditis. Further studies of the type done in glomerulonephritis must be done before myocarditis can be counted among the extrahepatic manifestations of viral hepatitis.

Neurologic Disease

A number of associations between neurologic symptoms and acute viral hepatitis have been made, and new reports continue to appear. Recently, a series of four cases of mononeuritis associated with viral hepatitis were reported by

Pelletier *et al.*[48] They describe two cases each of hepatitis A and hepatitis B in which the patients had protracted mononeuritis. Interestingly, mononeuritis appeared in both cases of hepatitis B prior to the onset of jaundice together with other prodromal symptoms of acute hepatitis. Better studied is the association between viral hepatitis and Guillain–Barré syndrome, a relationship that had been suggested many years ago. Other reports have noted Guillain–Barré syndrome in association with immune-complex nephritis[49] and with high levels of circulating immune complexes.[50] Two recent case reports make a strong case for a role of hepatitis B in some patients with Guillain–Barré. Huet *et al.*[51] report the case of a 27-year-old woman in whom Guillain–Barré syndrome developed after onset of jaundice due to hepatitis B. HB_sAg was initially detectable in the serum, but when paralysis began, the serum was HB_sAg negative. Cerebrospinal fluid (CSF) examination showed an elevated protein level without cells, and HB_sAg was detected by RIA. Immune complexes and other HBV antigens were not tested for either in serum or in CSF. In the second case, a 76-year-old man in whom Guillain–Barré syndrome developed after acute hepatitis B,[52] HB_sAg was still detectable in the serum 5 weeks after onset, as were HB_sAg-containing immune complexes. At this point, Guillain–Barré syndrome developed. CSF examination showed HB_sAg-containing immune complexes without free HB_sAg. Although the patient remained HB_sAg-positive in the serum, the HB_sAg–immune complexes disappeared after 5 weeks, and the patient recovered. Guillain–Barré syndrome in this patient correlated with development of HB_sAg-containing immune complexes in the serum as well as with the appearance of HB_cAg. An analysis of CSF–serum albumin–immunoglobulin ratios suggested that the immunoglobulin in the CSF was not produced there, but was present as a result of leakage through a disturbed blood–brain barrier (BBB). It seems possible that HBV antigen-containing immune complexes may have contributed to the damage to the BBB and that the coexistence of hepatitis B and Guillain–Barré syndrome were not merely coincidental.

The pathogenesis of the neurologic complications allegedly associated with hepatitis is not entirely clear, but immune complex-induced vasculitis may cause some of the peripheral neuropathies. A review of the neurologic complications of systemic vasculitis by Moore and Fauci[53] suggests that peripheral neuropathies are a complication of vasculitis, but CNS lesions were focal and there were no cases of Guillain–Barré syndrome. It is possible that multiple pathogenic mechanisms may be involved.

REFERENCES

1. Niermeijer P, Gips CH: Natural history of acute hepatitis B in previously healthy patients: A prospective study. *Acta Hepatogastroenterol (Stuttg)* 24:317–325, 1977.
2. Stewart JS, Farrow LJ, Clifford RE, et al: A three-year survey of viral hepatitis in West London. *QJ Med* 47:365–384, 1978.

3. Routenberg JA, Dienstag JL, Harrison WO, et al: Foodborne outbreak of hepatitis A: Clinical and laboratory features of acute and protracted illness. *Am J Med Sci* **278**:123–137, 1979.
4. Wands JR, Mann E, Alpert E, et al: The pathogenesis of arthritis associated with acute hepatitis B surface antigen positive hepatitis: Complement activation and characterization of circulating immune complexes. *J Clin Invest* **55**:930–936, 1975.
5. Dienstag JL, Rhodes AR, Bhan AK, et al: Urticaria associated with acute viral hepatitis type B: Studies of pathogenesis. *Ann Intern Med* **89**:34–40, 1978.
6. Weiss TD, Tsai CC, Baldassare AR, et al: Skin lesions in viral hepatitis: Histologic and immunologic findings. *Am J Med* **64**:269–273, 1978.
7. Gianotti F: Papular acrodermatitis of childhood: An Australia antigen disease. *Arch Dis Child* **48**794–799, 1973.
8. Claudy AL, Ortonne JP, Trepo C: Papular acrodermatitis with hepatitis B infection. *Arch Dermatol* **115**:931–932, 1979.
9. Coombes B, Shorey J, Barrera A, et al: Glomerulonephritis with deposition of Australia antigen–antibody complexes in glomerular basement membrane. *Lancet* **2**:234–237, 1971.
10. Brzosko W, Krawczynski K, Nazarewicz T, et al: Glomerulonephritis associated with hepatitis B surface antigen immune complexes in children. *Lancet* **2**:455–481, 1974.
11. Slusarczyk J, Michalak T, Nazarewicz-deMezer T, et al: Membranous glomerulopathy associated with hepatitis B core antigen complexes in children. *Am J Pathol* **98**:29–39, 1980.
12. Takekoshi Y, Shida N, Saheki Y, et al: Strong association between membranous nephropathy and hepatitis B surface antigenemia in Japanese children. *Lancet* **2**:1065–1068, 1978.
13. Levy M, Klenknecht C, Peix A: Membranous nephropathy and HBsAg. *Lancet* **1**:113, 1979.
14. Takekoshi Y, Tanaka M, Miyakawa Y, et al: Free "small" and IgG-associated "large" hepatitis B antigen in the serum and glomerular capillary walls of two patients with membranous glomerulonephritis. *N Engl J Med* **300**:814–198, 1979.
15. Ito H, Hattori S, Matusda I, et al: Hepatitis Be antigen-mediated membranous glomerulonephritis. *Lab Invest* **44**:214–220, 1981.
16. Cadrobbi P, Bartolotti F, Zacchello G, et al: Hepatitis B virus replication in acute glomerulonephritis with chronic acute hepatitis. *Arch Dis Child* **60**:583–585, 1985.
17. Mizushima N, Kanai K, Matsuda H: Improvement of proteinuria in a case of hepatitis B associated glomerulonephritis after treatment with interferon. *Gastroenterology* **92**:524–526, 1987.
18. Thomas HC, Potter BJ, Elias E, Sherlock S: Metabolism of the third component of complement in acute type B hepatitis, HBs antigen positive glomerulonephritis, polyarteritis nodosum, and HBs antigen positive and negative chronic liver disease. *Gastroenterology* **76**:673–679, 1979.
19. Gocke DJ, Morgan C, Lockshin M, et al: Association between polyarteritis and Australia antigen. *Lancet* **2**:1149–1153, 1970.
20. Gocke DJ, Hsu K, Morgan C, et al: Vasculitis in association with Australia antigen. *J Exp Med* **134**:330–339, 1971.
21. Trepo C, Thivolet J: Antigène Australie, hépatite à virus et periartérite noueuse. *Presse Med* **78**:1575, 1970.
22. Michalak T: Immune complexes of hepatitis B surface antigen in the pathogenesis of periarteritis nodosa. A study of seven necropsy cases. *Am J Pathol* **90**:619–628, 1978.
23. Drueke T, Barbanel C, Jimgers P, et al: Hepatitis B antigen associated periarteritis nodosa in patients undergoing long-germ hemodialysis. *Am J Med* **68**:86–90, 1980.
24. Travers RL, Alliston DJ, Brittle RP, et al: Polyarteritis nodosa: A clinical and angiographic analysis of 17 cases. *Semin Arthritis Rheum* **8**:184–199, 1979.
25. Gover RG, Sausker WF, Kohler PF, et al: Small vessel vasculitis caused by hepatitis B virus immune complexes. *J Allergy Immunol* **62**:222–228, 1978.
26. Kinderman G: Hepatitis B surface antigen and panarteritis. *Med Klin* **74**:1625–1628, 1979.

27. Bruckstein AH, Zimmon DS: Acute abdominal pain, vasculitis, and hepatitis B antigenemia. *NY State J Med* **197–199,** 1980.
28. Govindan S, Itarri AL, Garcia JH: Inflammation of the temporal artery associated with subacute bacterial endocarditis and hepatitis B antigen. *Arch Neurol* **37:**318, 1980.
29. Fainaru M, Friedman G, Friedman B: Temporal arteritis in Israel. A review of 47 patients. *J Rheumatol* **6:**330–335, 1979.
30. Barbado H, Gil-Aguado A, San Martin P, et al: Panarteritis nodosa with positive Australia antigen. *Med Clin (Barc)* **72:**149–153, 1979.
31. Dally S, Guillevin B, Maidenberg M, et al: Periarterite noueuse chez in toxicomane atteint d'hépatite B. *Ann Med Interne (Paris)* **130:**649–652, 1979.
32. Travers RL: Polyarteritis nodosa and related disorders. *Br J Hosp Med* **38–43,** 1979.
33. Sergent JS, Lockshin MD, Christian CL, et al: Vasculitis with hepatitis B antigenemia: Long-term observations in nine patients. *Medicine (Baltimore)* **55:**1–18, 1976.
34. Godeau P, Trepo C, Herreman G, et al: Periartérite noueuse et antigène Australia: Etude comparative à propos de 54 cas. *Sem Hop Paris* **53:**613–619, 1977.
35. Elkon KB, Hughes GRV, Catovsky D: Hairy-cell leukaemia with polyarteritis nodosa. *Lancet* **2:**280–282, 1979.
36. Ettlinger RE, Nelson AM, Burke EC, et al: Polyarteritis nodosa in childhood: A clinical pathologic study. *Arthritis Rheum* **22:**820–825, 1979.
37. Kawasaki disease—United States. *MMWR* **27:**9, 1978.
38. Levo Y, Gorevic PD, Kassab HJ, et al: Association between hepatitis B virus and essential mixed cryoglobulinemia. *N Engl J Med* **296:**1501–1504, 1977.
39. Realdi G, Alberti A, Rigoli A, et al: Immune-complexes and Australia antigen in cryoglobulinemic sera. *Z Immunitaetsforsch* **147:**114–126, 1974.
40. Bombardieri S, Ferri C, DiMunno E, et al: Liver involvement in essential mixed cryoglobulinemia. *Ric Clin Lab* **9:**361–368, 1979.
41. Galli M, Careddu F, D'Armino A, et al: Hepatitis B virus and essential mixed cryoglobulinaemia. *Lancet* **1:**1093, 1980.
42. Popp JW, Dienstag JL, Wands JR, et al: Essential mixed cryoglobulinemia without evidence for hepatitis B virus infection. *Ann Intern Med* **92:**379, 1980.
43. Sanghvi LM, Misra SN: Electrocardiograph abnormalities in epidemic hepatitis. *Circulation* **16:**88–94, 1957.
44. Bell H: Cardiac manifestations of viral hepatitis. *JAMA* **218:**387–391, 1971.
45. Sun NC, Smith VM: Hepatitis associated with myocarditis. *N Engl J Med* **274:**190–193, 1966.
46. Mahapaton RK, Ellis GH: Myocarditis and hepatitis B Angiology. 116–119, 1985.
47. Ursell PC, Habib A, Sharma P, et al: Hepatitis B virus and myocarditis. *Hum Pathol* **15:**481–484, 1984.
48. Pelletier G, Elghozi D, Trepo C, et al: Mononeuritis in acute viral hepatitis. *Digestion* **32:**53–56, 1985.
49. Behan PO, Stilmant M, Lowenstein LM, Sax DS: Landry–Guillain–Barré–Strohl syndrome and immune complex nephritis. *Lancet* **1:**850–854, 1973.
50. Tachovsky TA, Koprowski H, Lisak RP, et al: Circulating immune complexes in multiple sclerosis and other neurological disease. *Lancet* **2:**997–999, 1976.
51. Huet P-M, Layrargues G, Lebrun L-H, Ricker G: Hepatitis B surface antigen in the cerebrospinal fluid in a case of Guillain–Barré syndrome. *Can Med Assoc J* **122:**1157–1159, 1980.
52. Penner E, Maida E, Mamoli B, Gange A: Serum and cerebrospinal fluid immune complexes containing hepatitis B surface antigen in Guillain–Barré syndrome. *Gastroenterology* **82:**576–580, 1982.
53. Moore PM, Fauci AS: Neurologic manifestations of systemic vasculitis. *Am J Med* **71:**517–524, 1981.

The Serology of Viral Hepatitis
Making Sense out of Alphabet Soup

RONALD L. KORETZ

When I was a youngster, my mother told me to have a good hot lunch everyday. So there I was, eating some soup, when the letters

A, a, Ag, Anti, B, c, D, d, DNA, DNAP, e, G, H, HAV, HBV, Ig, M, NANB, r, s, w, y

came floating into my field of vision. I pushed them around with my spoon (since I never was a big fan of vegetable soup anyway) until they all were lined up in alphabetical order. For the rest of this chapter, I shall try to make some sense out of all of them.

Hepatitis viral serologic testing was an unknown entity until the 1960s, when Blumberg described the Australia antigen.[1] This antigenic substance, initially thought to be a genetic marker in Australian aborigines, and then a leukemia-associated factor, proved to be a component of the hepatitis B virus.[2,3] Its name has progressively changed—hepatitis-associated antigen (HAA), serum hepatitis (SH), Mir Serum 2 (MS-2), hepatitis B antigen (HBAg), and finally, hepatitis B surface antigen (HB_sAg)—as our knowledge of the virus has become more sophisticated. Its discovery set off a flurry of other investigations that resulted in the development of serologic tests for hepatitis A[4,5] as well as the recognition of the presence of other common hepatitis viruses for which no test has yet been developed, collectively called non-A, non-B (NANB).[6,7]

Before embarking on a discussion of each viral agent, a few definitions, abbreviations, and concepts must be clarified. The term antigen, abbreviated Ag,

RONALD L. KORETZ • Division of Gastroenterology, Olive View Medical Center, Sylmar, California 91342; and Department of Medicine, University of California School of Medicine, Los Angeles, California 90024;

refers to a component of the virus that the human host recognizes as foreign and to which an antibody (abbreviated anti) response is mounted. The antibody is a host-manufactured globulin that may be of either the immunoglobulin (Ig) G or M class. IgM antibody arises first and is relatively short-lived; the IgG antibody persists for many years and, in the case of an anamnestic response, is the type of antibody produced. Hepatitis A is referred to as HA and hepatitis B as HB. The specific viruses are the hepatitis A virus (HAV) and the hepatitis B virus (HBV).

SEROLOGY OF HEPATITIS A

The serology of hepatitis A is simpler than that of hepatitis B and is dealt with first. The virus has a short viremic phase; hepatitis A antigen (HAAg) can be found in the stool during the late incubation period, but it is usually cleared by the time the illness peaks clinically.[8] For these reasons, it is impractical to measure the presence of the virus directly (by demonstrating the presence of an antigen) either in stool or in blood.

Instead, the diagnosis of HA is established by finding IgM-specific antibody to HAAG (anti-HA). The antibody response to hepatitis A does occur early in the course of the illness, and anti-HA is demonstrable by the time the patient presents with symptoms.[9] Although anti-HA activity persists for many years (? lifelong), the IgM-specific anti-HA is classically thought to disappear in months.[10] Thus, the patient with clinically apparent acute hepatitis who has concomitant IgM-anti-HA positivity has hepatitis A by definition. If the serum is negative for anti-HA, or is only positive for IgG (or polyclonal)-anti-HA, non-A disease is present.

The advantage of this IgM-specific test is obvious. We do not have to collect both an acute and convalescent serum specimen and look for a rise in titer of anti-HA. This not only saves expense (the second blood test) but also allows for a determination of the illness at the time the disease appears. However, the validity of the test rests on the assumption that the IgM-specific anti-HA lasts only a short period, a time during which the patient is not likely to become exposed to, and manifest, a second hepatotoxic process.

Thus, it is important to ascertain how long the IgM-anti-HA test actually remains positive. The commercial assay no doubt undergoes periodic improvements in sensitivity (see later comments regarding antibody to HB_sAg), so it would be of interest to look at some recent data regarding persistence of IgM-anti-HA; these are summarized in Table I.[11-16] With the exception of one Italian study,[16] IgM-anti-HA appears to disappear in almost all patients within 1 year. Using the IgM-anti-HA test, one may occasionally misdiagnose acute hepatitis A (since an occasional patient with non-A liver disease might have been exposed to the HAV during the prior 12-month period and still carry IgM-anti-HA, but a positive test is going to be accurate in the majority of patients.

TABLE I. Persistence of IgM-Anti-HA

Number of patients	Number (%) positive at				Reference
	3 months	6 months	9 months	12 months	
7	7 (100%)	2 (29%)			Storch et al. (1982)[11]
7	6 (86%)	2 (29%)			Chara et al. (1983)[12]
47		6 (13%)		≧2 (≧4%)	Cornu et al. (1984)[13]
37	18 (49%)	8 (22%)	5 (14%)	1 (3%)	Kao et al. (1984)[14]
102	100 (98%)	18 (18%)			Hatzakis and Hadziyannis (1984)[15]
69		(93%)		(78%)	Caredda et al. (1984)[16]

SEROLOGY OF HEPATITIS B

Classic Considerations

Hepatitis B serology is more intimidating than hepatitis A serology because of the larger number of tests available. The virus itself has three separate antigens: surface (s), core (c), and e (e). The hepatitis B surface antigen (HB_sAg) is a component of the outer coat or surface of the HBV particle. This coat covers the nucleoprotein center (containing the DNA) of the virus and, in the circulation, the intact virus is referred to as the Dane particle.

Interestingly, for every intact virus, there are hundreds of empty coat particles in the circulation.[17] Teleologically, there may be good reason for this. The HBV infects the liver cell and turns it into a factory producing HBV-specific products. In particular, HBV DNA is made in the nucleus, where a DNA assembly line is already in place. The coat particles are manufactured in the cytoplasm. If only one coat particle were to be available for each HBV DNA produced, the two might never meet. By having a large excess of coat particles, each HBV DNA is sure to find a home. Since these materials ultimately escape from the hepatocyte, it is no small wonder that excess coat particles are found in the systemic circulation. (The preceding explanation is entirely my own speculation.)

HB_sAg is not a uniform protein. There appear to be subtype or strain variations of this antigen.[18] These subtypes are of some interest epidemiologically, since different subtypes predominate in different regions of the world; the different strains do not, however, behave any differently clinically. All HB_sAg contains the a serotype; in addition, it contains either a d or a y and either a w or an r. Thus, HB_sAg may be adr, adw, ayr, or ayw. (We shall return to the issue of subtypes later, when we examine the question of serum which tests positive for both HB_sAg and for its antibody.)

The host manufactures antibody to HB_sAg, anti-HB_s, which can be viewed as a convalescent phenomenon. When a person is infected with the HBV, HB_sAg appears; in those who recover from the illness (and the majority of patients do), HB_sAg disappears and anti-HB_s appears during the convalescent phase.[19] Anti-HB_s is then a marker of immunity against reinfection with hepatitis B; it is also a protective agent when administered exogenously to patients exposed to hepatitis B.[20]

The second antigen, hepatitis B core antigen (HB_cAg), is a component of the DNA nucleoprotein of the virus. This antigen never circulates freely, as it is always covered over by the coat. Therefore, we do not routinely test the blood for HB_cAg. It might be wondered how the body could then make antibody to it (anti-HB_c). Again, while the answer is not known conclusively, my speculation is that, at the level of the liver, occasional naked HB_cAg does escape from the hepatocyte. This antigen then immediately encounters the reticuloendothelial system (in the form of Kupffer cells) and stimulates the humoral response. The amount of HB_cAg that could reach the systemic circulation, however, is trivial.

Anti-HB_c, unlike anti-HB_s, is neither a marker of convalescence nor of immunity. In fact, it is found early in the course of the illness, arising within a few days or weeks of the appearance of HB_sAg in the circulation.[19,21,22] It persists whether or not the HBV infection resolves.[19] (A percentage of patients with HB develop a chronic infection and the chronic carrier state, in which HB_sAg is always demonstrable in the serum, and anti-HB_s never appears; more details about this phenomenon may be found in Chapter 12 of this volume).

The third antigen, hepatitis B e antigen (HB_eAg), is a degradation product of HB_cAg.[23,24] Unlike HB_cAg, however, it can be found free in the systemic circulation. It is seen early in the course of the infection and disappears before HB_sAg does. In acute HB (i.e., in which the HBV infection is cleared), HB_eAg may only be present for a few days or weeks; it is even possible to have it gone when the patient is first seen by a physician.[25] In chronic HBV carriers, HB_eAg may persist for years, but these patients often (perhaps always, if one waits long enough) lose this marker.[26] After HB_eAg disappears, its antibody (anti-HB_e) is demonstrable in the circulation. The HB_eAg–anti-HB_e system is not used in the serodiagnosis of hepatitis B, as it provides no further information than can be gleaned from the other three tests (HB_sAg, anti-HB_c, anti-HB_s). The e tests have been used for other information, a subject to which we shall also return.

The sequence of events in HB relates to the appearance of the antigens, followed by the development of the respective antibodies. Thus, the first serologic marker seen is HB_sAg, followed closely thereafter by HB_eAg and anti-HB_c (HB_cAg makes its appearance only at the level of the liver, not the systemic circulation). HB_eAg is usually lost before HB_sAg; anti-HB_e is commonly found even while HB_sAg is still present. If and when the infection resolves, HB_sAg

disappears and, after a period of time when there is no surface marker at all (days or many weeks, referred to as the serologic window), anti-HB$_s$ develops.

In theory, the antibodies last forever. In practice, this is not always the case. As we shall see, e testing is only an issue when the patient is HB$_s$Ag positive, so it is of no concern as to how long anti-HB$_e$ lasts in convalescence. Anti-HB$_c$ and anti-HB$_s$ persist for many years, perhaps even decades. Eventually, however, one or the other may disappear. If anti-HB$_c$ is lost first, the serologic picture is one of anti-HB$_s$ positivity only. This is the same serologic picture as one would see in a vaccinated patient (since the only antigenic exposure is to HB$_s$Ag). Note that both conditions (vaccination or a late convalescence) imply an immune state. If anti-HB$_s$ disappears first, the serologic status is identical to that seen during the serologic window. However, now the implications are different; it has been thought that some patients may still have active hepatitis B during the window phase,[21] whereas this is clearly not the situation very late in convalescence.

How can one tell, by serologic testing, what is going on in a patient who is positive only for anti-HB$_c$? In theory, if one knew that the antibody was recent in onset, the implication would be that the window phase was being observed. This observation can be made in practice by remembering the IgM–IgG globulin sequence. Tests for IgM-specific anti-HB$_c$ have been developed and might be useful in this situation.

In summary, three serologic tests can be used to diagnose HBV infection: HB$_s$Ag, anti-HB$_c$, anti-HB$_s$. Each test is either positive or negative; if one obtains a serologic panel, there are only eight possible combinations, i.e., 2^3. It would seem impossible to see concomitant HB$_s$Ag and anti-HB$_s$, since HB$_s$Ag should disappear before anti-HB$_s$ appears. Another rarely encountered situation would be HB$_s$Ag in the absence of anti-HB$_c$. Thus, there are only five predictably common combinations, which are summarized in Table II.

TABLE II. Common Combinations of Hepatitis B Serology[a]

HB$_s$Ag	Anti-HB$_c$	Anti-HB$_s$	Explanation
+	+	−	Active HBV infection
−	+	+	Convalescent hepatitis B
−	−	+	Late convalescence/vaccination
−	+	−	Late convalescence/window phase
−	−	−	No past/present HBV exposure

[a]The other three combinations would not be expected to be seen very often or at all; they include HB$_s$Ag+/anti-HB$_c$−/anti-HB$_s$−, HB$_s$Ag+/anti-HB$_c$+/anti-HB$_s$+, and HB$_s$Ag+/anti-HB$_c$−/anti-HB$_s$+.

False-Positive Anti-HB$_s$

The above discussion was labeled "classic considerations" and represents what I was taught, and subsequently taught others, through the mid-1980s. Unfortunately, some more recent information has forced me (and now you) to rethink. As a preamble, I will digress to tell you about three seemingly disparate observations, all of which point out the current problem.

Before 1980, it was rare to find a patient with concomitant anti-HB$_s$ and HB$_s$Ag in the same serum. This phenomenon was not seen in any of 303 HB$_s$Ag-positive blood donors.[27] However, such cases were occasionally seen and, by virtue of their uniqueness, reported.[28–32] Whenever these cases were evaluated, a subtype difference between the HB$_s$Ag and anti-HB$_s$ was found. This implied that at least some people developed incomplete immunity to the HBV, an implication that passed without much mention at the time.

After 1980, a series of reports appeared noting that concomitant anti-HB$_s$ was a common finding in large series of HB$_s$Ag-positive patients.[33–37] These data are summarized in Table III. What was a rare finding during the 1970s was a virtual epidemic during the 1980s.

The second observation was made by Hoofnagle et al.[38] In an effort to look for animal models of hepatitis B, animals (nonprimates) were tested for HBV markers. None was positive for HB$_s$Ag or anti-HB$_c$, but anti-HB$_s$ was found in some of them. This antibody was generally of low titer and IgM class. These animals are not recognized hosts of the human HBV.

Third, a number of reports exist describing the development of hepatitis B in individuals known to have preexistent anti-HB$_s$.[39–42] Although this phenomenon has been most often appreciated in individuals with low titers of preexistent anti-HB$_s$, this has not always been the case.[42]

All three observations describe the finding of anti-HB$_s$ where it does not belong or is not acting as a biologic antibody or both. Furthermore, it appears that the frequency of this finding increased dramatically after 1980. One might wonder whether the anti-HB$_s$ test is responsible, i.e., that it is identifying some

TABLE III. Frequency of Anti-HB$_s$ Positivity in HB$_s$Ag-Positive Persons

Patient population	Number HB$_s$Ag-positive individuals	Number (%) positive for anti-HB$_s$	Reference
Chronic hepatitis B	89	32 (36%)	Heijtink et al. (1982)[33]
Homosexual males	234	40 (17%)	Schreeder et al. (1982)[34]
Chronic hepatitis B	228	83 (32%)	Schiels et al. (1984)[35]
Hospital patients	269	64 (24%)	Tsang et al. (1986)[36]
Chronic hepatitis B	80	7 (9%)	Sjogren et al. (1986)[37]

non-anti-HB_s substance as antibody; in laboratory parlance, we would call this a false-positive result. It has been reported that the commercial anti-HB_s test has become more sensitive but less specific.[43,44]

The anti-HB_s test is a radioimmunoassay (RIA) in which positivity or negativity is determined by the ratio of the amount of radioactivity in the unknown serum compared to that in the negative control. In general, a ratio > 2.1 is considered positive. This ratio roughly correlates with the actual titer of antibody, and a serum to negative control, or sound to noise (S–N) ratio of $2.1–10$ is now called low titer. Although false-positive tests may exist in higher titer (the early reports of concomitant HB_sAg and anti-HB_s, reference 42) the major clinical problem is with the interpretation of the low titer positives.

The prevalences of anti-HB_s in populations of healthy health care workers are summarized on Table IV.[45–51] Between 6 and 13% of them had anti-HB_s; about one third to one half had anti-HB_s in the absence of anti-HB_c. Of note, 65–85% of those who had anti-HB_s as the only hepatitis B serologic marker were found to have this anti-HB_s present in low titer. When such patients were challenged with one dose of hepatitis B vaccine, anamnestic responses were only seen in 0%,[45] 40%,[46] 23%,[48] and $\leq$33%[52] of them. Thus, low-titer anti-HB_s is a common finding in healthy populations (at least in healthy populations of health care workers), and if an anamnestic response is to be taken as evidence of true anti-HB_s, most low-titer anti-HB_s represents a false-positive test result.

Armed with this information about the serologic tests, we can now look at the other three serologic combinations not considered in Table II, which are summarized in Table V. Concomitant HB_sAg and anti-HB_s should be interpreted as active HBV infection with a false-positive anti-HB_s test (not as incomplete immunity). HB_sAg in the absence of anti-HB_c would represent early HBV infec-

TABLE IV. Frequency of Low Titer Anti-HB_s in Health Care Workers[a]

| Population (N) | Percentage of population with | | | Reference |
	Anti-HB_s	Only anti-HB_s	LT anti-HB_s	
HCW (1626)	12	3.8	2.5	Hadler et al.[45]
Students (813)[b]	6	3.8	3.1	Perrillo et al.[46]
HCW (908)	12	4.2	3.5	Kessler et al.[47]
HCW (2109)	13	6.0	4.0	Werner et al.[48]
HCW (192)[c]	(100)	(47)	(30)	Hanson and Polesky[49]
HCW (620)	6	4.2	3.2	Warner et al.[50]
HCW (825)	11	5.5	4.4	Storch et al.[51]

[a]HCW, health care workers; LT, low titer.
[b]Medical/dental students.
[c]Only anti-HB_s positive workers considered.

TABLE V. Less Common Combinations of Hepatitis B Serologies

HB$_s$Ag	Anti-HB$_c$	Anti-HB$_s$	Explanation
+	−	−	Very early HBV infection or vaccinemia
+	+	+	Active HBV infection and false-positive anti-HB$_s$
+	−	+	Very early HBV infection or vaccinemia with false-positive anti-HB$_s$

tion (before the development of anti-HB$_c$). (Although there would be no reason in practice to do these tests at the time, this combination might also be seen if blood were obtained from a very recently vaccinated patient.)

Clinical Value of HB$_e$Ag/Anti-HB$_e$

In patients with acute hepatitis B, e tests do not add any information to the diagnostic evaluation (since either test may be positive when the patient is first seen). There is no reason to obtain these tests at that time. In practice, the clinical value of these tests is limited to the HB$_s$Ag chronic carrier.

It is clear that chronic carriers who are HB$_e$Ag positive are more likely to be infective; its presence correlates strongly with disease transmission.[53-56] However, this correlation is not 100%; not all HB$_e$Ag-positive exposures result in transmission, and some anti-HB$_e$-positive patients have spread disease. From a practical perspective, we treat all HB$_s$Ag exposures the same, regardless of the e status of the exposor (with regard to prophylaxis for the exposee). For this reason, there is not a great demand for e testing.

Patients with chronic hepatitis B who are HB$_e$Ag positive tend to have more severe inflammatory disease than do those who are anti-HB$_e$ positive with regard to histology[57] and to aminotransferase levels.[58-60] Again, this correlation is not 100%; HB$_e$Ag will not uniformly predict the presence of chronic active hepatitis, nor will anti-HB$_e$ always be associated with chronic persistent (or less severe) hepatitis. Cirrhosis is associated with anti-HB$_e$ positivity.[61] (This latter association may not be directly due to HB$_e$Ag seroconversion, however; both cirrhosis and anti-HB$_e$ are later phenomena of chronic HBV infection.)

In addition to more active disease, the presence of HB$_e$Ag correlates (again, not completely) with other markers of HBV replication, such as the presence of Dane particles,[62] DNA polymerase,[63] HB$_s$Ag titer,[64] and HBV DNA.[64,65] In fact, one might wonder whether the degree of replication is responsible for the severity of the inflammatory response.[66] On the basis of the assumption that this is true, various trials of antiviral agents (e.g., interferon) have used HB$_e$Ag seroconversion (to anti-HB$_e$) as a therapeutic end point. If this assumption turns out to be true, and if antiviral therapy proves effective, this would be one area in which e testing could have practical clinical value.

One final comment with regard to HB_eAg is the occasional report of it being found in the absence of HB_sAg.[67,68] It is unclear whether these observations represent false-positive tests for HB_eAg, false-negative tests for HB_sAg, or a true, but rare, situation. From a practical point of view, it does not matter, not only because it is rarely seen, but, more importantly, because e status only has clinical relevance in the HB_sAg-positive person.

Clinical Value of IgM-Specific Anti-HB$_c$

If anti-HB$_c$ goes through the same IgM–IgG sequence as other antibodies, the IgM-anti-HB$_c$ test would be a useful way to diagnose acute hepatitis B as well as to separate that process from a non-B disease in an HB_sAg chronic carrier. In fact, the lack of demonstration of IgM-anti-HB$_c$ has been widely accepted as the definition of non-B disease in carriers.[69–72]

If IgM-anti-HB$_c$ arose early in and only lasted for a relatively short period during, the initial HBV infection and then disappeared forever, this would be an appropriate use of the assay. In acute hepatitis B, the IgM-anti-HB$_c$ has been reported to last for only 5 weeks after the peak aminotransferase has been reached[73]; unfortunately, other investigators have found this antibody to last much longer,[74–76] even as long as 6 years.[77] Furthermore, it has been found in patients with chronic hepatitis B.[73,75,76,78] It has even been found to recur (i.e., the patient again becomes IgM-anti-HB$_c$ positive) in acute exacerbations of chronic hepatitis B.[79–81]

Part of the confusion with this test has to do with the fact that different assay systems are used. Unfortunately, even if data using only the commercially available tests are considered, confusion still abounds. Persons inadvertently diagnosed at a very early stage of infection (HB_sAg positive, anti-HB$_c$ negative) who were followed for several weeks all developed anti-HB$_c$; the IgM-anti-HB$_c$ test only was positive when the total anti-HB$_c$ was present in high titer.[82] Infants developing hepatitis B were never positive for IgM-anti-HB$_c$.[83] Two of 24 cases of acute hepatitis B (clearly acute by other criteria) were HB_sAg positive but IgM-anti-HB$_c$ negative.[84] In an outbreak of hepatitis B (in cancer patients) related to a HBV-contaminated serum, at least two patients (7%) failed to demonstrate IgM-anti-HB$_c$ during the first 2 weeks of clinical illness, and at least 10% remained positive for this IgM antibody (even though the hepatitis resolved) for at least 1 year.[85] The commercial IgM-anti-HB$_c$ test may be positive in chronic hepatitis B; its presence may correlate with high aminotransferase levels.[86,87] Thus, the commercial assay may be falsely negative in about 10% of cases of adult acute hepatitis B; it may also be falsely positive in an indeterminate (but probably relatively low) percentage of chronic infections.

What about its use in defining the window phase of HBV infections? Even here, the IgM-anti-HB$_c$ has become nondetectable in some patients (? about 50%) before anti-HB$_s$ has appeared.[85,88] If the test were to be positive in a patient with anti-HB$_c$ as the only hepatitis B serologic marker, it would be reasonable to assume that this did represent the window phase.

SEROLOGY OF HEPATITIS NANB

The NANB agents are so named because we do not have any specific serologic tests for them. It is unclear to me (and most others) why we have not yet been able to identify these agents. Cytomegalovirus and Epstein–Barr virus, agents known to cause hepatitis, are not the culpable parties in most cases of NANB disease. In a chapter I wrote in 1978, I boldly stated: "In the near future an assay for hepatitis C and possibly other hepatitis viruses will be developed."[57] It is obvious that my "near future" has to be taken in the cosmic sense rather than as a small fraction of one lifetime.

One could speculate as to the reasons why NANB tests have been so long in coming, in spite of probably hundreds of attempts. We may have been fortunate with hepatitis B, in that the antigen load in the serum was so high, a situation not occurring in other infections. If the NANB infections are associated with large numbers of antigen–antibody immune complexes, these complexes may interfere with standard immunologic reactions.[89] It is also possible that the virus circulates inside another cell, such as a lymphocyte; as such, its antigenic sites would be no more available for immunologic reaction than is HB$_c$Ag.[90]

It has been speculated that NANB is actually a *forme fruste* of the HBV.[91] The diseases do share epidemiologic similarities. Tissue (hepatic) HBV markers have been observed in patients without serologic markers of past or present hepatitis B infection.[92,93] Electron microscopic similarities to hepatitis B were reported in specimens of NANB disease,[94] although this histologic finding was subsequently attributed to a non-B process.[95] A monoclonal antibody has allegedly detected HB$_s$Ag in the sera of patients with putative NANB hepatitis.[96] An HB$_e$Ag-like product has also been found in such patients.[97]

These observations have not been widely accepted because the findings could not be validated. HBV DNA has not been found.[98,99] When these putative *formes frustes* of HBV have been given to chimpanzees, hepatitis occurred without any change in the baseline hepatitis B serologies.[96,97] For the present, we will presume that the NANB agents are separate and distinct from hepatitis B.

Delta is an RNA virus that is incomplete, that is, it cannot infect man unless there is active (acute or chronic) HBV infection. This virus has been recognized only in the past few years and, presumably because of its Greek name, has been called hepatitis D. I personally object to this nomenclature, because the virus cannot exist by itself (therefore, why give it a capital letter?) and because it will interrupt the alphabetic sequence of the complete viruses (since we know that at least three other NANB agents exist). For this reason, in this chapter it will be referred to as δ.

Classically, active δ infection has been thought to be present if the antibody, anti-δ, is present.[100,101] Although HδAg has occasionally been found in the circulation, it is usually absent[101]; it may be found histologically (in hepatocytes), however.[101] The problem in defining active infection by an antibody test is in being sure that this antibody will disappear shortly after the infection does. In the case of δ, this appears not to be the case; the anti-δ has been observed for years,[101] and was recently noted to persist for 5 years after HB_sAg was no longer detectable.[102]

Analogously to IgM-anti-HB_c, we are now seeing investigators using high-titer IgM-specific anti-δ as the definition of active δ infection.[103,104] Also analogously to the IgM-anti-HB_c test, we now are finding out that the level of this IgM antibody is also related to the activity of the disease[102] and that this IgM antibody is not always found in the early phases of many (? most) δ infections.[105]

CONCLUSION: THE BOTTOM OF THE BOWL

Having stirred the "soup" for awhile, with what useful points can we be left?

1. A positive IgM-anti-HA test is the standard definition of acute hepatitis A; the absence of this IgM-specific antibody implies the absence of a recent (active) HAV infection.
2. Active HBV infection is usually defined by the presence of HB_sAg; it may also be present in patients who have anti-HB_c as their only hepatitis B serologic marker and in whom the IgM-anti-HB_c test is positive.
3. A person who has acute hepatitis (on clinical grounds) and who is positive for HB_sAg but negative for IgM-anti-HB_c will usually (but not always) be a chronic HB_sAg carrier with a superimposed non-B process.
4. Patients with anti-HB_s as their only hepatitis B serologic marker, especially if this anti-HB_s is low titer, will often be found to have non-biologic antibody (i.e., they are unprotected against hepatitis B).
5. Patients with clinical evidence of hepatitis epidemiologically consistent with a viral exposure should be considered to have NANB viral disease if they lack serologic evidence of active HAV or HBV infection.
6. We are currently unsure exactly how to diagnose δ hepatitis, although a high titer of IgM-specific anti-δ may be the best test.

Bon appetit!

REFERENCES

1. Blumberg BS, Alter HJ, Visnich S: A "new" antigen in leukemia sera. *JAMA* **191:**101–106, 1965.
2. Blumberg BS, Gerstley BJS, Hungerford DA, et al: A serum antigen (Australia antigen) in Downs' syndrome, leukemia, and hepatitis. *Ann Intern Med* **66:**924–931, 1967.
3. Prince AM: An antigen detected in the blood during the incubation period of serum hepatitis. *Proc Natl Acad Sci USA* **60:**814–821, 1968.
4. Feinstone SM, Kapikian AZ, Purcell RH: Hepatitis A: detection by immune electron microscopy of a viruslike antigen associated with acute illness. *Science* **182:**1026–1028, 1973.
5. Provost PJ, Ittensohn OL, Villarejos VM, et al: A specific complement-fixation test for human hepatitis A employing CR 326 virus antigen: Diagnosis and epidemiology. *Proc Soc Exp Biol Med* **148:**961–968, 1975.
6. Hollinger FB, Mosley JW, Szmuness W, et al: Transfusion-transmitted viruses study: Experimental evidence for two non-A, non-B hepatitis agents. *J Infect Dis* **142:**400–407, 1980.
7. Bradley DW, Maynard JE, Cook EH, et al: Non-A, non-B hepatitis in experimentally infected chimpanzees: Cross challenge and electron microscopic studies. *J Med Virol* **6:**185–201, 1980.
8. Dienstag JL: Viral hepatitis type A: Virology and course. *Clin Gastroenterol* **9:**135–154, 1980.
9. Bradley DW, Maynard JE, Hindman SH, et al: Serodiagnosis of viral hepatitis A: Detection by acute-phase immunoglobulin M anti-hepatitis A virus by radioimmunoassay. *J Clin Microbiol* **5:**521–530, 1977.
10. Schafer DF, Hoofnagle JH: Serological diagnosis of viral hepatitis. *Viewpoints Dig Dis* **14:**5–8, 1982.
11. Storch, GA, Bodicky, C, Parker M, et al: Use of conventional and IgM-specific radioimmunoassays for anti-hepatitis A antibody in an outbreak of hepatitis A. *Am J Med* **73:**663–668, 1982.
12. Ohara, H, Naruto H, Watanabe W, et al: An outbreak of hepatitis A caused by consumption of raw oysters. *J Hyg* **91:**163–165, 1983.
13. Cornu C, Lamy ME, Geubel A, et al: Persistence of immunoglobulin M antibody to hepatitis A virus and relapse of hepatitis A infection. (Letter.) *Eur J Clin Microbiol* **3:**45–46, 1984.
14. Kao HW, Ashcavi, M, Redeker AG: The persistence of hepatitis A IgM antibody after acute clinical hepatitis. *Hepatology* **4:**933–936, 1984.
15. Hatzakis A, Hadziyannis S: Sex-related differences in immunoglobulin M and in total antibody response to hepatitis A virus observed in two epidemics of hepatitis A. *Am J Epidemiol* **120:**936–942, 1984.
16. Caredda F, D'Arminio Monforte A, Rossi E, et al: Prolonged course and relapses of acute type A separarl hepatitis. *Boll Ist Sieroter Milan* **63:**34–36, 1984.
17. Einarsson M, Kaplan L, Utter G: Purification of hepatitis B surface antigen by affinity chromatography. *Vox Sang* **35:**224–233, 1978.
18. Courouce-Pauty A-M, Soulier JP: Further data on HBs antigen subtypes—Geographical distribution. *Vox Sang* **27:**533–549, 1974.
19. Krugman S, Overby LR, Mushahwar IK, et al: Viral hepatitis, type B. *N Engl J Med* **300:**101–106, 1979.
20. Seeff LB, Koff RS: Passive and active immunoprophylaxis of hepatitis B. *Gastroenterology* **86:**958–981, 1984.
21. Krugman S, Hoofnagle JH, Gerety RJ, et al: Viral hepatitis, type B. *N Engl J Med* **290:**1331–1335, 1974.
22. Courouce A, Drouet J, LeMarrec N, et al: Blood donors positive for HBsAg and negative for anti-HBc antibody. *Vox Sang* **49:**26–33, 1985.
23. Takahashi K, Akahane Y, Gotanda T, et al: Demonstration of hepatitis B e antigen in the core of Dane particles. *J Immunol* **122:**275–279, 1979.

24. Slusarczyk J, Hess G, Meyer zum Buschenfelde K-H: Association of hepatitis B e antigen (HBeAg) with the core of the hepatitis B virus. *Liver* **5:**48–53, 1985.
25. Frosner GG, Brodersen M, Papaevangelou G, et al: Detection of HBeAg and anti-HBe in acute hepatitis B by a sensitive radioimmunoassay. *J Med Virol* **3:**67–76, 1978.
26. Sanchez-Tapias JM, Vilar JH, Costa J, et al: Natural history of chronic persistent hepatitis B. *J Hepatol* **1:**15–27, 1984.
27. Vyas GN, Roberts I, Peterson DL, et al: Nonspecific test reactions for antibodies to hepatitis B surface antigen in chronic HBsAg carriers. *J Lab Clin Med* **89:**428–432, 1977.
28. Tabor E, Gerety RJ, Smallwood LA, et al: Coincident hepatitis B surface antigen and antibodies of different subtypes in human serum. *J Immunol* **118:**369–370, 1977.
29. Courouce-Pauty A-M, Drouet J, Kleinknecht D: Simultaneous occurrence in the same serum of hepatitis B surface antigen and antibody to hepatitis B surface antigen of different subtypes. *J Infect Dis* **140:**975–978, 1979.
30. Brandt K-H, Katchaki JN, Bronkhorst FB, et al: Co-occurrence of hepatitis Bs-antigen and heterotypic anti-HBs in the same serum. *Neth J Med* **23:**233–236, 1980.
31. Le Bouvier GL, Capper RA, Williams AE, et al: Concurrently circulating hepatitis B surface antigen and heterotypic anti-HBs antibody. *J Immunol* **117:**2262–2264, 1976.
32. Sasaki T, Ohkubo Y, Yamashita Y, et al: Co-occurrence of hepatitis B surface antigen of a particular subtype and antibody to a heterologous subtypic specificity in the same serum. *J Immunol* **117:**2258–2259, 1976.
33. Heijtink RA, Van Hattum J, Schalm S, et al: Co-occurrence of HBsAg and anti-HBs. *J Med Virol* **10:**83–90, 1982.
34. Schreeder MT, Thompson SE, Hadler SC, et al: Hepatitis B in homosexual men: Prevalence of infection and factors related to transmission. *J Infect Dis* **146:**7–12, 1982.
35. Shiels MT, Taswell HF, Czaja AJ, et al: Concurrent HBsAg and anti-HBs in acute and chronic hepatitis B. *Hepatology* **4:**1035, 1984 (abst).
36. Tsang TK, Blei AT, O'Reilly D, et al: Clinical significance of concurrent hepatitis B surface antigen and antibody positivity. *Dig Dis Sci* **31:**620–624, 1986.
37. Sjogren MH, Bancroft WH, Hoofnagle JH, et al: Clinical significance of low molecular weight (7–8 S) immunoglobulin M antibody to hepatitis B core antigen in chronic hepatitis B virus infection. *Gastroenterology* **91:**168–173, 1986.
38. Hoofnagle JH, Schafer DF, Ferenci P, et al: Antibody to hepatitis B surface antigen in nonprimate animal species. *Gastroenterology,* **84:**1478–1482, 1982.
39. Koziol DE, Alter HJ, Kirchner JP, et al: The development of HBsAg-positive hepatitis despite the previous existence of antibody to HBsAg. *J Immunol* **117:**2260–2262, 1976.
40. Swenson, PD, Escobar MR, Carithers RL, et al: Failure of pre-existing antibody against hepatitis B surface antigen to prevent subsequent hepatitis B infection. *J Clin Microbiol* **18:**305–309, 1983.
41. Sherertz RJ, Spindel E, Hoofnagle JH: Antibody to hepatitis B surface antigen may not always indicate immunity to hepatitis B virus infection. (Letter.) *N Engl J Med* **309:**1519, 1983.
42. Linnemann CC, Askey PA: Susceptibility to hepatitis B despite high titer anti-HBs antibody. *Lancet* **1:**346–347, 1984.
43. Koretz RL: Hepatitis: Serious papers, funny papers, in Gitnick GL (ed): *Current Hepatology,* Vol. VI. Chicago, Year Book Medical, 1986, pp. 1–63.
44. Leibowitz AI, Vladutiu AO: Concomitant hepatitis B surface antigen and antibody. (Letter.) *Ann Intern Med* **100:**615, 1984.
45. Hadler SC, Murphy BL, Schable CA, et al: Epidemiological analysis of the significance of low-positive test results for antibody to hepatitis B surface and core antigen. *J Clin Microbiol* **19:**521–525, 1984.
46. Perrillo RP, Parker MC, Campbell C, et al: Prevaccination screening of medical and dental students. *JAMA* **250:**2481–2484, 1983.

47. Kessler HA, Harris AA, Payne JA, et al: Antibodies to hepatitis B surface antigen as the sole hepatitis B marker in hospital personnel. *Ann Intern Med* **103**:21–26, 1985.
48. Werner BG, Dienstag JS, Kuter BJ, et al: Isolated antibody to hepatitis B surface antigen and response to hepatitis B vaccination. *Ann Intern Med* **103**:201–205, 1985.
49. Hanson M, Polesky HF: Prevalence of anti-HBc in anti-HBs positive individuals: Implications for selecting vaccine candidates. *Am J Clin Pathol* **82**:716–719, 1984.
50. Warner HA, MacSween HM, MacLeod JE, et al: Hepatitis B immune status of health workers: Survey of a regional hospital in New Brunswick. *Can J Public Health* **75**:314–317, 1984.
51. Storch GA, Perillo RP, Miller JP, et al: Prevalence of hepatitis B antibodies in personnel at a children's hospital. *Pediatrics* **76**:29–35, 1985.
52. MacLeod JE, MacSween HM, Warner HA, et al: Should individuals with anti-HBs as the only marker of infection with hepatitis B receive hepatitis B vaccine? *Can J Public Health* **76**:229–232, 1985.
53. Alter HJ, Seeff LB, Kaplan PM, et al: Type B hepatitis: The infectivity of blood positive for e antigen and DNA polymerase after accidental needlestick exposure. *N Engl J Med* **295**:909–913, 1976.
54. Shikata T, Karasawa T, Abe K, et al: Hepatitis B e antigen and infectivity of hepatitis B virus. *J Infect Dis* **136**:571–576, 1977.
55. Koretz RL: Hepatitis: Same time, same station, in Gitnick GL (ed): *Current Hepatology*. Vol. III. Wiley, New York, 1983, pp. 1–47.
56. Weiner BG, Grady GF: Accidental hepatitis-B-surface-antigen-positive inoculations. *Ann Intern Med* **97**:367–369, 1982.
57. Koretz RL: Acute and chronic hepatitis, in Gitnick GL (ed): *Current Gastroenterology and Hepatology*. Boston, Houghton-Mifflin, 1979, pp. 234–275.
58. Reesing HW, Wesdorp ICE, Grijm R, et al: Follow-up of blood donors positive for hepatitis B surface antigen. *Vox Sang* **38**:136–146, 1980.
59. DeFranchis R, D'Arminio A, Vecchi M, et al: Chronic asymptomatic HBsAg carriers: Histologic abnormalities and diagnostic and prognostic value of serologic markers of the HBV. *Gastroenterology* **79**:521–527, 1980.
60. Sasaki T, Hattori T, Mayumi M: A large-scale survey on the prevalence of HBeAg and anti-HBe among asymptomatic carriers of HBV. *Vox Sang* **37**:216–221, 1979.
61. Realdi G, Alberti A, Rugge M, et al: Seroconversion from hepatitis B e antigen to anti-HBe in chronic hepatitis B virus infection. *Gastroenterology* **79**:195–199, 1980.
62. Trepo C, Bird RG, Zuckerman AJ: Correlations between the detection of e antigen or antibody and electron microscopic pattern of hepatitis B surface antigen (HBsAg) associated particles in the serum of HBsAg carriers. *J Clin Pathol* **30**:216–220, 1977.
63. Heijtink RA, Schalm SW: Quantitative assay of hepatitis B surface antigen and DNA polymerase activity. *N Engl J Med* **301**:165, 1979.
64. Kam W, Rall LB, Smuckler EA, et al: Hepatitis B viral DNA in liver and serum of asymptomatic carriers. *Proc. Natl Acad Sci USA* **79**:7522–7526, 1982.
65. Overby LR: Serology of liver diseases, in Gitnick GL (ed): *Current Hepatology*. Vol. VII. Chicago, Year Book Publishers, 1986, pp. 35–67.
66. Sjogren M, Hoofnagle JH: Immunoglobulin M antibody to hepatitis B core antigen in patients with chronic type B hepatitis. *Gastroenterology* **89**:252–258, 1985.
67. Tabor E, Ziegler JL, Gerety RJ: Hepatitis B e antigen in the absence of hepatitis B surface antigen. *J Infect Dis* **141**:289–292, 1980.
68. Tabor E, Krugman S, Weiss EC, et al: Disappearance of hepatitis B surface antigen during an unusual case of fulminant hepatitis B. *J Med Virol* **8**:277–282, 1981.
69. Kryger P, Mathiesen LR, Aldershvile J, et al: Presence and meaning of anti-HBc IgM as determined by ELISA in patients with acute type B hepatitis and healthy HBsAg carriers. *Hepatology* **1**:233–237, 1981.

70. Perrillo RP, Chau KH, Overby LR, et al: Anti-hepatitis B core immunoglobulin M in the serologic evaluation of hepatitis B virus infection and simultaneous infection with type B, delta agent, and non-A, non-B viruses. *Gastroenterology* **3**:163–167, 1983.

71. Hoofnagle JH: Serodiagnosis of acute viral hepatitis. *Hepatology* **3**:267–268, 1983.

72. Chau KH, Hargie MP, Decker RH, et al: Serodiagnosis of recent hepatitis B infection by IgM class anti-HBc. *Hepatology* **3**:142–149, 1983.

73. Niermeijer P, Gips CH, Huizenga JR, et al: Anti-HBc titers and anti-HBc immunoglobulin (M/G) classes in acute, chronic, and resolved hepatitis B. *Hepatogastroenterology* **27**:271–276, 1980.

74. Hawkes RA, Broughton CR, Ferguson V, et al: Use of immunoglobulin M antibody to hepatitis B core antigen in diagnosis of viral hepatitis. *J Clin Microbiol* **11**:581–583, 1980.

75. Aldershvile J, Nielson JD: HBeAg, anti-HBe, and anti-HBc IgM in patients with hepatitis B. *J Virol Methods* **2**:97–105, 1980.

76. Tedder RS, Wilson-Croome R: IgM-antibody response to the hepatitis B core antigen in acute and chronic hepatitis B. **86**:163–172, 1981.

77. Widell A, Hansson BG, Lofgren B, et al: IgM antibody to the hepatitis B core antigen in acute hepatitis determined by SPRIA-diagnostic value. *Acta Pathol Microbiol Scand B* 90:79—84, 1982.

78. Feinman SV, Overby LR, Berris B, et al: The significance of IgM antibodies to hepatitis B core antigen in hepatitis B carriers and hepatitis-B associated chronic liver disease. *Hepatology* **2**:795–799, 1982.

79. Davis GL, Hoofnagle JH: Reactivation of chronic type B hepatitis presenting as acute viral hepatitis. *Ann Intern Med* **102**:762–765, 1985.

80. Liaw YF, Yang S-S, Chen T-J, et al: Acute exacerbations in hepatitis B e antigen positive chronic type B hepatitis. *J Hepatol* **1**:227–233, 1985.

81. De Cock K, Govindarajan S, Sandford N, et al: Fatal reactivation of chronic hepatitis B. *JAMA* **256**:1329–1331, 1986.

82. Courouce A, Drouet J, LeMarrec N, et al: Blood donors positive for HBsAg and negative for anti-HBc antibody. *Vox Sang* **49**:26–33, 1985.

83. Chen DS, Sung JL, Lai MY, et al: Inadequacy of immunoglobulin M hepatitis B core antibody in detecting acute hepatitis B virus infection in infants of HBsAg carrier mothers. *J Med Virol* **16**:309–314, 1985.

84. Hoofnagle JH, Ponzetto A, Mathiesen LR, et al: Serological diagnosis of acute viral hepatitis. *Dig Dis Sci* **30**:1022–1027, 1985.

85. Lindsay KL, Nizze JA, Koretz R, et al: Diagnostic usefulness of testing for anti-HBc IgM in acute hepatitis B. *Hepatology* **6**:1325–1328, 1986.

86. Shiels MT, Czaja AJ, Taswell HF, et al: Frequency and significance of IgM antibody to hepatitis B core antigen in severe HBsAg (+) chronic active hepatitis. *Hepatology* **5**:1052, 1985. (abst)

87. Nowicki MJ, Tong MJ, Nair PV, et al: Detection of anti-HBc IgM following prednisone treatment in patients with chronic active hepatitis B virus infection. *Hepatology* **6**:1129–1133, 1984.

88. Koretz RL: Acute hepatitis papers: The sports section, in Gitnick GL (ed): *Current Hepatology*, Vol. VII. Chicago, Year Book Medical, 1987, pp. 1–34.

89. Dienstag JL, Bhan AK, Alter HJ, et al: Circulating immune complexes in non-A, non-B hepatitis. *Lancet* **1**:1265–1267, 1979.

90. Hellings JA, Van Der Veen-DuPrie J, Snelting-Van Densen R, et al: Preliminary results of transmission experiments of non-A, non-B hepatitis by mononuclear leucocytes from a chronic patient. *J Virol Methods* **10**:321–326, 1985.

91. Dienstag JL: Non-A, non-B hepatitis. II. Experimental transmission, putative virus agents and markers, and prevention. *Gastroenterology* 743–768, 1983.

92. Vergani D, Locasciulli A, Masera G, et al: Histological evidence of hepatitis-B-virus infection with negative serology in children with acute leukemia who develop chronic liver disease. *Lancet* **1**:361–364, 1982.
93. Weigand K, Zimmerman A, Scheurer U, et al: Hepatitis B virus infection with negative HBV-serology. (Letter.) *Lancet* **2**:551–552, 1982.
94. De Vos R, de Wolf-Peeters C, Favery J, et al: Non-A, non-B hepatitis in man: Further evidence in favor of hepatitis-B like particles. *Liver* **1**:298–300, 1981.
95. De Vos R, de Wolf-Peeters C, van Stapel MJ, et al: New ultrastructural marker in hepatocytes in non-A, non-B viral hepatitis. *Liver* **2**:35–44, 1982.
96. Woods JR, Lieberman HM, Muchmore E, et al: Detection and transmission in chimpanzees of hepatitis B virus-related agents formerly designated "non-A, non-B" hepatitis. *Proc Natl Acad Sci USA* **79**:7552–7556, 1982.
97. Trepo C, Degos F, Degotte C, et al: Serial transmission of hepatitis and associated markers to chimpanzees successfully immunized against HBV. *Dev Biol Stand* **54**:443–449, 1983.
98. Fields HA, Berninger M, Nath N, et al: Unrelatedness of factor VIII-derived non-A/non-B hepatitis and hepatitis B virus. *J Med Virol* **11**:59–65, 1983.
99. Yap SH, Hellings JA, Rijntjes PJM, et al: Absence of detectable hepatitis B virus DNA in sera and liver of chimpanzees with non-A, non-B hepatitis. *J Med Virol* **15**:343–350, 1985.
100. Farci P, Smedile A, Lavarini C, et al: Delta hepatitis in inapparent carriers of hepatitis B surface antigen. *Gastroenterology* **85**:669–673, 1983.
101. Rizetto M: The delta agent. *Hepatology* **3**:729–737, 1983.
102. Farci P, Gerin JL, Aragona M, et al: Diagnostic and pregnostic significance of the IgM antibody to the hepatitis delta virus. *JAMA* **255**:1443–1446, 1986.
103. De Cock KM, Govindarajan S, Chin KP, et al: Delta hepatitis in the Los Angeles area: A report of 126 cases. *Ann Intern Med* **105**:108–114, 1986.
104. Rizzetto M, Verme G: Delta hepatitis-present status. *J Hepatol* **1**:187–193, 1985.
105. Buti M, Esteban R, Jardi R, et al: Serological diagnosis of acute delta hepatitis. *J Med Virol* **18**:81–85, 1986.

Modern Concepts of Hepatitis A

STEPHEN M. FEINSTONE and IAN D. GUST

INTRODUCTION

Recent developments in virology, immunology, and molecular biology have greatly expanded our knowledge of hepatitis A. These advances have the potential for leading in the forseeable future to preventive measures for hepatitis A virus (HAV) infections and possibly even to treatments for people who are already infected. This chapter reviews hepatitis A by answering the major questions important to physicians interested in liver disease in general and in hepatitis in particular. Hepatitis A is often relegated to poor relative status among hepatologists who find that the complexities of hepatitis B, the uniqueness of delta hepatitis, and the mystery of non-A, non-B hepatitis all provide more grist for the intellectual mill. We hope that this chapter will provide not only useful information but will also spark heightened curiosity about what we believe is an interesting medical and virologic problem.

WHAT IS HEPATITIS A?

Hepatitis A is probably an ancient disease noted from time to time by political as well as medical historians. Hepatitis A has long been recognized as a problem during wars and at times of social or political upheaval.[1] The modern era for viral hepatitis research began during World War II, when infectious hepatitis was a major cause of morbidity throughout the war among both Allied

STEPHEN M. FEINSTONE • Laboratory of Infectious Diseases, National Institute of Allergy and Infectious Diseases, National Institutes of Health, Bethesda, Maryland 20892.   IAN D. GUST • Macfarlane Burnet Centre for Medical Research, Fairfield Hospital, Melbourne, Australia 3078.

and Axis forces.[2,3] In some areas of the Pacific theater, the incidence of infectious hepatitis (presumed HA) exceeded 80 cases per 1000 per year. Such attack rates as well as the outbreak of hepatitis B related to the yellow fever vaccine, which had been stabilized with pooled human serum, prompted both the British and American armies to sponsor research in human volunteers aimed at determining ways to control the disease.

These studies accomplished several goals: (1) clearly separated infectious hepatitis from serum hepatitis, (2) showed that the infectious agent could pass bacterial filters, (3) demonstrated that the common route of transmission was fecal oral, and (4) defined the incubation period and the duration of infectivity.[2,4] These wartime studies were followed by the pioneering work of Krugman, Giles, Ward, and colleagues at the Willowbrooke State School.[5] The Willowbrooke studies were most important for the development of reagents known to contain infectious hepatitis A or B viruses or antibodies to them,[6,7] and these greatly accelerated the development of diagnostic tests. In 1973 the virus particle of HAV was first identified,[9] in 1979 HAV was first cultivated *in vitro*,[10] and in 1983 the viral genome was molecularly cloned.[11]

Although this is an exceptionally brief history, we believe it is important to understand that recent developments in hepatitis research, as with all of science, were possible because of a deep foundation laid by many investigators over a long period.

Hepatitis A is an acute infectious disease that exhibits varying degrees of symptomatology. Many infected persons experience no symptoms whatsoever, while in rare cases fulminant hepatitis, coma, and death may ensue. Age has been shown to be the single most important determinant of the clinical expression of illness. For instance, in the Greenland epidemic of 1970–1974, Skinhoj *et al.*[11] reported that hepatitis was detected in only about 1% of susceptible children under 1 year of age but increased to about 24% in children 15 years of age. By contrast, a serologic analysis of the 1969 hepatitis outbreak among the Holy Cross football team indicated that all the young adults and adults at risk who had serologic evidence of HAV infection were jaundiced, while those who were asymptomatic or who had nonspecific symptoms such as nausea showed no serologic evidence of infection.[12]

The incubation period for hepatitis A, defined as the time from exposure to the onset of symptoms, ranges between 15 and 50 days, with a mean of about 28 days.[13,14] It is not known precisely what determines the duration of the incubation period, but in experimental infections of primates the incubation period has been shown to vary inversely with the dose of administered virus. We showed in marmosets that 10^8 infectious doses administered intravenously produced evidence of liver disease in about 1 week, while one infectious dose resulted in disease in about 7 weeks (Fig. 1). The severity of illness, however, was not directly related to dose.

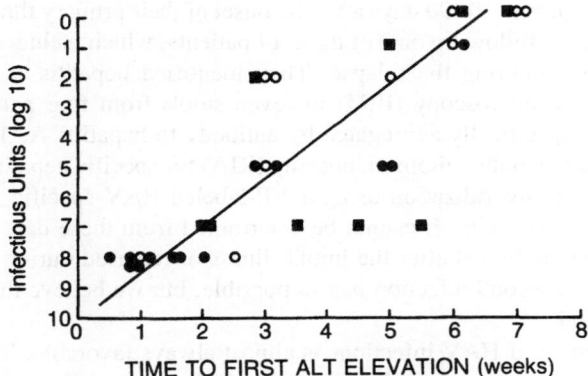

FIGURE 1. Inverse relationship between dose of HAV and incubation period in marmosets and chimpanzees measured from the time of intravenous inoculation to the first elevation of serum isocitrate dehydrogenase or alanine amino transferase.

Clinically apparent hepatitis A usually begins with a short prodromal illness lasting a few days to a week. Typical symptoms during this stage include fatigue, malaise, loss of appetite, nausea and vomiting, low-grade fever, and mild head-ache. These symptoms are rarely of sufficient severity to cause the patient to seek medical attention. The first objective sign that usually brings the patient to a physician is the onset of dark urine followed by pale stools and noticeable jaundice.

It is not the purpose of this chapter to detail the entire clinical picture of hepatitis A; however, the important points are that by the time the patient seeks medical attention, the complete picture of hepatitis is usually evident and in fact may already have reached its peak. Transaminase levels occasionally continue to rise after the onset of jaundice, but usually at this time they begin to fall toward normal and symptoms begin to resolve, providing attending physicians with justified satisfaction in their healing skills. By the third week, most patients feel well, and their liver function tests have returned to near-normal.

Cholestasis has been associated with hepatitis A, but the precise incidence has not been reported.[16] The patient may remain icteric for 12–18 weeks with the typical symptoms of cholestatic hepatitis. Even though the resolution of this complication is universal, however, both the severity and duration of symptoms may be reduced by a short, rapidly tapered course of corticosteroids.

Relapses in HA have occasionally been reported and recently some cases have been relatively well documented. Sjogren and colleagues[17] found 17 cases of relapse among 256 patients with serologically confirmed hepatitis A in Rosario, Argentina. These patients developed symptoms and significant increases in ALT levels 30–90 days after the onset of their primary illness. Sjogren *et al.* had detailed follow-up on 7 of these 17 patients, which included serial stool samples obtained during the relapse. They identified hepatitis A particles by immune electron microscopy (IEM) in seven stools from four patients. These particles were specifically aggregated by antibody to hepatitis A. These results were confirmed by both radioimmunoassay (RIA) for specific hepatitis A antigen and by molecular hybridization using a ^{32}P-labeled HAV-specific complementary DNA (cDNA) probe. It cannot be determined from these data whether the HAV shedding continued after the initial illness or recurred during reactivation of the illness. A second infection is also possible, but we believe that immunity to HAV is solid.

The outcome of HAV infections is almost always favorable, but fulminant hepatitis A has been reported. In a series of 2174 consecutive virologically or serologically confirmed hospitalized cases of HA, three deaths (0.14%) occurred.[18] Therefore, the death rate among all infected persons (including asymptomatic and nonhospitalized symptomatic patients) must be low. Interestingly, two of the three deaths in this series occurred in patients under 20 years of age.

While occasional patients may have mildly elevated serum levels of liver enzymes for several months following infection, chronic liver disease has never been associated with HAV infection. In marmosets experimentally infected with HAV, HAV antigen has frequently been observed by immunofluorescence to persist in the liver for up to 6 months after resolution of the acute disease[19] (Gust and Feinstone, unpublished observations). All these animals have serum antibody to HAV, do not have detectable virus in their feces, and have no biochemical or histologic evidence of liver disease. The persistence of antigen has generally not been seen in experimentally infected chimpanzees. Since hepatologists rarely perform liver biopsies on patients with hepatitis A, we do not know how long HAV or HAV antigens may persist in infected humans.

HOW IS HEPATITIS A DIAGNOSED?

Following infection with HAV, virus can be detected in the stools during the incubation period by a variety of immunologic detection methods. The techniques that have been most used are IEM (Fig. 2),[8] solid-phase RIA,[20,21] and enzyme immunoassay (EIA).[22] Molecular hybridization using cloned cDNA probes has recently been applied to the detection of HAV in stools.[23,24] By the time the patient seeks medical attention, the peak shedding of HAV has usually passed and serum antibody has appeared. Therefore, while HAV can be detected by one of the methods mentioned, only about 45% of patients still have detectable virus within the first week after the onset of dark urine and only 11% in the

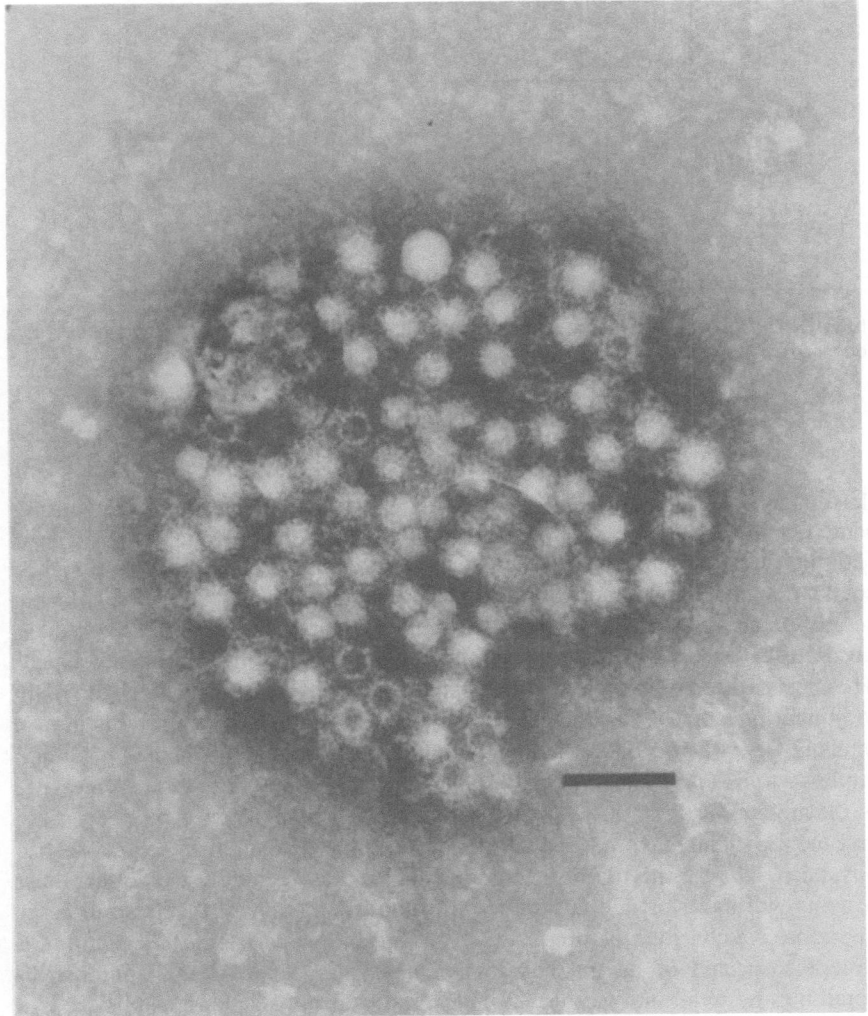

FIGURE 2. Electron micrograph of hepatitis A virus aggregated by antibody. Scale bar:
100 nm.

second week. Molecular hybridization may improve these numbers,[25] but the
proportion of false-negative results would still remain too high for virus detection
to be useful as a sole diagnostic tool. Serum antibody is usually detectable by
RIA by the time the patient presents to the physician (Fig. 3). However, since as
many as 50% of adult Americans have been exposed to HAV and therefore have

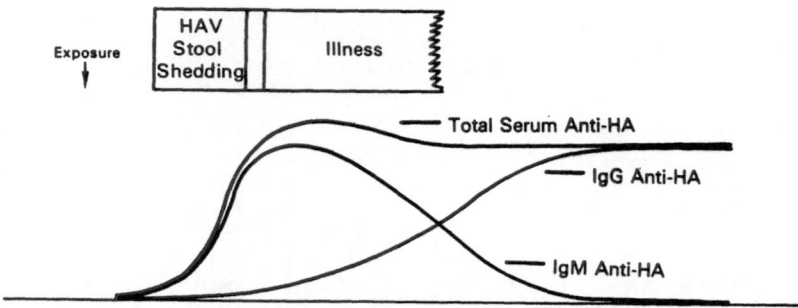

FIGURE 3. Diagrammatic representation of the clinical, virologic, and serologic events that occur in HAV infections.

detectable serum antibody, the total antibody test is not useful for diagnosing acute hepatitis A. While it is sometimes possible to demonstrate rising titers of antibody in serum specimens taken several weeks apart, this time lapse makes such a diagnostic method of little clinical value. Indeed, acute and convalescent sera often show little difference in total antibody titer. For these reasons, diagnostic tests based on IgM class-specific antibody to HAV have been developed. The most successful of these tests are capture RIA or EIA tests in which antibody to human IgM on the solid phase captures IgM from the test serum; this in turn binds HAV, which is then detected by radiolabeled or enzyme-labeled IgG class antibody to HAV.[26] The amount of the labeled IgG bound is an indirect measure of the amount of IgM anti-HAV in the test serum. These assays can be sensitive, and most patients have detectable IgM at the time of their first contact with a physician. The sensitivity of the commercial test has been adjusted so that most patients will have lost all detectable IgM within 3 months of the acute disease. Therefore we consider the presence of IgM-specific anti-HAV in the serum of a patient suspected of having HA to be diagnostic. There is little purpose in obtaining the total antibody test to aid the diagnosis of acute hepatitis A. If a diagnosis of HA is suspected and the IgM test is negative, the test should be repeated, as we have occasionally seen patients early in the course of their illness who have negative IgM anti-HAV levels, as measured by commercial tests. The total antibody test has its greatest values in epidemiologic investigations and in determining which potential contacts are at risk and which have preexisting antibody as well as screening travelers prior to offering immune serum globulin. A contact of a patient with HA who has anti-HA by a total antibody test must be further tested by the IgM test in order to determine whether the patient has an acute HAV infection.

IS HEPATITIS A IMPORTANT?

Since HA is generally self-limited, rarely causes severe liver disease, and never causes chronic liver disease, is this really a problem with which physicians and public health officials should be concerned? A review of the epidemiology of HA provides an answer to this question.

The important points to consider in understanding the epidemiology of HA are that (1) the local conditions largely determine the epidemiologic situation, and (2) the epidemiologic patterns existing in some parts of the world are rapidly changing. Figure 4 shows three distinct patterns of age-stratified prevalence of antibody to HAV.[27] These are in general the patterns for many enteric infections; that is, like other enteric diseases, HA is in most parts of the world a disease of childhood, but as sanitation and other living conditions improve, fewer and fewer children are infected. Older age groups (who were infected as children) have higher antibody prevalence rates than do the present children.

The first pattern is seen generally in developing countries, especially in the tropics, where HA is hyperendemic. In these parts of the world, HA is essentially universal among children who rarely exhibit clinical disease. In these countries, HA is not considered a major health problem, but it is really not known whether HA contributes significantly to the overall morbidity of the childhood population. While HA is rarely diagnosed in the local adult population, outside visitors to these areas, such as missionaries, Peace Corps workers, and tourists, are at risk.

The second pattern is seen commonly in more highly developed countries with large, open populations. In these countries, there is a general increase in

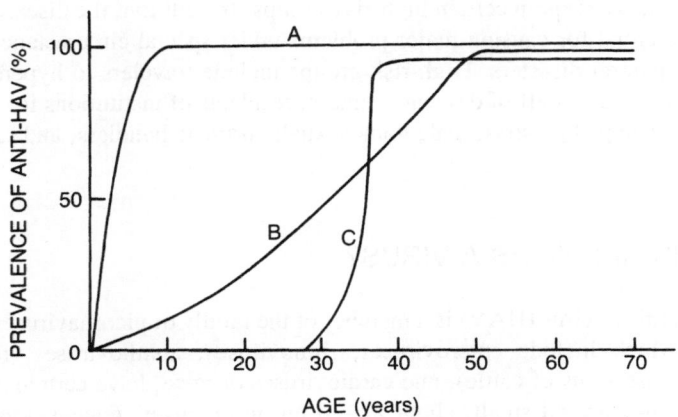

FIGURE 4. Diagrammatic representation of three epidemiologic patterns of age-specific prevalence of anti-HAV.[27]

antibody prevalence with age that results in a straight-line or sigmoidal curve, depending on the recent HA prevalence in children and the maximal prevalence in the older age groups.

The third pattern is seen in highly developed countries with relatively small homogeneous populations as well as in some small closed populations, such as certain island nations in the Pacific. In such areas, HA once existed but, because of rapidly improved sanitary or living conditions, the disease has essentially been eradicated. Although no cases may have occurred in children for more than two decades, the prevalence curve in people over 20 years of age resembles either of the first two patterns.

In countries in which the second pattern exists, sporadic cases and epidemics may occur, usually imported cases by travelers and breakdowns in the sanitary barrier, such as sewage contamination of water supplies or shellfish harvesting areas.

The major HA public health problem in the world is not seen in developing countries in which universal childhood exposure occurs. The major problem is in countries that are emerging or that have recently emerged from the developing status. In these areas, there is a growing nonimmune adult population. At the same time, breaches in the sanitary barrier and the continued presence of the virus in the environment result in relatively common outbreaks of HA, some of which can be rather large in terms of the number of infected people.

Large areas of the world are in, or will soon be in, this epidemiologic situation. The Mediterranean basin, the Middle East, and many areas of Asia, including China, fit this category, and control of the disease in these areas has become a major concern.

In North America and western Europe, hepatitis A has become a relatively minor problem except in certain high-risk groups. In addition, the disease always has the potential for causing major problems under special circumstances, such as war or natural disasters. High-risk groups include travelers to hyperendemic areas, children and staff of day-care centers, residents of institutions for intellectually handicapped persons, male homosexuals, primate handlers, and sanitation workers.

WHAT IS HEPATITIS A VIRUS?

Hepatitis A virus (HAV) is a member of the family of picornaviruses. These viruses, which include enteroviruses, rhinoviruses, aphthoviruses (foot and mouth disease virus of cattle), and cardioviruses of mice, have certain common features. They are all small, about 27–30 nm in diameter, nonenveloped, icosahedral viruses with a single-stranded message (plus) sense RNA genome. These viruses replicate entirely within the cytoplasm; the viral RNA (vRNA) acts both as a message for protein translation and as the template for negative-strand RNA synthesis, which in turn is the template for new messenger RNA (mRNA) and vRNA. The vRNA of picornaviruses is 7000–8000 bases in length and contains a single open reading frame initiated by an AUG codon about 750 bases from the 5' end of the RNA. Neither the vRNA nor the viral mRNA has a 5' cap structure typical of eukaryotic mRNA, but instead has a small viral-coded protein VPg covalently bound to the 5' end of the RNA. The vRNA does have a polyadenylic acid [poly(A)] tract at its 3' end as is generally found in mRNAs. This poly(A) is present in the vRNA and is not added by a host enzyme. The RNA is translated into a single polyprotein that then undergoes a series of proteolytic cleavages to form the mature viral proteins necessary for viral replication as well as the structural proteins that form the viral capsid. These cleavages are all believed to be carried out by viral-coded proteases. The details of the replication of picornaviruses are beyond the scope of this chapter and have been well reviewed recently.[28]

Classically, the picornaviruses have been classified by certain virologic, biochemical and biophysical features that seem to separate them into genera. The enteroviruses, which include polio-, coxsackie, and echoviruses, replicate initially in the alimentary tract, are resistant to acid, and have a buoyant density of about 1.34 g/cm^3 in cesium chloride. The rhinoviruses replicate in the upper respiratory tract, are acid labile, and have a buoyant density of 1.4 g/cm^3. Cardioviruses of mice resemble enteroviruses in these characteristics, while aphthoviruses (foot and mouth disease virus) are acid labile and have a density of ~1.45 g/cm^3. Both cardio- and aphthoviruses can be further distinguished from entero- and rhinoviruses by the presence of the genetic coding capacity for an extra peptide termed the "leader" peptide that has an unknown function. HAV resembles enteroviruses in that it is resistant to acid, has a density in cesium chloride of about 1.32–1.34, and probably replicates in the alimentary tract. However, HAV has one characteristic that distinguishes it from all other picornaviruses. HAV survives heating to 60°C, a temperature at which all other members of this virus family are inactivated by this treatment.

Molecular cloning techniques have recently permitted a detailed analysis of HAV that was previously impossible because of the limited quantities of virus available.[10,31,32] The RNA genome of HAV is 7478 nucleotides in length (Fig. 5). Beginning at its 5' end, there is a small viral protein, VPg, covalently attached followed by a noncoding region of 734 bases. There are two potential AUG translation initiation codons at bases 735-7 and 741-3. We do not know which of these is the active site. The initiation codon, a single open reading frame of 6681 nucleotides, is terminated by a nonsense codon at position 7417 followed by 63 noncoding bases at the 3' end and terminating with the poly(A) tract. The coding region of picornaviruses is divided into three regions (P1, P2, and P3), according to where the initial cleavages in the polyprotein occur. The

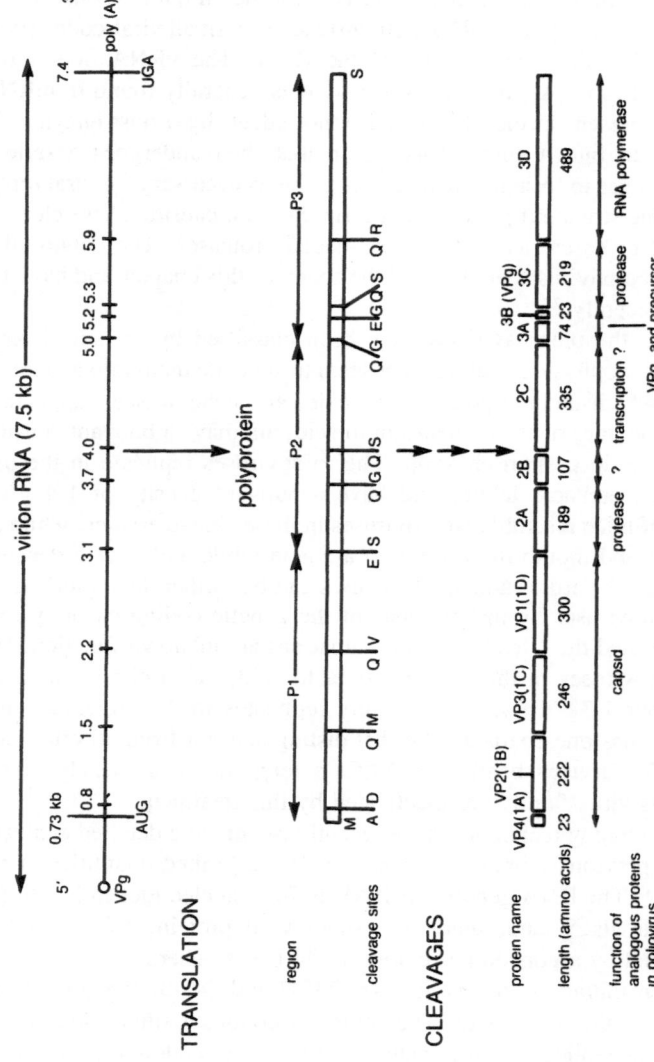

FIGURE 5. Diagrammatic representation of the HAV genome organization (translation product) and the protein cleavage sites (tentative) that result in the viral peptides.[33]

proteins coded by the genome and cleaved from the polyprotein are named in order from the 5' end of the genome. For example, the proteins coded by the P1 region are called 1A, 1B, 1C, and 1D. The capsid-coding region is at the 5' end of the genome and by analysis of nucleic acid and predicted amino acid sequence the coding regions for many of the other viral peptides have been located either generally or precisely.

This analysis shows that HAV has essentially the same gene order as other picornaviruses. However, HAV has some peculiarities. Picornaviruses all have four capsid proteins classically termed VP1, VP2, VP3, and VP4 in order of decreasing molecular size. The gene order for these peptides from 5' to 3' is 1A (VP4), 1B (VP2), 1C (VP3), and 1D (VP1). First, it appears that VP4 is only about 2500 M_r, while VP4 in other picornaviruses is 7000–8500 M_r. Second, VP2 (1B) has a predicted molecular weight of 24,700 while VP3 (1C) is 27,300 M_r. In other words, 1B is smaller than 1C, while in enteroviruses 1B (VP2) is larger than 1C (VP3).

All the picornaviral peptides are processed from the polyprotein by viral coded proteases. These proteases recognize very specific dipeptide cleavage sites. There are at least 10 such sites in each picornavirus (EMCV and FMDV have 11 because they have the additional leader protein). HAV shares only four of these dipeptide cleavage sites with EMCV but no more than two with any of the other picornaviruses.

Finally, computer comparisons of both nucleic acid and predicted amino acid sequences of HAV and other picornaviruses show little homology except in most conserved regions of protein 3D, the viral polymerase. Actual molecular hybridization experiments carried out by Ticehurst using cloned HAV probes shows essentially no homology between HAV and other picornaviruses, even at very low stringency of hybridization conditions.[33]

Thus, while HAV has a molecular structure that is in all general respects similar to other picornaviruses, it seems to be only distantly related to the other members of this viral family at the level of nucleotide and amino acid sequence.

HOW DOES HEPATITIS A VIRUS CAUSE DISEASE?

We do not fully understand the pathogenesis of HAV. We know that the virus is infectious by the fecal oral route, but we do not know how it gets to the liver from the gastrointestinal (GI) tract. There is limited evidence for both oropharangeal and a gut phase of replication in the small intestine.[34] Indeed, gut physiologists may explain that the virus can pass from the intestinal lumen to the portal circulation without replicating in any cell in the intestinal wall. By whatever means HAV reaches the liver when it does, it binds to specific receptors on the surface of hepatocytes and is then internalized and uncoated by other unknown processes. HAV, like other picornaviruses, is organ specific. The only cell in which the virus is known to replicate is the hepatocyte. Hepatitis A antigen has been observed in other cells, particularly reticuloendothelial cells, by immunohistology, but it is difficult to assess whether the virus is actually replicating in these cells.[35] No extrahepatic pathology is recognized in hepatitis A. HAV grows *in vitro* in a variety of cell substrates of primate origin, including both epithelial and fibroblastic cells. In cell culture, HAV is generally not cytopathic, although a few exceptions are reported with viral strains that have been adapted to cell culture and grown under special conditions.[36,37] We do not know what happens in the liver, but we do have some clues from animal experiments. When we inoculate marmosets (*Saguinus mystax* or *S. labiatus*) with HAV, we can often observe HA antigen in almost all the hepatocytes by immunofluorescence. On histologic examination, there is a prominent portal inflammatory infiltrate and some individual hepatocytes exhibit ballooning degeneration, while others appear shriveled and eosinophilic. Certainly we do not observe necrosis of the entire liver and in fact necrosis is not the major histopathologic finding. When we inoculated marmosets with a large dose (10^8 infectious doses) of HAV, we observed an interesting phenomenon (Fig. 6). Normally, HA in marmosets has an incubation period of at least 3 weeks, but in these animals we observed distinct enzyme elevations within 1 week, and these abnormal serum liver tests were accompanied by HAV antigen in the liver detected by immunofluorescence and in the stool as detected by RIA. The enzyme levels stabilized or even declined a little until 3 weeks after inoculation when, coincident with the appearance of serum antibody, they rose again, this time higher than during the first elevation. Little inflammation was noted in liver biopsies taken during the first episode, but inflammation was prominent during the latter phase. The obvious explanation is that the early hepatic injury was a direct viropathic effect and that the second was due to an immunopathic effect. In the typical lower-dose HAV infection, it takes longer for the viropathic effect to become noticeable, and it cannot be separated in time from the immunologically mediated disease. Krawczynski *et al.*[38] were unable to detect deposits of immunoglobulin or complement components in liver biopsies of HAV-infected marmosets. However, Kurane and colleagues showed that mononuclear cells with characteristics of natural killer (NK) cells from nonimmune donors will lyse HAV-infected tissue culture cells[39] and Flehmig *et al.*[40] show that lymphocytes from convalescent patients produced cytotoxic changes in their own epidermal cell lines infected with HAV.

While the hypothesis is far from proven, it seems likely that HAV infections produce a generally mild cytopathic effect in hepatocytes but that the major hepatic injury is a result of a cell-mediated immune response. Circulating antibody may be most important for limiting the spread of virus and other factors such as interferon may be important for recovery.

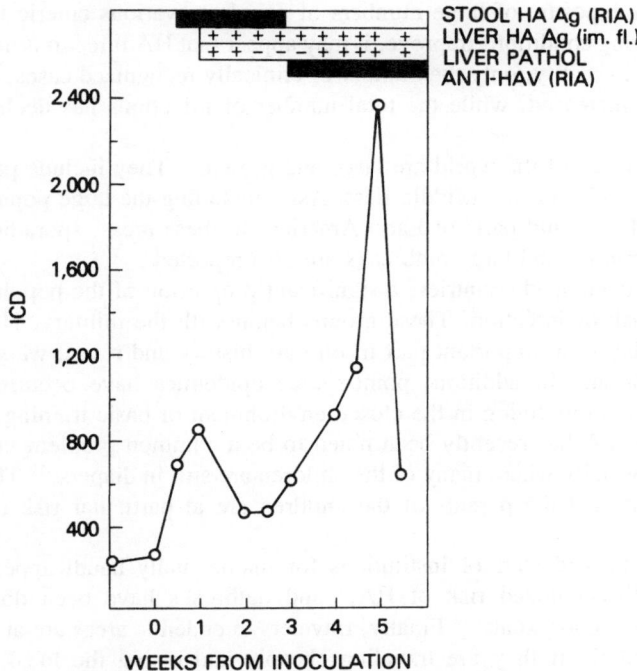

FIGURE 6. Biphasic enzyme elevations in a marmoset inoculated with 10^8 infectious units of HAV. The second enzyme elevation occurs at about the same time as the appearance of serum antibody.

SHOULD HA BE PREVENTED?

Hepatitis A is generally mild and self-limited (see the sections on the clinical aspects of HAV). In addition, in areas of the world where it is a nearly universal infection of childhood, clinical cases among the local population are almost unknown. In developed countries, high standards of living, hygiene, and sanitation have largely eliminated HAV infections among both children and adults. What then is the justification for an effort to develop a vaccine to prevent HAV infection?

From the global point of view, the largest hepatitis A problem comes from the now vast areas of the world in which rapidly improving living standards are resulting in a growing nonimmune adult population. However, it is in these same areas that occasional breakdowns of sanitation systems are most likely to occur, resulting in exposure of large numbers of people to various enteric infections. Thus, as living conditions improve, it may appear that HA infections are actually increasing. In reality, only the number of clinically recognized cases, usually in adults, has increased, while the total number of infections has declined enormously.

These areas of the world are large and growing. They include parts of the Mediterranean basin, the Middle East, Asia, including the huge populations of China and India, and parts of Latin America. In these areas, sporadic cases of HA are common, and large outbreaks are also reported.

In the developed countries, a significant proportion of the population is at increased risk of infection. These groups begin with the military. HA has for centuries played an important part in military history and recent wars have not been exceptions. In addition, point-source epidemics have occurred among peace-time recruits living in the closed environment of basic training.[41]

Hepatitis A has recently been noted to be a common problem in day-care centers, especially where many of the children are still in diapers.[42] The staff of these centers and the parents of the children are at particular risk of clinical disease.

Residents and staff of institutions for intellectually handicapped persons have a well-recognized risk of HA,[7] and outbreaks have been documented among male homosexuals.[43] Finally, travelers to endemic areas are at increased risk, particularly if they are traveling cheaply and eating the local food and drinking the local water. These people frequently return home incubating the disease and spread it to their families.[11] If these groups are considered candidates for HAV vaccine, especially everyone entering the military and all children and staff in day-care centers, a significant proportion of the U.S. population would eventually be vaccinated. If the eventual vaccine proved to be highly safe and effective in providing lifelong immunity, a case for universal vaccination in the United States could be made. Depending on the nature of the vaccine, it could perhaps be included with ration 1, 2, 3 and given early in life with either. measles, mumps, and rubella in childhood.

HOW CAN HAV INFECTION BE PREVENTED?

The first and the major effective means to prevent HAV infection is to provide a safe supply of water and the proper disposal of feces. Intrafamily and intrahospital spread is generally prevented by proper hygiene, especially hand-washing. Hospitalized patients with HA need not be isolated unless they are unable to control their bowels. Precautions should be taken to prevent direct contact with patients' feces.

Both pre- and postexposure prophylaxis with immune-serum globulin (ISG) is often effective in prevention of infection or in preventing or reducing the severity of clinical disease. Close contacts of patients with HA (usually only family members) should receive ISG. Some individuals exposed to HAV may develop passive/active immunity following ISG immunization. However, in most recipients, the protection of ISG is only temporary, lasting about 3 months. Travelers to endemic areas are also advised to take ISG.

A great deal of effort is directed toward the development of vaccines against HAV, mostly following the classic lines that led to the development of both killed and live poliovirus vaccines. Since HAV can now be grown in cell culture, it is possible to produce sufficient quantities of virus, inactivate it, and use the resultant killed virus as a vaccine.[44,45] This approach has been studied and seems to work, although only low antibody titers have been achieved. The use of adjuvants or a higher vaccine dose may improve the antibody response. However, the information from passive immunization studies indicates that large quantities of serum antibody are not required for protection. Provost and co-workers demonstrated that marmosets with very low levels of antibody following killed vaccine were protected from challenge with live HAV.

Killed vaccines have certain inherent problems. Because the virus does not replicate in the host, the immunizing dose must be relatively large. Although HAV replicates in cell culture, it does not grow to as high a titer as poliovirus, which may make a killed vaccine relatively expensive, especially if multiple booster inoculations were required to stimulate and maintain an adequate immune response. If immunization requires multiple inoculations, a killed vaccine will have little practical use in the developing countries, where it is most needed.

The alternative to a killed viral vaccine is a live attenuated vaccine. At least two such vaccines are under study. The group at Merck Institute and the group at the National Institutes of Health (NIH) showed that HAV that had been passaged many times in cell culture retained its ability to infect chimpanzees and marmosets but that these cell culture-adapted viruses exhibited reduced virulence in these animals and some passage levels produced essentially no detectable disease in the infected animals. In addition, these animals developed an antibody response and were protected from infection and disease when challenged with wild type virulent HAV.[46-48]

Provost and colleagues at Merck recently studied two cell culture-adapted HAV variants of their original CR326 strain.[47] Both variants, called F and F′ were passaged 15 times in FRhk6 cells and a further 8 (F) or 15 (F′) times in human diploid fibroblasts (MRC5). The F variant stimulated high-titered antibody response in 12 of 12 marmosets but produced mild enzyme elevations in 3. The F′ variant caused no biochemical evidence of liver disease in the 12 marmosets inoculated, while 10 of the 12 developed an antibody response. All the animals were protected in an intravenous challenge with $10^5 ID_{50}$ of wild-type HAV. No biochemical evidence of hepatitis was found when either F or F′ was inoculated into chimpanzees, although mild histologic changes were observed in some chimpanzees that received the less attenuated F variant.

A range of doses of the F and F' variants were administered to human volunteers (F variant at $10^{3.6}$, $10^{4.6}$, or $10^{5.6}$ $TCID_{50}$, and F' $10^{6.8}$ $TCID_{50}$) in 1-ml volumes subcutaneously. The results of this experiment are summarized in Table I. The F variant produced an antibody response in most recipients, but a significant proportion of the vaccinees had mild ALT elevations. The F' variant induced antibody response in 6 of 11 vaccinees by a standard RIA and 10 out of 11 by a modified more sensitive RIA. None of the F' vaccinees developed ALT elevations. This strain has been chosen for more extensive study in marmosets and for phase II clinical studies in them.

At the NIH, Karron et al.[48] studied cell culture-adapted variants of the HM175 strain of HAV in marmosets and chimpanzees. After 21 passages in primary African green monkey kidney cells, the virus showed reduced virulence in chimpanzees but not in marmosets. After 32 passages there was reduced virulence in both species and 100% seroconverted by a standard RIA test (HAVAB). Karron et al.[48] showed that there was a reduced expression of HAV in the livers of these animals and reduced shedding of the virus in the stools. This strain is being adapted to human diploid fibroblasts and will undergo further testing as a live vaccine candidate. The results of the Merck and NIH groups indicate that a live attenuated HAV vaccine is feasible, but further work may be required to produce a strain that meets the necessary safety and immunogenicity criteria.

Molecular cloning of the HAV genome has opened several possibilities for the development of vaccines through recombinant DNA technology. The expression or synthesis of viral capsid peptides may produce useful immunogenic antigens. However, many picornavirus antigens are conformational, and more than one of the structural proteins may contribute to a single epitope. Therefore, simple peptides may not confer a protective immune response. Insertion of HAV sequences into other viral vectors, most notably vaccinia virus, is a possible.

TABLE I. Results of Trial with F and F¹ Vaccines in Man

Vaccine	Dose	ALT elevation	Seroconversion
F	$10^{5.6}$	3/9	9/9
	$10^{5.6}$	2/11	6/11
	$10^{4.6}$	3/9	6/9
	$10^{3.6}$	1/8	2/8
F¹	$10^{6.3}$	0/11	6/11[a]

[a]10/11 positive when more sensitive "modified" RIA used.

means of delivering immunizing antigens, but this approach also may not deliver the appropriate antigen. It may be possible to use recombinant DNA technology to synthesize all the viral proteins necessary for assembly of the viral capsid without the genome. If large quantities of empty capsids could be synthesized, they may be an excellent vaccine. Finally, Racaniello et al.[49] originally demonstrated that when full-length cloned poliovirus cDNA was transfected into appropriate cell culture, infectious poliovirus was produced. This has now been accomplished for other picornaviruses. Recently, Cohen et al.[50] at NIH have synthesized full-length infectious cDNA or RNA transcribed from cDNA of HAV. This achievement permits the creation of specific site-directed mutations within the cDNA that can then be transferred into the virion genome. It may be possible to create HAV mutants with this technique that have just the attenuation and immunogenicity characteristics desired.

CAN HAV INFECTION BE TREATED?

In most instances, treatment of HAV infections is not required. However, in severe cases or to reduce the duration of illness or even to eliminate the clinical expression of illness treatment may be indicated. As of now, we have no specific therapy for HAV infections. However, there is tremendous interest in the development of antiviral agents, and much of this effort is directed toward picornaviruses. Some of these agents developed for other picornaviruses may display activity against HAV but, as HAV is so distantly related to other picornaviruses, it does not necessarily follow that a drug that inhibits rhinovirus replication for instance would do the same for HAV. Recently, the crystallographic structures of rhinovirus 14,[51] poliovirus 1,[52] and mengovirus have been solved.[53] This type of analysis may permit the synthesis of highly specific drugs that could bind to precise areas of the viral capsid and inhibit such viral functions as binding to the cellular receptor or uncoating.[54] If the crystallographic structure of HAV can be solved, this approach could be applied.

WHAT ARE THE UNANSWERED QUESTIONS CONCERNING HAV?

We have learned a tremendous amount about HAV during the past 14 years and some of this knowledge may even have practical application. Several important questions remain. HAV is a picornavirus, but it has several unique features. First, why does the virus fail to have a cytopathic effect in cell culture? Second, why does HAV not affect the host macromolecular synthesis as most other picornaviruses do? Third, are the first two questions related? Finally, how does HAV cause disease?

REFERENCES

1. Bachman L: Infectious hepatitis in Europe, in Rodenwalt E (ed): *World Atlas of Epidemic Diseases.* Hamburg, Falk-Verlag, 1952, pp. 1–67.
2. Havens WP Jr: Viral hepatitis, in Anderson RS (ed): *Internal Medicine in World War II*, Vol. 3. Washington, DC, Office of the Surgeon General, Department of the Army, 1968.
3. Gutzeit KR: Die Hepatitis Epidemica. *MMW* **92:**1161, 1950.
4. Paul JR, Gardner HT: *Viral Hepatitis in Preventive Medicine in World War II*, Vol. 4. Coates JB, Hoff EC, Hoff PM (eds): Washington, DC, U.S. Government Printing Office, 1960.
5. Ward R, Krugman S, Giles JP, et al: Infectious hepatitis: Studies of its natural history and prevention. *N Engl J Med* **258:**407–416, 1958.
6. Krugman S, Giles JP, Hammond J: Infectious hepatitis: Evidence for two distinctive clinical, epidemiological and immunological types of infection. *JAMA* **200:**365–373, 1967.
7. Krugman S: The Willowbrooke hepatitis studies revisited: Ethical aspects. *J Infect Dis* **8:**157–162, 1986.
8. Feinstone SM, Kapikian AZ, Purcell RH: Hepatitis A: Detection by immune electron microscopy of a virus-like particle associated with acute illness. *Science* **182:**1026–1028, 1973.
9. Provost PJ, Hilleman MR: Propagation of human hepatitis A virus in cell culture *in vitro. Proc Soc Exp Biol Med* **160:**213–221, 1979.
10. Ticehurst JR, Racaniello VR, Baroudy BM, et al: Molecular cloning and characterization of hepatitis A virus cDNA. *Proc Natl Acad Sci USA* **80:**5885–5889, 1983.
11. Skinhoj P, Gluud C, Ramsoe K: Traveler's hepatitis. Origin and characteristics of cases in Copenhagen 1976–1978. *Scand J Infect Dis* **13:**1–4, 1981.
12. Friedman LS, O'Brien TF, Morse LJ, et al: Revisiting the Holy Cross football team hepatitis outbreak (1969) by serologic analysis. *JAMA* **254:**774–776, 1985.
13. Havens WP Jr: Hepatitis. *Medicine (Baltimore)* **27:**279–307, 1948.
14. Krugman S, Ward R, Giles, JP, et al: Infectious hepatitis: Detection of virus during the incubation period and clinically inapparent infections. *N Engl J Med* **261:**729–734, 1959.
15. Purcell RH, Feinstone SM, Ticehurst JR, et al: Hepatitis A virus, in Vyas GN, Dienstag JL, Hoofnagle, JH (eds): *Viral Hepatitis and Liver Disease.* Orlando, Grune & Stratton, 1984, pp. 9–22.
16. Gordon SC, Reddy KR, Schiff L, Schiff ER: Prolonged intrahepatic cholestasis secondary to acute hepatitis A. *Ann Intern Med* **101:**635–637, 1984.
17. Sjogren MH, Tanno H, Fay O, et al: Hepatitis in stool during clinical relapse. *Ann Intern Med* **106:**221–226, 1987.
18. McNeil M, Hoy JF, Richards MJ, et al: Etiology of fatal hepatitis in Melbourne. *Med J Aust* **2:**637–640, 1984.
19. Mathiesen LR, Feinstone SM, Purcell RH, Wagner JA: Detection of hepatitis A antigen by immunofluorescence. *Infect Immun* **18:**524–530, 1977.
20. Hollinger FB, Bradley DW, Maynard JE, et al: Detection of hepatitis A viral antigen by antigen by radioimmunoassay. *J Immunol* **115:**1464–1466, 1975.
21. Purcell RH, Wong DC, Moritsugu Y, et al: A microtiter solid phase radioimmunoassay for hepatitis A antigen and antibody. *J Immunol* **116:**349–356, 1976.
22. Mathiesen LR, Feinstone SM, Wong DC, et al: Enzyme-linked immunosorbent assay for detection of hepatitis A antigen in stool and antibody to hepatitis A antigen in sera: Comparison with

solid-phase radioimmunoassay, immune electron microscopy and immune adherence hemagglutination assay. *J Clin Microsc* **7**:184–193, 1978.

23. Jansen RW, Newbold JE, Lemon SM: Combined immunoaffinity cDNA–RNA hybridization assay for detection of hepatitis A virus in clinical specimens. *J Clin Microsc* **221**:984–989, 1985.

24. Ticehurst JR, Feinstone SM, Chestnut T, et al: Detection of hepatitis A virus by extraction of viral RNA and molecular hybridization. *J Clin Microsc* **1822**:25, 1987.

25. Tassopoulos NC, Papavangelou GJ, Ticehurst JR, Purcell RH: Fecal excretion of Greek strains of hepatitis A virus in patients with hepatitis A and in experimentally infected chimpanzees. *J Infect Dis* **154**:231–237, 1986.

26. Locarnini SA, Coulepis AG, Stratton AM, et al: Solid-phase enzyme immunoassay for detection of hepatitis A specific immunoglobulin M. *J Clin Microsc* **9**:459–465, 1979.

27. Gust ID: The epidemiology of viral hepatitis, in Vyas GN, Dienstag JL, Hoofnagle JN (eds): *Viral Hepatitis and Liver Disease*. Orlando, Grune & Stratton, 1984, pp. 417–421.

28. Rueckert RR: Picornaviruses and their replication, in Fields BN (ed): *Fundamental Virology*. New York, Raven, 1988, pp. 357–390.

29. Siegl G, Frosner GG, Gauss-Muller V, et al: The physicochemical properties of infectious hepatitis A virion. *J Gen Virol* **57**:331–341, 1981.

30. Siegl G: The biochemistry of hepatitis A virus, in Gerety RJ, (ed): *Hepatitis A*. Orlando, Academic Press, 1984, pp. 12–32.

31. Najarian R, Caput D, Gee W, et al: Primary structure and gene organization of human hepatitis A virus. *Proc Natl Acad Sci USA* **82**:2627–2631, 1985.

32. Cohen JI, Ticehurst JT, Purcell RH, et al: Complete nucleotide sequence of wild type hepatitis A virus: Comparison with different strains of hepatitis A virus and other picornaviruses. *J Virol* **61**:50–59, 1987.

33. Ticehurst JR: Hepatitis A virus: Clones, cultures and vaccines. *Semin Liver Dis* **6**:46–55, 1986.

34. Karayiannis P, Jowett T, Enticott MJ, et al: Hepatitis A virus (HAV) replication in tamarins and host immune response in relation to pathogenesis of liver cell damage in acute HAV infection. *J Med Virol* **18**:261–276, 1986.

35. Mathiesen LR, Drucker J, Lorenz D, et al: Localization of hepatitis A antigen in marmoset organs during acute infection with hepatitis A virus. *J Infect Dis* **138**:369–377, 1978.

36. Anderson DS: Cytopathology, plaque assay and heat inactivation of hepatitis A virus strain HM175. *J Med Virol* **22**:35–44, 1987.

37. Cromeans T, Sobsey MD, Fields HA: Development of a plaque assay for a cytopathic, rapidly replicating isolate of hepatitis A virus. *J Med Virol* **22**:45–56, 1987.

38. Krawczynski KS, Bradley DW, Murphy BL, et al: Pathogenic aspects of hepatitis A virus infection in enterally inoculated marmosets. *Am J Clin Pathol* **76**:698–706, 1981.

39. Kurane I, Binn LN, Bancroft WH, Ennis FA: Human lymphocyte responses to hepatitis A virus-infected cells: Interferon production and lysis of infected cells. *J Immunol* **135**:2140–2144, 1985.

40. Vallbracht A, Gabriel P, Maier K, et al: Cell mediated cytotoxicity in hepatitis A virus infection. *Hepatology* **6**:1308–1314, 1986.

41. Dienstag JL, Routenberg JA, Purcell, RH, et al: Food handler-associated outbreak of hepatitis type A. *Ann Intern Med* **83**:647–650, 1975.

42. Hadler SC, Erben JJ, Francis DP, et al: Risk factors for hepatitis A in day-care centers. *J Infect Dis* **145**:255–261, 1982.

43. Corey L, Holmes KK: Sexual transmission of hepatitis A in homosexual men. *N Engl J Med* **302**:435–438, 1980.

44. Provost PJ, Hughes JV, Miller WJ, et al: An inactivated hepatitis A viral vaccine of cell culture origin. *J Med Virol* **19**:23–31, 1986.

45. Binn LN, Bancroft WH, Lemon SM, et al: Preparation of a prototype inactivated hepatitis A virus vaccine from infected cell cultures. *J Infect Dis* **153:**749–756, 1986.
46. Provost PJ, Banker FS, Giesa PA, et al: Progress towards a live attenuated human hepatitis A vaccine. *Proc Soc Exp Biol Med* **170:**8–14, 1982.
47. Provost PJ, Bishop RP, Gerety RJ, et al: New findings in live attenuated hepatitis A vaccine development. *J Med Virol* **20:**165–175, 1986.
48. Karron RA, Daemer R, Ticehurst J, et al: Studies of prototype live HAV vaccines in primate models. *J Infect Dis* **338:**157, 1988.
49. Racaniello VR, Baltimore D: Cloned poliovirus complementary DNA is infectious in mammalian cells. *Science* **214:**916–919, 1981.
50. Cohen, JI, Ticehurst JR, Feinstone SM, et al: Hepatitis A virus cDNA and its RNA transcripts are infectious in cell culture. *J Virol* **61:**3035–3039, 1987.
51. Rossmann MG, Arnold E, Erickson JW, et al: Structure of a human common cold virus and functional relationship to other picornaviruses. *Nature (Lond.)* **317:**145–153, 1985.
52. Hogle JM, Chow M, Filmany DJ: Three-dimensional structure of poliovirus at 2.8A resolution. *Science* **229:**1358–1365, 1985.
53. Luo M, Vriend G, Kamer G, et al: The structure of mengovirus at atomic resolution. *Science* **235:**182–191, 1987.
54. Smith JJ, Kremer MJ, Luo M, et al: The site of attachment in human rhinovirus 14 for antiviral agents that inhibit uncoating. *Science* **233:**1286–1293, 1986.

Acute Viral Hepatitis
Hepatitis B

V. J. DESMET

INTRODUCTION

Every gastroenterologist knows that acute uncomplicated viral hepatitis B is a self-limited disease and that biopsy is not of much help in guidance for therapy. This explains why histologic confirmation is sought much less frequently in acute than in chronic hepatitis. It follows that the sequence of histologic changes and immunohistochemical features is less documented in acute viral hepatitis type B (AVHB) than in the chronic variants of the disease. This is not to say that no information is available. Several excellent reviews, which can hardly be improved, are scattered in the literature of the last 10 years.[1-18]

This chapter concentrates on some basic components of the histopathologic lesions and their possible pathogenesis and on the prognostic value of some histologic features in predicting possible transition to chronicity.

HISTOPATHOLOGIC FEATURES OF ACUTE HEPATITIS B

General Overview of Histopathologic Lesions

In fully developed AVHB, changes indicating parenchymal cell damage, inflammation, and regeneration dominate the histologic picture. Hepatocellular damage is reflected in cytologic alterations, cholestasis, and cell necrosis.

Cellular alterations are variable: some hepatocytes show shrinkage and in-

V. J. DESMET • Laboratory of Cytochemistry and Histochemistry, University Hospital St. Raphael, Catholic University, Leuven, B-3000 Leuven, Belgium.

creased eosinophilia (acidophil condensation), while others appear pale and swollen (ballooning) (Fig. 1). These changes are more marked in the centrilobular region (according to the lobular concept of liver architecture) or acinar zone 3 (according to the acinar concept of liver architecture)[19] (Fig. 2).

Cholestasis is observed to a variable extent. Histologically, cholestasis is recognized by accumulation of bile pigment, either as inclusions in hepatocytes and Kupffer cells or as inspissated bile plugs in intercellular canaliculi. Thus, in

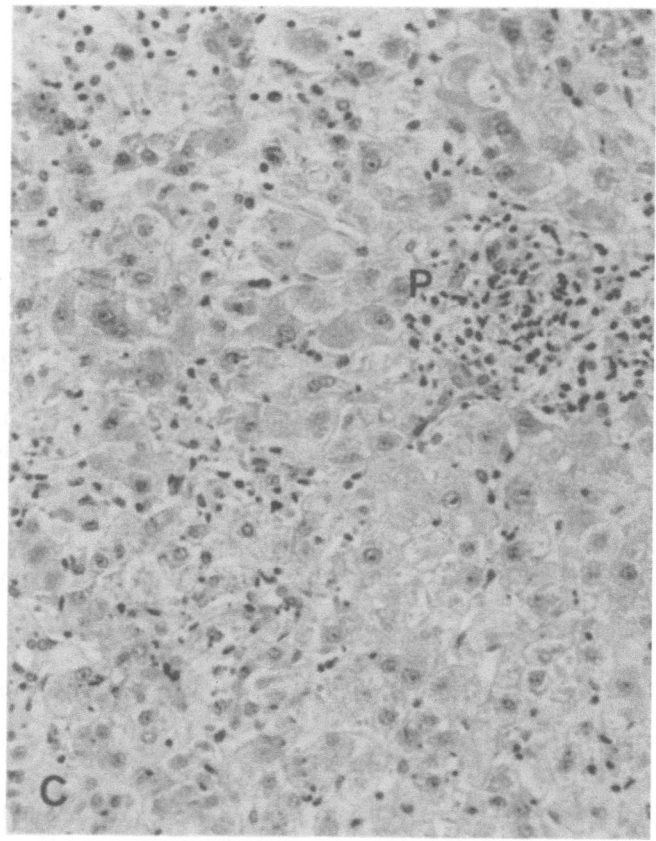

FIGURE 1. Overview of portal tract (P) and lobular parenchyma. The portal tract shows lymphoid infiltration; the parenchymal cells display heterogeneous morphology (liver cell pleomorphism) and irregular arrangement of liver cell plates (lobular disarray); mononuclear inflammatory cells infiltrate the parenchyma, especially in the centrilobular area (C). (H&E, ×250.)

AVHB, impairment in bile secretory function of zone 3 hepatocytes is identified more by bilirubinostasis than by so-called cholatestasis.[1,20]

Hepatocellular necrosis occurs in different forms: acidophil necrosis of single hepatocytes and lytic necrosis. Inflammation is manifested by infiltration of various cell types in numerous locations.

The portal connective tissue appears loosely textured by edema; it is infiltrated by a variable number of inflammatory cells (see Fig. 1). These include mainly lymphocytes, fewer plasma cells, occasionally a few neutrophil poly-

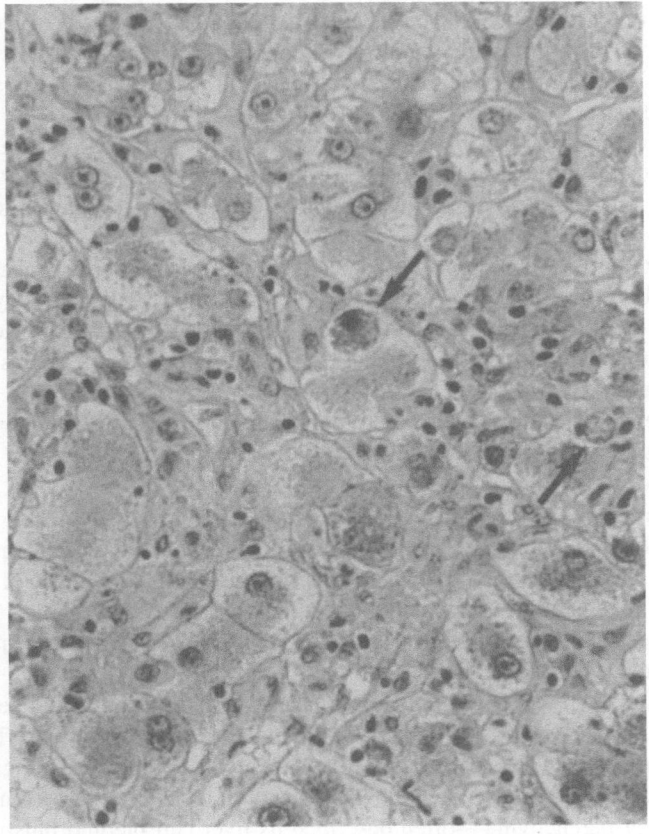

FIGURE 2. Centrolobular area in acute viral hepatitis B. Detail of liver cell pleomorphism, lobular disarray and spotty necrosis. Parenchymal cells have focally disappeared and are replaced by inflammatory cells (middle right). A couple of acidophilic bodies (arrows) are intermingled with ballooned hepatocytes. (H&E, ×400.)

morphs, some macrophages, and a number of poorly defined mesenchymal cells often indicated with the vague term histiocytes. Generally, the cellular infiltrate is confined within the limits of the portal connective tissue. When a few mononuclear cells occasionally extend beyond the portal tract into the surrounding parenchyma, without causing hepatocellular damage or necrosis, this is described as cell spillover.

Inflammatory cells are found also in parenchymal areas, where they cause increased cellularity of the sinusoids. Parenchymal inflammation is more pronounced in acinar zone 3, where hepatocellular damage prevails. Composed of different cell types, it includes hyperplastic (increased number) and hypertrophic (increased volume) Kupffer cells, which react as macrophages; these cells phagocytose the cellular debris from necrotizing hepatocytes. These scavenger cells acquire a bulky cytoplasm, loaded with coarsely granular inclusions; the latter are diastase resistant and stainable with periodic acid-Schiff (PAS) stain: PAS positive-diastase resistant (DPAS) ceroid inclusions.

Such ceroid-loaded macrophages occur mainly in areas of focal liver cell dropout; they tend to form clusters and are often in close contact with plasma cells (Fig. 3). The meaning of this plasma cell–ceroid macrophage association is unknown.

Scattered between damaged hepatocytes and ceroid macrophages lay variable numbers of lymphocytes; many show close contact with parenchymal cells; they may even be found inside the latter, surrounded by a narrow clear halo; a feature termed emperipolesis.[21] What happens exactly in emperipolesis requires further study.

Recent studies drew attention to participation in the inflammatory infiltrate of various subtypes of plasma cells[22-23] as well as mast cells.[24] The functional meaning of these observations remains unknown.

Parenchymal regeneration quickly follows parenchymal loss in uncomplicated AVHB. Parenchymal regeneration reflects itself in liver cell mitoses, binucleated hepatocytes, and thickened liver cell plates. Around areas of confluent necrosis, regeneration may also be evident as zones of smaller basophilic hepatocytes. In young children, parenchymal regeneration may occur in the form of multinucleated parenchymal giant cells.

Parenchymal regeneration is important for liver restoration and healing.[25] It may lead to extensive renewal of parenchyma after acute hepatitis.[7] The simultaneous presence of these various changes creates a complex histologic picture, which clearly departs from the homogeneous outlook and regular arrangement of normal liver parenchyma—often described as liver cell pleomorphism and lobular disarray (see Figs. 1 and 2). The most important features from the complex histologic scenery described above are hepatocellular necrosis and inflammation. The following section considers them in greater detail.

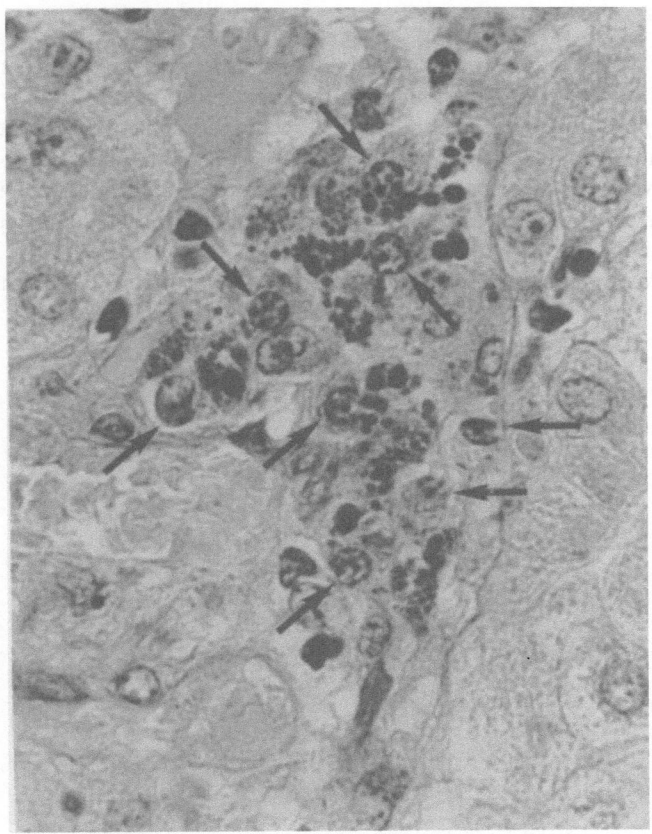

FIGURE 3. Cluster of periodic acid-Schiff (PAS)-positive, granular ceroid macrophages in close contact with several plasma cells (arrows). (PAS diastase stain, ×1000.)

Hepatocellular Necrosis and Inflammation

Inflammatory cells are found in close association with damaged and necrotizing hepatocytes. Three main types of inflammatory necrosis can be distinguished: spotty necrosis, confluent necrosis, and piecemeal necrosis. All three deserve special consideration in AVHB.

Spotty Necrosis

Three forms of necrosis of individual hepatocytes (spotty necrosis) are recognized: acidophilic, apoptotic, and cytolytic.[26]

Acidophil necrosis is the end stage of acidophil condensation, the nucleus becomes smaller and hyperchromatic (pyknosis) and finally disappears (Fig. 4). When necrotic, the cell is extruded from the liver cell plate and is phagocytosed by Kupffer cells.[27] The precise mechanism of single-cell acidophil necrosis is unknown, but it appears to include dehydration of the cell.[28,29]

Apoptosis represents a special form of cell death, different from classic

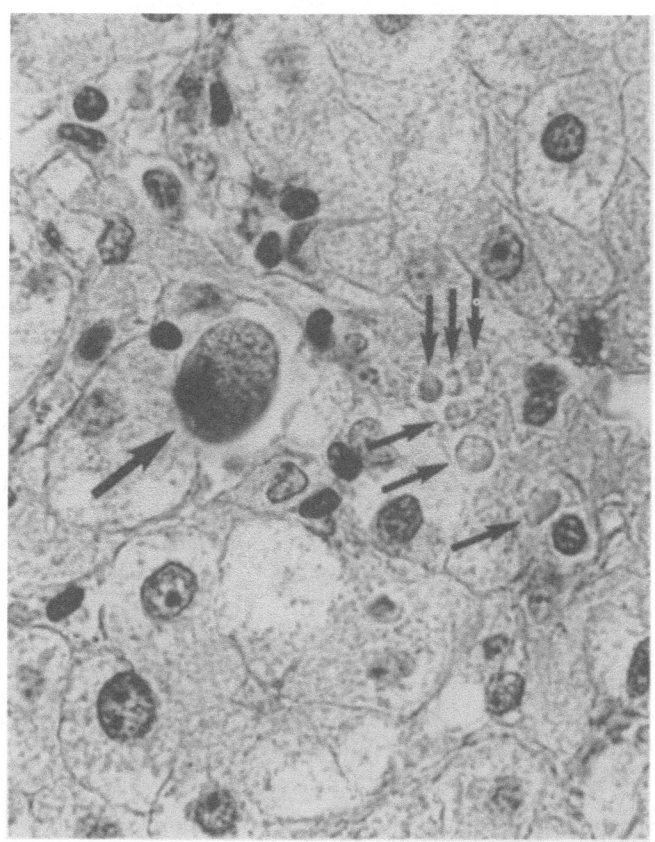

FIGURE 4. Detail of spotty acidophil necrosis, showing larger acidophilic body with pyknotic nucleus (large arrow) and six smaller acidophilic fragments, possibly phagocytosed by neighboring cells (small arrows). This area is infiltrated by several lymphocytes (small dark nuclei). (H&E, ×1000.)

(e.g., ischemic) cell necrosis.[30] Apoptosis corresponds to programmed cell death and plays a role in physiologic cell turnover. However, apoptosis may also be triggered by cell injury.[31] The ultrastructural features of apoptosis are well studied.[30] The cytoplasm becomes condensed by loss of intracellular fluid. The nuclear chromatin marginates into peripheral dense masses. Cytoplasmic organelles, like mitochondria and ribosomes, become arranged in compact formations. Subsequently, the cell breaks up into several membrane-bound fragments of unequal size, containing a variety of cytoplasmic organelles; some include nuclear fragments. The cell fragments are subsequently phagocytosed by neighboring macrophages and parenchymal cells.

Under the light microscope, apoptotic cells are not very conspicuous; they consist of portions of intensely eosinophilic-staining cytoplasm, sometimes containing small, densely basophilic (pyknotic) nuclear fragments. Apoptosis in normal or endocrine-accelerated cell turnover is not accompanied by inflammatory cells.

However, it is of interest that immunologically mediated cell death, as caused by cytotoxic T lymphocytes, killer and natural killer (NK) cells, also has the morphology of apoptosis,[30,32,33] although it is described as "lysis" of target cells.[34,35] In apoptosis switched on by immunologic signals (K, NK, and cytotoxic T lymphocytes), the apoptotic bodies are accompanied by lymphocytic infiltration[33] (Fig. 4).

In liver histopathology, it is not yet clear whether single-cell acidophil necrosis, also described as Councilman-like bodies,[28,29] always corresponds to the special, and possibly immunologically mediated, mode of cell death called apoptosis. At least in light microscopy, Councilman-like bodies resemble larger apoptotic cell fragments (Fig. 4). Definite distinction between acidophil necrosis and apoptosis would require ultrastructural investigation of liver biopsies in acute hepatitis. Although ultrastructural proof is lacking, it seems reasonable to assume that at least part of the spotty necrosis of the single-cell acidophilic type in AVHB corresponds to apoptosis induced by cell-mediated immunologic attack.[36]

Cytolysis in its morphologic definition refers to lytic necrosis of the hepatocyte (hepatocytolysis).[8,25,27] It is considered the end stage of ballooning or hydropic swelling of the cell.[26] Lytic necrosis is a rapid mode of cell death, caused by primary damage of the cell membrane.[37] Virtually no cell remnants remain, and lytic necrosis is recognized by the disappearance (dropout) of the affected cells. This type of necrosis is seen as the absence of cells. Lytic necrosis of single hepatocytes is difficult to recognize. It is easier to identify when it affects groups of cells (see further under Confluent Necrosis). It is not known to what extent this rapid explosive type of necrosis is mediated by cell-mediated immune mechanisms. By contrast, humoral immune mechanisms involving complement components have been shown to cause rapid cytolysis by primary damage to the cell membrane.[38,39]

The pathogenesis of spotty necrosis in viral hepatitis B has mainly been studied in the chronic variants of the disease.[26,40–52]

The general conclusion is that in chronic hepatitis B, spotty necrosis of virus-infected hepatocytes is caused by specific, HLA class I-restricted, cytotoxic T lymphocytes. The viral antigens to which the cell-mediated lymphocytic attack is mounted appear to correspond to the nucleocapsid proteins of the hepatitis B virus (HB_cAg and HB_eAg) expressed on the cell membrane of infected cells.[52]

In acute hepatitis B, the pathogenetic mechanisms of hepatocellular necrosis remained less well known,[53] until recent functional immunologic studies started to generate more data. One study suggested cytotoxic T-cell attack to HB_cAg localized in the plasma membrane.[54] Another study revealed that cellular immunity to pre-S antigens is the first detectable immune response during the early incubation phase of AVHB, appearing 30 days before the first rise in serum aminotransferases. T-cell sensitization to HB_cAg follows, with IgM and anti-HB_c appearing 10 days later. A cellular immune response to HB_sAg is the last to appear, 10 days before the onset of liver damage.[54a] Continued liver cell necrosis after the fourth week may be associated with T cell responses to HB_sAg.[54b]

From morphologic studies, it is reasonable to assume that HLA class I-restricted T-cell cytotoxicity plays a role, because the stage seems to be set for such reactions to occur. The predominant lymphocyte subset present in the intrahepatic inflammatory infiltrate corresponds to the OKT8$^+$ suppressor/cytotoxic category of lymphocytes.[55,56]

Specific T-cell cytotoxicity requires expression of the target viral antigen on the cell membrane in conjunction with the HLA class I (A,B,C) histocompatibility antigens. Normal hepatocytes do not express HLA class I antigens; however, these glycoproteins are markedly enhanced on the surface of liver parenchymal cells in various pathological conditions of the liver, including AVHB.[50,51,57–62] The expression of HLA class I proteins is apparently induced by interferon.[50,51,63–64] The latter is produced by intrahepatic leukocytes and fibroblasts.[65] This mechanism of HLA-restricted T-cell cytotoxicity in causing liver cell damage was beautifully demonstrated in a recently developed and elegant animal model of viral hepatitis.[66]

A further requirement for T-cell-mediated immune attack would be expression of target viral antigen(s) on the hepatocellular membrane. This requirement is not as amply documented in acute as in chronic hepatitis B. Whereas both HB_sAg[67,68] and HB_cAg[69,70] have been demonstrated in the plasma membrane of hepatocytes by morphologic study of tissue sections from liver biopsies of patients with chronic hepatitis B, similar observations are more scanty in the acute phase of the disease.[71,72] Originally, HB_sAg was found to be localized in the plasma membrane of isolated hepatocytes prepared by mechanical disruption of liver specimens from patients with AVHB.[73] This observation suggested that HB_sAg may represent a target antigen in acute hepatitis.[40,73,74] A recent study also demonstrated HB_cAg on the membrane of mechanically isolated hepatocytes.[54] It should be kept in mind, however, that isolation of parenchymal cells by mechanical disruption causes considerable membrane damage and potential exposure of intracellular components.[75]

In studies using tissue sections, very little or no viral antigens (HB_sAg, HB_cAg) are detectable by immunohistochemical means in liver specimens taken at the peak of transaminase elevation.[53] Only in the early presymptomatic phase of experimental[71,72,76] and human[77,78] AVHB are viral antigens more easily demonstrable. This finding supports the concept that AVHB is an elimination type of hepatitis; that is, at the time of fully developed disease, most or all of the virus-infected cells have been efficiently eliminated.[5,7,79]

For this very reason, and because liver biopsies are not often taken in the presymptomatic early phase, the morphologic substrate of whatever immunologic mechanism that occurs is not well known. Other target antigens have been considered to be involved in immune-mediated hepatocytolysis: Dane particle-associated antigen and host cell antigens known as liver-specific protein (LSP) and liver membrane antigen (LMA).[53,80] The humoral and cellular immune reactions to such host antigens appear to be due to deficient suppressor T-cell function.[41,42]

The immune response to AVHB is modulated through secretion of immunoregulatory molecules by altered or virus-infected cells; such components have been labeled liver immunoregulatory protein (LIP)[81,82] and rosette inhibitory factor (RIF).[43,80,83]

Furthermore, liver cell necrosis itself causes the release of a soluble factor, termed liver extract (Lex), which inhibits lymphocytes at the site of action; this results in focal restriction of hepatocellular damage. The release of such bioregulatory molecules may explain the spotty and focal localization of liver cell necrosis.[83]

Further studies are needed to define the precise morphologic substrate of T cell-mediated cytotoxicity, whether it corresponds to spotty lytic necrosis, spotty acidophil necrosis, and/or apoptosis. The immunologic mechanism in AVHB is not restricted to OKT8$^+$ T cell-mediated cell necrosis. Some morphologic[84] and functional[47-49,54] studies also emphasized the participation of natural NK lymphocytes.

Other immune-mediated mechanisms (antibody-dependent cellular cytotoxicity; macrophage-induced cytotoxicity; immune complex-mediated liver cell damage) are neither proved nor excluded.[53] The lobular disarray and liver cell pleomorphism observed by light microscopy in liver biopsy sections indeed suggest that multiple mechanisms operate synchronously: The variable morphologic appearance of hepatocytes is not readily explained as different stages of a single mechanism; rather, it suggests that a variety of initial damaging factors hits the parenchymal cells.

Furthermore, the extent to which different mechanisms participate may vary in individual patients. For example, the occurrence of chronic active hepatitis in occasional patients with agammaglobulinemia[85] is often invoked to indicate that humoral mechanisms are not an absolute requisite for liver cell necrosis. The same may hold true for some aspects of cell-mediated cytotoxicity, as illustrated by acute self-limiting hepatitis B in an exceptional patient with cellular immune deficiency.[86]

Variability in the participation of the different components of the immunologic orchestra in individual patients would help explain the variation in histologic complexity from one biopsy to the next. Whatever the range of mechanisms involved, it is clear that uncomplicated AVHB results in complete eradication of viral infection (so-called elimination type of viral hepatitis B).[5,7,79]

Confluent Necrosis

Patterns. Confluent lytic necrosis of hepatocytes in more severe cases of AVHB does not display a random topography. To the contrary, it occurs in well-defined territories of the parenchyma, which correspond to the microcirculatory periphery of parenchymal units. The anatomic distribution of confluent necrosis is best explained on the basis of the acinar concept of liver architecture.[19,87] With increasing severity and extent of necrosis, the loss of liver cells progressively affects portions of parenchyma that lie closer to the vascular supply (Fig. 5). Thus, milder forms of confluent necrosis cause dropout of liver cells in the most extreme periphery of the complex acinus. This pattern corresponds to areas of necrosis surrounding the terminal hepatic venules (or so-called central veins): perivenular (or centrilobular) zonal confluent necrosis. More extensive necrosis occupies the entire periphery of the complex acinus. This pattern corresponds to stretches of necrosis between adjacent central veins; this pattern is termed central–central bridging necrosis (Fig. 5).

Further increase in the extent of confluent necrosis corresponds to the peripheral portions of the simple acinus: the so-called acinar zone 3. This pattern creates necrotic bridges between portal tracts and central veins: portal–central bridging necrosis (Figs. 5–7). In the framework of the classic lobular concept of liver architecture, this pattern appears as starfish-shaped areas of necrosis, radiating from the central vein (terminal hepatic venule)[19] (Figs. 5 and 6).

Not only does this pattern represent a higher magnitude of parenchymal loss; it acquires additional biologic significance by creating links or bridges between the afferent vessels in the portal tracts and the efferent veins (Fig. 7). As such, portal–central necrosis creates the blueprint for potential subsequent development of portal–central (i.e., portocaval) vascular shunts.

Dropout of still larger masses of parenchyma by confluent lytic necrosis involves acinar zone 2, leaving only narrow rims (zone 1) of surviving parenchyma around the terminal portal tracts.

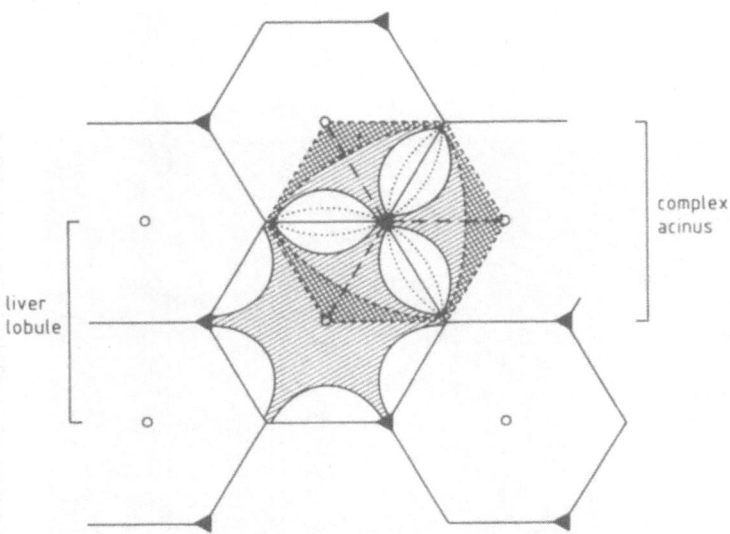

FIGURE 5. Schematic representation of different degrees of confluent necrosis at the acinar and lobular level. For explanation, see text. (▲) portal tracts; (○) central veins; (▨) central–central bridging necrosis; (▨) portal–central bridging necrosis.

Panlobular necrosis refers to a situation in which the parenchymal cells of all acinar zones have disappeared. Multilobular necrosis indicates total parenchymal loss in several adjacent liver acini (Fig. 8). Presumably, it corresponds to complete parenchymal necrosis of an acinar agglomerate.[19] It is remarkable that multilobular necrosis may show irregular distribution throughout the liver. This indicates that some, but not all, acinar agglomerates are involved in confluent necrosis at the same time and suggests that humoral factors, originating from the blood supply, play a role in its pathogenesis.[88] Multilobular necrosis in its variable degrees corresponds to submassive and massive necrosis from older terminologies.

Confluent lytic necrosis that causes bridging between various hepatic architectural landmarks is indicated by the general term bridging hepatic necrosis[89] and by the older terminology of subacute hepatic necrosis.[90] Areas of confluent lytic necrosis may become repopulated by hepatocytes, provided that the necrotic area is not too large (e.g., perivenular zonal necrosis) and that the adjacent surviving hepatocytes have preserved sufficient regenerative power. The serum of patients with severe necrotizing hepatitis contains a growth factor for hepatocytes that may stimulate regeneration.[91,92]

In case of more extensive lytic necrosis (e.g., some cases with portal–

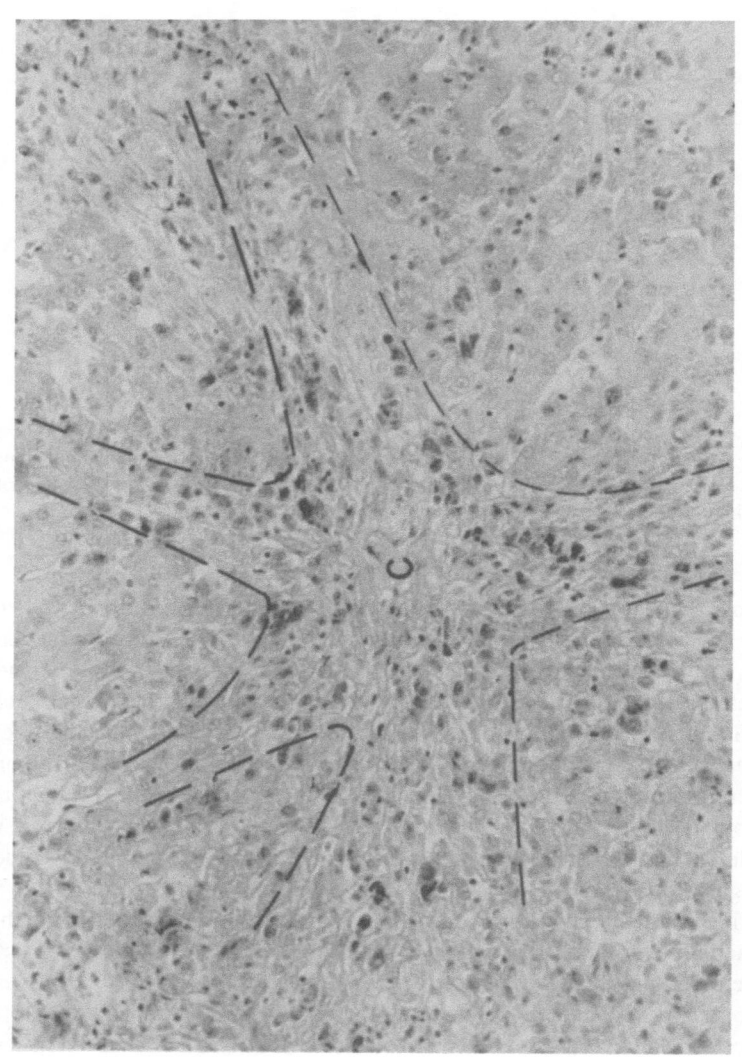

FIGURE 6. Confluent lytic necrosis in acute viral hepatitis B. The central vein (c) is surrounded by a star-shaped area, in which hepatocytes have disappeared. Ceroid macrophages and some lymphocytes are scattered between the condensing reticulin framework. Compare with Fig. 5. (PAS-diastase stain, ×250.)

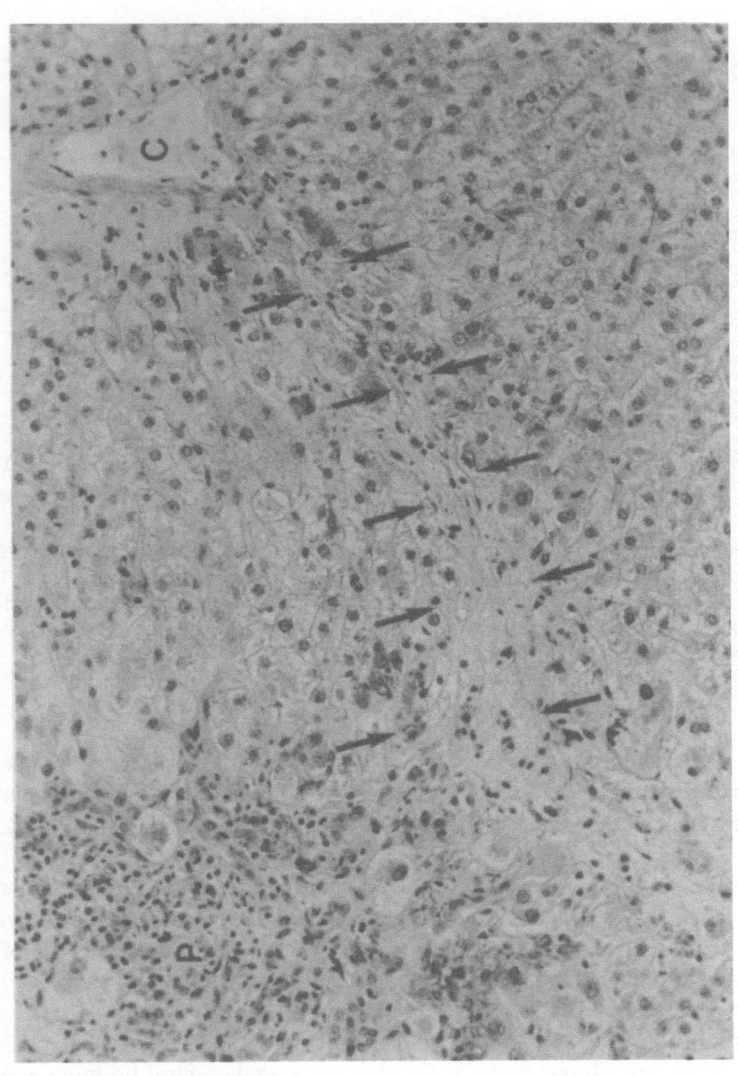

FIGURE 7. Portal–central bridging necrosis. The portal tract (P) is infiltrated by lymphoid cells. A curved bridge of lytic necrosis (arrows) links P with the central vein (c). There is partial collapse of the reticulin framework in the necrotic bridge. (H&E, ×250.)

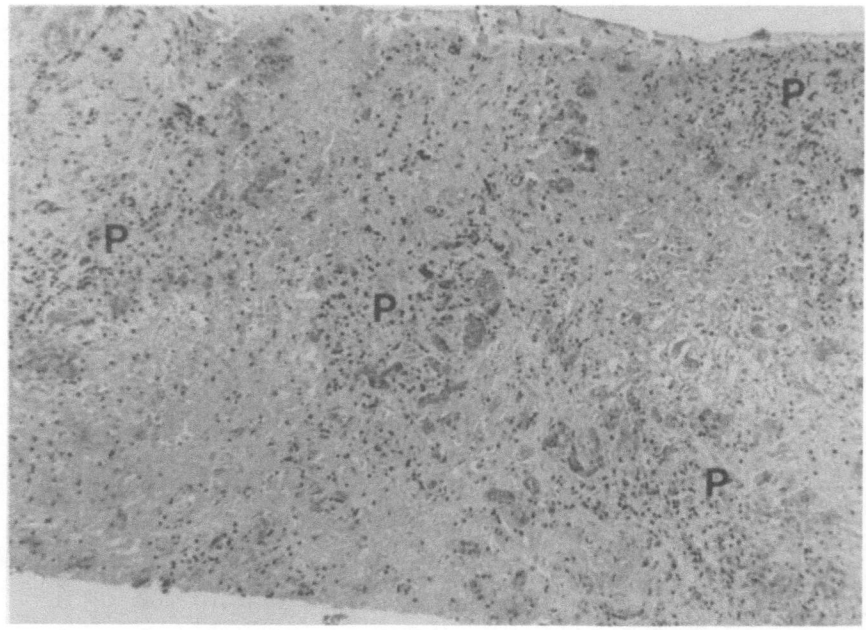

FIGURE 8. Postmortem needle biopsy from patient with fulminant hepatitis B. The portal tracts (P) show moderate lymphoid infiltration. Except for a few clusters of acinar zone 1 hepatocytes, all parenchymal cells have disappeared in several adjacent lobules (multi-lobular necrosis). Ghost lobules are infiltrated with scattered lymphocytes. The reticulin framework has not yet collapsed (recent necrosis). (H&E, ×100.)

central bridging necrosis and higher degrees of parenchymal loss), or when the remaining parenchyma is itself severely altered, regeneration is delayed. Under these circumstances, the necrotic areas with denuded reticulin framework collapse.

Activation of the more resistant mesenchymal cells results in progressive deposition of increasing amounts of collagen, which contribute to the formation of a fibrous scar. The pattern of the fibrous scar is determined by the pattern of the preceding confluent necrosis: central–central septa, portal–central septa, and multilobular postnecrotic scars.

Some sinusoids remain open in the collapsing areas and ensure vascularization of the developing fibrous scars. It follows that portal–central bridging and higher degrees of necrosis result in the establishment of portal–central vascular shunts. These enable a fraction of the intrahepatic blood flow to bypass the parenchyma. Intrahepatic shunting is an important component of the derangement of intrahepatic blood flow in cirrhosis.

Histologic Features and Pathogenesis. Confluent necrosis is characterized by lysis of hepatocytes and is identified as the absence of parenchymal cells. In the early stages, it produces an empty reticulin framework in which the sinusoids remain identifiable and in which the inflammatory cells and reactive Kupffer cells remain enmeshed. Ceroid macrophages and lymphocytes lie scattered as single cells throughout the necrotic area. In some cases, numerous neutrophil polymorphs are scattered throughout the denuded area.[53]

With progressive collapse, ceroid macrophages group in clusters, often mixed with lymphocytes and plasma cells. Increasing amounts of collagen can be demonstrated with connective tissue stains; older scars can be identified by their increasing elastin content.[93,94]

The pathogenesis of confluent lytic necrosis is not elucidated. It is not known whether the explosive loss of larger parenchymal territories is caused by lymphocyte-mediated or humoral immunologic mechanisms. The anatomic pattern suggests at least partial involvement of humoral factors.[88] Possible mechanisms include activation of the complement system by circulating endotoxins due to Kupffer cell failure[95] or a Schwarzman-like reaction to the liver.[96] The observation in some cases of neutrophil polymorphs in areas of extensive confluent necrosis is consistent with, but not proof of, involvement of the complement cascade.[53]

In fulminant hepatitis B, antibodies to HB_sAg may appear early, while HB_sAg is not demonstrable in the blood, suggesting formation of immune complexes that might be cytotoxic.[97]

Piecemeal Necrosis

Piecemeal necrosis is a typical feature of chronic active hepatitis, but it may also be observed in early[78] and late[87] AVHB. Morphologically, piecemeal necrosis[98] represents an interphase hepatitis, meaning mononuclear leukocytic infiltration associated with liver cell necrosis at the interphase between connective tissue stroma (portal tracts and septa) and parenchyma (Fig. 9). The slow destruction of hepatocytes leads to irregular erosion of the limiting plate and an imprecise delineation of the portal perimeter. The most important cell types participating in periportal piecemeal necrosis are antigen-presenting reticulum cells[99] and T lymphocytes.[100] OKT4 + helper/inducer lymphocytes predominate in the central part of the portal area, whereas OKT8 + suppressor/cytotoxic lymphocytes are located mainly in the peripheral connective tissue–parenchymal interphase.[100]

The mechanism of cell death in piecemeal necrosis corresponds to apoptosis.[101] Authentic piecemeal necrosis must be differentiated from minimal spillover of inflammatory cells not associated with liver cell damage.[87]

True piecemeal necrosis should not be confused with biliary piecemeal necrosis,[102] which also produces a blurred connective tissue–parenchymal in-

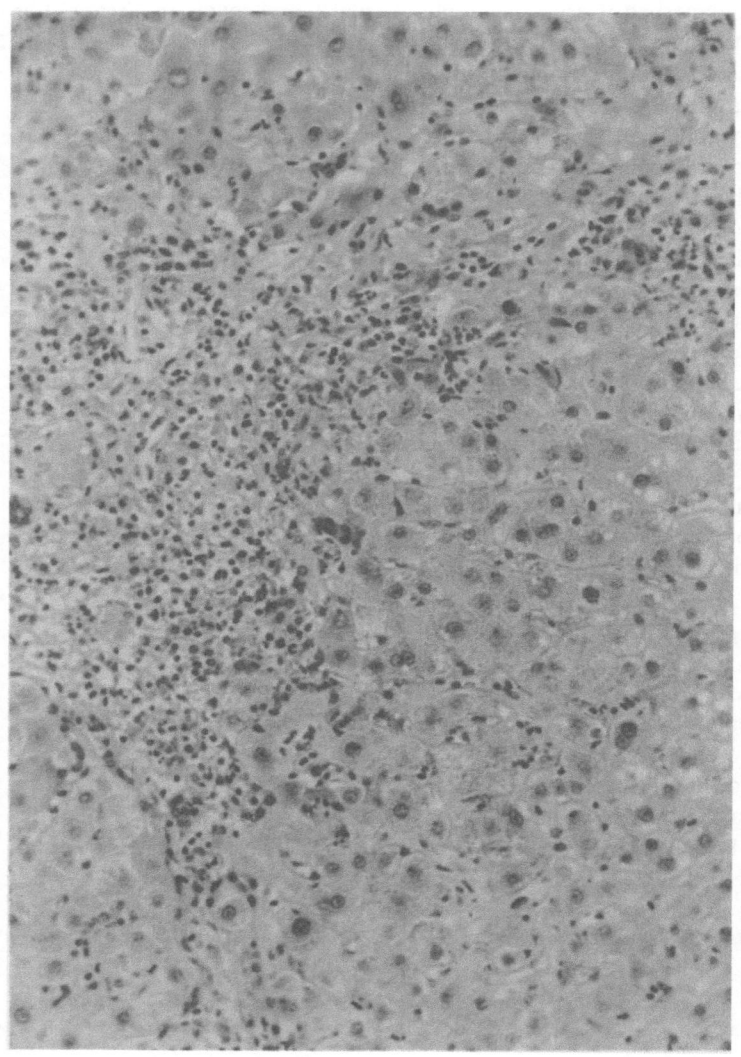

FIGURE 9. Piecemeal necrosis in acute viral hepatitis. The portal tract (upper portion) is infiltrated by mononuclear cells, mostly lymphocytes. The inflammatory infiltrate extends into the surrounding acinar zone 1 parenchyma, associated with disappearance of hepatocytes in that area. This leads to destruction of the limiting plate and an unsharp portal–parenchymal interphase. (H&E, ×250.)

terphase. The biliary type of piecemeal necrosis comprises more ductular reaction, polymorphonuclear leukocyte infiltration, and cholatestasis of acinar zone 1 hepatocytes and is seen in chronic cholestatic diseases.[20]

Classic piecemeal necrosis is difficult to differentiate from the periportal necrosis seen in viral hepatitis type A.[13,26,103] The latter type of periportal necrosis includes more B lymphocytes and plasma cells and probably involves different mechanisms than true piecemeal necrosis.[104] On routine liver histology, however, differentiation is not easy. Were it not an awkward term, periportal necrosis in hepatitis A might be phrased pseudo-piecemeal necrosis.

The pathogenesis of piecemeal necrosis is not well understood. Most of the available information suggests an antibody-dependent cellular cytotoxicity reaction. The target antigen may be autoantigens of the LSP or liver membrane antigen (LMAg) complex.[26,100] It must be kept in mind, however, that these features were investigated in chronic, not in acute variants of viral hepatitis B. The prognostic implications of piecemeal necrosis in AVHB are considered in the section on piecemeal necrosis as a predictor of chronicity.

Variants and Stages of Acute Hepatitis

The clinical variants of acute hepatitis B roughly correlate with the histopathologic features in liver biopsies. Anicteric and mild icteric AVHB is characterized mainly by spotty necrosis and focal–zonal confluent necrosis. More severe cases show features of bridging confluent necrosis. Fulminant hepatitis is associated with the more extensive (submassive and massive) forms of necrosis. Cholestatic variants of acute hepatitis reveal more striking features of bilirubinostasis in the parenchyma and even in the portal ductules.[7,105]

The individual components of the complex histologic picture of AVHB also vary during the course of the disease.[5,7,8,87,105] Microscopic analysis of liver biopsy features permits approximate estimation of early, fully developed, late, and residual stages of the disease.

HISTOLOGIC PREDICTION OF CHRONICITY

In 5–10% of patients with AVHB, chronic hepatitis develops.[106] Numerous studies have attempted to identify which features of acute histologic injury would permit prediction of a chronic outcome. The histologic alterations suggested as indicators of possible transition to chronicity include bridging hepatic necrosis,[107] piecemeal necrosis,[87] impaired regeneration,[25] abundance of plasma cells,[108] peculiar hepatitic bile duct lesions,[109] and presence of ground-glass hepatocytes.[78] The main discussion has centered on confluent bridging necrosis and piecemeal necrosis.

Bridging Hepatic Necrosis as a Predictor of Chronicity

This series of studies was triggered in 1970. From a retrospective analysis of 170 patients with acute hepatitis, Boyer and Klatskin[107] concluded that bridging hepatic necrosis in the acute stage of viral hepatitis heralded an unfavorable outcome; cirrhosis developed in 37% of their patients. This conclusion was supported by other retrospective[110,111] and prospective[113,112] studies. By contrast, other investigations resulted in the opposite conclusion that bridging hepatic necrosis has no ominous implications for long-term prognosis.[78,106,114–116]

This apparent controversy is at least partly resolved when one considers other factors than just bridging hepatic necrosis.[106] These include: etiology of the acute hepatitis, age of the patient, and the timing of the biopsy during the course of the disease. Hepatitis A does not lead to chronic disease, irrespective of the presence of bridging necrosis.[106] Comparisons with other studies must consider that in the original report[107] 63% of patients were over 40 years of age, and the liver biopsy was apparently taken relatively late in the course of the disease.

It appears that bridging hepatic necrosis observed in early biopsies (within 4–6 weeks after the onset of symptoms) from patients with AVHB, especially when younger than 40 years, has no prognostic meaning for subsequent development of chronic hepatitis and cirrhosis.[106]

Bridging hepatic necrosis indicates a more severe form of hepatitis and, as such, may have significance for more immediate prognosis. This is especially true for older patients with impaired regenerative capacity of the liver.[25] Nevertheless, patients with severe bridging hepatic necrosis may recover without important sequelae.[117,118] The prognosis may be less favorable when bridging hepatic necrosis is detected in older patients and during later stages of the acute illness.[106]

In recent years, it became clear that superinfection with delta hepatitis virus in patients infected with HBV is an additional factor causing severely necrotizing liver disease with bridging necrosis.[119–122]

Piecemeal Necrosis as a Predictor of Chronicity

An international group of pathologists suggested that "there are cases (of acute hepatitis), often of unusually long duration, in which the histological appearances suggest the *possibility* of transition to chronic aggressive hepatitis."[123] The bad histologic sign in such liver biopsies is periportal piecemeal necrosis. This claim about the prognostic value of piecemeal necrosis was questioned,[124] and even contradicted,[125] whereas other studies[108] supported the original claim.

A prospective study of 24 patients with AVHB in medical personnel of renal dialysis units showed that piecemeal necrosis in the early stage of the disease (at the peak of transaminase elevation) has no predictive value for transition to chronicity.[78] Piecemeal necrosis, as well as portal–central bridging necrosis, appears to be a common feature of early AVHB in humans.[78] A further retrospective study[126] reconfirmed the value of piecemeal necrosis in predicting a chronic outcome in acute hepatitis B. However, in this study most of the biopsies were taken in a later stage, beyond the first 4–6 weeks after the onset of symptoms.

The tentative conclusion that emerges from these studies is that piecemeal necrosis is a common feature without prognostic value in the early stage of the disease, up to the time of maximum transaminase levels. The same applies to bridging hepatic necrosis.[78]

However, the persistence of piecemeal necrosis carries a poor prognosis. Thus, this histologic lesion has strong predictive value for transition into chronic hepatitis when it is observed in a liver biopsy taken 2 months after the onset of the disease.[78,126] But it must be remembered that it is crucial to differentiate piecemeal necrosis from the periportal necroinflammatory lesion present in acute hepatitis A.[126] This confusion may explain the contradictory results of some studies.[125] When application of appropriate immunohistochemical techniques demonstrates persistence of HB_sAg or HB_cAg in scattered hepatocytes in the liver biopsy taken after 2 months, this finding most strongly suggests a chronic outcome.[3,67,72,78,126]

The final conclusion about the prognostic value of histologic lesions in the liver biopsy is that until now no single lesion (neither bridging hepatic necrosis nor piecemeal necrosis) has predictive value when observed in the early stage. Liver biopsy thus is not indicated for prognostic evaluation during the first few weeks after onset of symptoms in acute hepatitis B. By contrast, later biopsies (after 2 months) may yield prognostic information in the form of piecemeal necrosis, possibly in the presence of confluent necrosis, and definitely when viral antigens can be demonstrated in the tissue. The moral of the story is that piecemeal necrosis must be evaluated most carefully in order to avoid overdiagnosis of chronic liver disease.

The final message to the histopathologist is always to examine liver biopsies without knowledge of clinical data in order to ensure objectivity, but *never* to report a final diagnosis without checking microscopic impressions with the clinical data.

REFERENCES

1. Bianchi L: Liver biopsy interpretation in hepatitis. Part I. Presentation of critical morphologic features used in diagnosis. (Glossary.) *Pathol Res Pract* **178:**2–19, 1983.
2. Bianchi L: Liver biopsy interpretation in hepatitis. Part II. Histopathology and classification of acute and chronic viral hepatitis. Differential diagnosis. *Pathol Res Pract* **178:**180–213, 1983.

3. Bianchi L, Gudat F: Immunopathology of hepatitis B, in Popper H, Schaffner F (eds): *Progress in Liver Diseases*, Vol. VI. New York, Grune & Stratton, 1979, pp. 371–392.

4. Bianchi L, Gudat F: Viral antigens in liver tissue and type of inflammation in hepatitis B, in Bianchi L, Gerok W, Sickinger K, Stalder GA (eds): *Virus and the Liver*. Lancaster, MTP Press, 1980, pp. 197–204.

5. Bianchi L, Gudat F: Histo- and immunopathology of viral hepatitis, in Deinhardt F, Deinhardt J (eds): *Viral Hepatitis: Laboratory and Clinical Sciences*. New York, Dekker, 1983, pp. 335–382.

6. Bianchi L, Spichtin H-P: Histopathological studies of hepatitis B, in Gerety RJ (eds): *Hepatitis B*. Orlando, Academic, 1985, pp. 269–302.

7. Bianchi L, Zimmerli-Ning M, Gudat F: Viral hepatitis, in MacSween RNM, Anthony PP, Scheuer PJ (eds): *Pathology of the Liver*. Edinburgh, Churchill Livingstone, 1979, pp. 164–191.

8. MacSween NMR: Pathology of viral hepatitis and its sequelae. *Clin Gastroenterol* **9**:23–46, 1980.

9. Phillips MJ, Poucell S: Modern aspects of the morphology of viral hepatitis. *Hum Pathol* **12**:1060–1084, 1981.

10. Popper H: Pathology of viral hepatitis, in Overly LR, Deinhardt F, Deinhardt J (eds): *Viral Hepatitis*. New York, Dekker, 1983, pp. 11–18.

11. Popper H. Lessons from the pathology of viral hepatitis in animal models, in Callea F, Zorzi M, Desmet VJ (eds): *Viral Hepatitis*. Berlin, Springer-Verlag, 1986, pp. 64–71.

12. Popper H, Dienstag JL, Feinstone SM, et al: Lessons from the pathology of viral hepatitis in chimpanzees, in Bianchi L, Gerok W, Sickinger K, Stalder GA (eds): *Virus and the Liver*. Lancester, MTP Press, 1980, pp. 137–150.

13. Popper H, Dienstag JL, Feinstone SM, et al: The pathology of viral hepatitis in chimpanzees. *Virchows Arch [A]* **387**:91–106, 1980.

14. Scheuer PJ: Pathological aspects of viral hepatitis, in Brunner H, Thaler H (eds): *Hepatology, A Festschrift for Hans Popper*. New York, Raven, 1985, pp. 109–117.

15. Scheuer PJ: The pathology of acute viral hepatitis, in Callea F, Zorzi M, Desmet VJ (eds): *Viral Hepatitis*. Berlin, Springer-Verlag, 1986, pp. 29–31.

16. Thung SN, Gerber MA, Popper H: Basic morphologic patterns of viral hepatitis A, B, non-A, non-B and delta agent in animal and man, in Chisari FV (ed): *Advances in Hepatitis Research*. New York, Masson Publishing USA, 1984, pp. 293–302.

17. Uchida T, Kronborg I, Peters RL: Acute viral hepatitis: Morphologic and functional correlations in human livers. *Hum Pathol* **15**:267–277, 1984.

18. Wright R, Millward-Sadler GH, Bull FG: Acute viral hepatitis, in Wright R, Millward-Sadler GH, Alberti KGMM, Karran S (eds): *Liver and Biliary Disease*, 2nd Ed. London, Baillière Tindall–WB Saunders, 1985, pp. 677–767.

19. Rappaport AM: The microcirculatory acinar concept of normal and pathological hepatic structure. *Beitr Pathol* **157**:215–243, 1976.

20. Desmet VJ: Current problems in diagnosis of biliary disease and cholestasis. *Semin Liver Dis* **6**:233–245, 1986.

21. Bechtelsheimer H, Gedigk P, Müller R, Klein H: Aggressive Emperipolese bei chronischen Hepatitiden. *Klin Wochenschr* **54**:137–140, 1976.

22. Mietkiewski JM, Scheuer PJ: Immunoglobulin-containing plasma cells in acute hepatitis. *Liver* **5**:84–88, 1985.

23. Bardadin KA, Scheuer PJ: Plasma cells in acute hepatitis: An ultrastructural study. *Virchows Arch [A]* **408**:1–13, 1985.

24. Bardadin KA, Scheuer PJ: Mast cells in acute hepatitis. *J Pathol* **149**:315–325, 1986.

25. Peters RL, Omata M, Aschavai M, Liew CT: Protracted viral hepatitis with impaired regenera-

tion, in Vyas GN, Cohen SN, Schmid R (eds): *Viral Hepatitis*. Philadelphia, Franklin Institute Press, 1978, pp. 79–84.
26. Bianchi L. Necroinflammatory liver diseases. *Semin Liver Dis* **6:**185–198, 1986.
27. Ishak KG: Light microscopic morphology of viral hepatitis. *Am J Clin Pathol* **65:**787–827, 1976.
28. Klion F, Schaffner F: The ultrastructure of acidophilic "Councilman-like" bodies in the liver. *Am J Pathol* **48:**755–767, 1966.
29. Biava C, Mukhlova-Montiel M: Electron miscroscopic observations in Councilman-like acidophilic bodies and other forms of acidophilic changes in human liver cells. *Am J Pathol* **46:**775–802, 1965.
30. Wyllie AH: Cell death: A new classification separating apoptosis from necrosis, in Bowen ID, Lockshin RA (eds): *Cell Death in Biology and Pathology*. London, Chapman & Hall, 1981, pp. 9–34.
31. Wyllie AH, Kerr JRF, Currie AR: Cell death—The significance of apoptosis. *Int Rev Cytol* **68:**251–306, 1980.
32. Searle J, Kerr JFR, Bishop CJ: Necrosis and apoptosis: Distinct modes of cell death with fundamentally different significance. *Pathol Annu* **17:**229–259, 1982.
33. Stacey NH, Bishop CJ, Halliday JW, et al: Apoptosis as the mode of cell death in antibody-dependent lymphocytotoxicity. *J Cell Sci* **74:**169–179, 1985.
34. Matter A. Microcinematographic and electron microscopic analysis of target cell lysis induced by cytotoxic T lymphocytes. *Immunology* **36:**179–190, 1979.
35. Russell SW, Rosenau W, Lee JC: Cytolysis induced by human lymphotoxin. Cinematographic and electron microscopic observations. *Am J Pathol* **69:**103–118, 1972.
36. Searle J, Harmon BV, Bishop CJ, Kerr JFR: The significance of cell death by apoptosis in hepatobiliary disease. *J Gastroenterol Hepatol* **2:**77–96, 1987.
37. Desmet VJ, De Vos R: Structural analysis of acute liver injury, in Keppler D, Bianchi L, Reutter w (eds): *Mechanisms of Hepatocyte Injury and Death*. Lancaster, MTP Press, 1984, pp. 11–30.
38. Bhakdi S, Tranum-Jensen J: Membrane damage by channel-forming proteins. *Trends Biochem Sci* **8:**134–136, 1983.
39. Tranum-Jensen J, Bhakdi S: Freeze-fracture analysis of the membrane lesion of human complement. *J Cell Biol* **87:**618–626, 1983.
40. Alberti A, Trevisan A, Fattovich G, Realdi G: The role of hepatitis B virus replication and hepatocyte membrane expression in the pathogenesis of HBV-related hepatic damage, in Chisari FV (ed): *Advances in Hepatitis Research*. New York, Masson Publishing USA, 1984, pp. 134–143.
41. Mondelli M, Naumov N, Eddleston ALWF: The immunopathogenesis of liver cell damage in chronic hepatitis B virus infection, in Chisari FV (ed): *Advances in Hepatitis Research*. New York, Masson Publishing USA, 1984, pp. 144–151.
42. Mondelli M, Eddleston ALWF: Mechanisms of liver cell injury in acute and chronic hepatitis B. *Semin Liver Dis* **4:**47–58, 1984.
43. Chisari FV: Hepatic immunoregulatory molecules and the pathogenesis of hepatocellular injury in viral hepatitis, in Chisari FV (ed): *Advances in Hepatitis Research*. New York, Masson Publishing USA, 1984, pp. 168–178.
44. Thomas HC, Pignatelli M, Goodall A, et al: Immunologic mechanisms of cell lysis in hepatitis B virus infection, in Vyas GN, Dienstag JL, Hoofnagle (eds): *Viral Hepatitis and Liver Disease*. Orlando, Grune & Stratton, 1984, pp. 167–177.
45. Van den Oord JJ, De Vos R, Desmet VJ: In situ distribution of major histocompatibility complex products and viral antigens in chronic hepatitis B virus infection: Evidence that HBc-containing hepatocytes may express HLA-DR antigens. *Hepatology* **6:**981–989, 1986.

46. Thomas HC, Pignatelli M, Scully LJ: Viruses and immune reactions in the liver. *Scand J Gastroenterol* **20**(suppl):105–117, 1985.

47. Dienstag JL, Bhan AK, Klingenstein RJ, Savarese AM: Immunopathogenesis of liver disease associated with hepatitis B, in Szmuness W, Alter HJ, Maynard JE (eds): *Viral Hepatitis.* Philadelphia, Franklin Institute Press, 1982, pp. 221–236.

48. Dienstag JL: Studies of cell-mediated immunity in chronic hepatitis B virus infection: The elusive goal of virus and host antigen specificity, in Chisari FV (ed): *Advances in Hepatitis Research.* New York, Masson Publishing USA, 1984, pp. 163–167.

49. Klingenstein RJ, Dienstag JL: Immunopathogenesis of acute and chronic hepatitis B, in Gerety RJ (ed): *Hepatitis B.* Orlando, Academic, 1985, pp. 221–245.

50. Thomas HC, Lever AML: Has immunology become important to hepatologists? in Popper H, Schaffner F (eds): *Progress in Liver Diseases,* Vol. VIII. Orlando, Grune & Stratton, 1986, pp. 179–189.

51. Pignatelli M, Waters J, Brown D, et al: HLA-Class I antigens on the hepatocyte membrane during recovery from acute hepatitis B virus infection and during interferon therapy in chronic hepatitis B virus infection. *Hepatology* **6**:349–353, 1986.

52. Pignatelli M, Waters J, Lever A, et al: Cytotoxic T-cell responses to the nucleocapsid proteins of HBV in chronic hepatitis. Evidence that antibody modulation may cause protracted infection. *J Hepatol* **4**:15–21, 1987.

53. Bianchi L: The immunopathology of acute type B hepatitis. *Springer Semin Immunopathol* **3**:421–438, 1981.

54. Mondelli MU, Bortolotti F, Pontisso P, et al: Definition of hepatitis B virus (HBV)-specific target antigens recognized by cytotoxic T cells in acute HBV infection. *Clin Exp Immunol* **68**:242–250, 1987.

54a. Vento S, Ranieri S, Williams R, et al: Prospective study of cellular immunity to hepatitis-B-virus antigens from the early incubation phase of acute hepatitis B. *Lancet* **ii**:119–122, 1987.

54b. Mohite BJ, Rath S, Bal V, et al: Mechanisms of liver cell damage in acute hepatitis B. *J Med Virol* **22**:199–210, 1987.

55. Govindarajan S, Uchida T, Peters RL: Identification of T lymphocytes and subsets in liver biopsy cores of acute viral hepatitis. *Liver* **3**:13–18, 1983.

56. Miller JD, Dwyer JN, Klatskin G: Identification of lymphocytes in percutaneous liver biopsy cores. *Gastroenterology* **72**:1199–1203, 1977.

57. Montano L, Miescher GC, Goodall AL, et al: Hepatitis B virus and HLA antigen display in the liver during chronic hepatitis B virus infection. *Hepatology* **2**:557–561, 1982.

58. De Vos R, De Wolf-Peeters C, Van den Oord J, Desmet V: Ultrastructural immunocytochemical demonstration of MHC class I antigens in human pathological liver tissue. *Hepatology* **5**:1071–1075, 1985.

59. Thomas HC, Pignatelli M: Is modulation of HLA display by interferon important in preventing the development of the chronic carrier state of hepatitis B virus in adults? (Editorial) *Gastroenterol Clin Biol* **9**:287–289, 1985.

60. Nagafuchi Y, Scheuer PJ: Expression of bèta-2-microglobulin in hepatocytes in acute and chronic type B hepatitis. *Hepatology* **6**:20–23, 1986.

61. Fukusato T, Gerber MA, Thung SN, et al: Expression of HLA class I antigens on hepatocytes in liver disease. *Am J Pathol* **123**:264–270, 1986.

62. Van den Oord JJ, Desmet VJ: Verteilungsmuster der Histokompatibilitäts-Hauptantigene im normalen und pathologischen Lebergewebe. *Leber Magen Darm* **14**:244–254, 1984.

63. Ikeda T, Pignatelli M, Lever AML, Thomas HC: Relationship of HLA protein display to activation of 2-5 A synthetase in HBe-antigen or anti-HBe positive chronic HBV infection. *Gut* **27**:1498–1501, 1986.

64. Peters M, Davis GL, Dooley JS, Hoofnagle JH: The interferon system in acute and chronic viral hepatitis, in Popper H, Schaffner F (eds): *Progress in Liver Diseases*, Vol. VIII. Orlando, Grune & Stratton, 1986, pp. 453–467.

65. Jilbert AR, Burrell CJ, Gowans EJ, et al: Cellular localization of alpha-interferon in hepatitis B-virus-infected liver tissue. *Hepatology* 6:957–961, 1986.

66. Zinkernagel RM, Haenseler E, Leist T, et al: T cell-mediated hepatitis in mice infected with lymphocytic choriomeningitis virus. Liver cell destruction by H-2 class I-restricted virus-specific cytotoxic T cells as a physiological correlate of the ^{51}Cr-release assay? *J Exp Med* 164:1075–1093, 1986.

67. Callea F, Facchetti F, Bonera E, et al: Prognostic significance of viral antigens in liver tissue, in Callea F, Zorzi M, Desmet VJ (eds): *Viral Hepatitis*. Berlin, Springer-Verlag, 1986, pp. 41–54.

68. Gerber MA, Thung SN: Molecular and cellular pathology of hepatitis B. *Lab Invest* 52:572–590, 1985.

69. Kojima T, Desmet VJ: Hepatitis B core antigen (HBcAg) in liver cell plasma membrane: Immunoelectron microscopic study. *Hepatology* 4:780, 1984.

70. Kojima T, Bloemmen J, Desmet VJ: Immune electron microscopic demonstration of hepatitis B core antigen (HBcAg) in liver cell plasma membranes. *Liver* 7:191–200, 1987.

71. Berquist KR, Peterson JM, Murphy BL, et al: Hepatitis B antigens in serum and liver of chimpanzees acutely infected with hepatitis B virus. *Infect Immunol* 12:602–605, 1975.

72. Ray MB: *Hepatitis B Virus Antigens in Tissues*. Lancaster, MTP Press, 1979.

73. Alberti A, Realdi G, Tremolada F, Spina GP: Liver cell surface localization of hepatitis B antigen and of immunoglobulins in acute and chronic hepatitis and in liver cirrhosis. *Clin Exp Immunol* 25:396–402, 1976.

74. Gudat F, Bianchi L: HBsAg: A target antigen on the liver cell? in Popper H, Bianchi L, Reutter W (eds): *Membrane Alterations as Basis of Liver Injury*. Lancaster, MTP Press, 1977, pp. 171–178.

75. Lenzi M, Preda P, Bianchi FB, et al: Mechanically isolated hepatocytes are unsuitable to detect antibodies directed against plasma membrane determinants. *Liver* 5:212–220, 1985.

76. Barker LF, Chisari FV, McGrath PP, et al: Transmission of type B viral hepatitis to chimpanzees. *J Infect Dis* 127:648–662, 1973.

77. Arnold W, Meyer zum Buschenfelde KH, Hess G, Knolle J: The diagnostic significance of intrahepatocellular hepatitis B surface antigen (HBsAg), hepatitis B core antigen (HBcAg) and IgG for the classification of inflammatory liver diseases. *Klin Wochenschr* 53:1069–1074, 1975.

78. Houthoff HJ, Niermeijer P, Gips CH, et al: Hepatic morphologic findings and viral antigens in acute hepatitis B. *Virchows Arch [A]* 389:153–166, 1980.

79. Gudat F, Bianchi L, Sonnabend W, et al: Pattern of core and surface expression in liver tissue reflects state of specific immune response in hepatitis B. *Lab Invest* 32:1–9, 1975.

80. Chisari FV, Edgington TS, Routenberg JA, Anderson DS: Cellular immune reactivity in HBV-induced liver disease, in Vyas GN, Cohen SN, Schmid R (eds): *Viral Hepatitis*. Philadelphia, Franklin Institute Press, 1978, pp. 245–266.

81. Brattig NW, Berg PA: Immunosuppressive serum factors in viral hepatitis. I. Characterization of serum inhibition factor(s) as lymphocyte antiactivator(s). *Hepatology* 3:638–646, 1983.

82. Brattig NW, Schrempf-Decker GE, Brockl CW, Berg PA: Immunosuppressive serum factors in viral hepatitis. II. Further characterization of serum inhibition factor as an albumin-associated molecule. *Hepatology* 3:647–655, 1983.

83. Levy GA, Chisari FV: The immunopathogenesis of chronic HBV induced liver disease. *Springer Semin Immunopathol* 3:439–460, 1981.

84. Eggink HF, Houthoff HJ, Huitema S, et al: Cellular and humoral immune reactions in chronic active liver disease. II. Lymphocyte subsets and viral antigen in liver biopsies of patients with acute and chronic hepatitis B. *Clin Exp Immunol* **56:**121–128, 1984.

85. Tong MJ, Nies KM, Redeker AG: Rapid progression of chronic active type B hepatitis in a patient with hypogammaglobulinemia. *Gastroenterology* **73:**1418–1421, 1977.

86. Ceuppens JL, Stevens E, Fevery J, Schurmans J: Complete recovery from hepatitis B and associated hemolysis in a patient with underlying T-cell deficiency. *Gastroenterology* **86:**937–940, 1984.

87. Bianchi L, De Groote J, Desmet VJ, et al: Acute and chronic hepatitis revisited. *Lancet* **2:**914–919, 1977.

88. Desmet VJ: Morphogenese der chronischen Hepatitis. *MMW* **120:**1523–1530, 1978.

89. Conn HO: Chronic hepatitis: Reducing an iatrogenic enigma to a workable puzzle. *Gastroenterology* **70:**1182–1184, 1976.

90. Tisdale WA: Clinical and pathologic features of subacute hepatitis. *Medicine (Baltimore)* **45:**557–563, 1966.

91. Diaz-Gil JJ, Sanchez G, Santamaria L, et al: Liver DNA synthesis promotor activity detected in human plasma from subjects with hepatitis. *Hepatology* **6:**658–661, 1986.

92. Gohda E, Tsubouchi H, Nakayama H, et al: Human hepatocyte growth factor in plasma from patients with fulminant hepatic failure. *Exp Cell Res* **166:**139–150, 1986.

93. Scheuer PJ, Maggi G: Hepatic fibrosis and collapse: Histological distinction by orcein staining. *Histopathology* **4:**487–490, 1980.

94. Thung SN, Gerber MA: The formation of elastic fibers in livers with massive hepatic necrosis. *Arch Pathol Lab Med* **106:**468–469, 1982.

95. Liehr H, Grün M: Endotoxins in liver disease. *Prog Liver Dis* **6:**313–316, 1979.

96. Mori W, Shiga J, Irie H: Schwarzman reaction as a pathogenetic mechanism in fulminant hepatitis. *Semin Liver Dis* **6:**267–276, 1986.

97. Tabor E, Krugman S, Weiss EG, Gerety RJ: Disappearance of hepatitis B surface antigen during an unusual case of fulminant hepatitis B. *J Med Virol* **8:**277–282, 1981.

98. Popper H, Paronetto F, Schaffner F: Immune processes in the pathogenesis of liver disease. *Ann NY Acad Sci* **124:**781–799, 1965.

99. Bardadin KA, Desmet VJ: Interdigitating and dendritic reticulum cells in chronic active hepatitis. *Histopathology* **8:**657–667, 1984.

100. Desmet VJ: New aspects of piecemeal necrosis, in Bianchi L, Gerok W, Popper H (eds): *Trends in Hepatology.* Lancaster, MTP Press, 1985, pp. 183–200.

101. Kerr JFR, Cooksley WGE, Searle J, et al: Hypothesis: The nature of piecemeal necrosis in chronic active hepatitis. *Lancet* **2:**827–828, 1979.

102. Popper H: Changing concepts of the evolution of chronic hepatitis and the role of piecemeal necrosis. *Hepatology* **3:**758–762, 1983.

103. Teixeira MR Jr, Weller IVD, Murray AM, et al: The pathology of hepatitis A in man. *Liver* **2:**53–60, 1982.

104. Sciot R, Van den Oord JJ, De Wolf-Peeters C, Desmet VJ: In situ characterisation of the (peri)portal inflammatory infiltrate in acute hepatitis A. *Liver* **6:**331–336, 1986.

105. Desmet VJ, De Groote J: Histological diagnosis of viral hepatitis. *Clin Gastroenterol* **3:**337–354, 1974.

106. Carithers RL Jr, Fallon HJ: When does acute hepatitis become chronic? in Cohen S, Soloway RD (eds): *Chronic Active Liver Disease.* New York, Churchill Livingstone, 1983, pp. 189–206.

107. Boyer, JL, Klatskin G: Pattern of necrosis in acute viral hepatitis. Prognostic value of bridging (subacute hepatic necrosis). *N Engl J Med* **283:**1063–1071, 1970.

108. Dietrichson O, Juhl E, Christoffersen P, et al: Acute viral hepatitis: Factors possibly predicting chronic liver disease. *Acta Pathol Microbiol Scand [A]* **83**:183–188, 1975.
109. Poulsen H, Christoffersen P: Abnormal bile duct epithelium in chronic aggressive hepatitis and cirrhosis. A review of morphology and clinical, biochemical and immunologic features. *Hum Pathol* **3**:217–225, 1972.
110. Ware AJ, Eigenbrodt EH, Combes B: Prognostic significance of subacute hepatic necrosis in acute hepatitis. *Gastroenterology* **68**:519–524, 1975.
111. Spitz RD, Keren DF, Boitnott JK, Maddrey WC: Bridging hepatic necrosis—Etiology and prognosis. *Am J Dig Dis* **23**:1076–1078, 1978.
112. Gregory PB, Knauer M, Kempson RL, Miller R: Steroid therapy in severe viral hepatitis: A double-blind, randomized trial of methyl-prednisolone versus placebo. *N Engl J Med* **294**:681–687, 1976.
113. Nisman RM, Ganderson AP, Vlahcevic ZR, Gregory DH: Acute viral hepatitis with bridging hepatic necrosis. An overview. *Arch Intern Med* **139**:1289–1291, 1979.
114. Ware AJ, Cuthbert JA, Shorey J, et al: A prospective trial of steroid therapy in severe viral hepatitis: The prognostic significance of bridging necrosis. *Gastroenterology* **80**:219–224, 1981.
115. Schmid M, Pirovino M, Altorfer J, et al: Acute viral hepatitis B with bridging necrosis: A follow-up study. *Liver* **1**:222–229, 1981.
116. Theodor E, Niv Y: The clinical course of subacute hepatic necrosis. *Am J Gastroenterol* **70**:600–606, 1978.
117. Desmet VJ, De Groote J, Van Damme B: Acute hepatocellular failure. A study of 17 patients treated with exchange transfusion. *Hum Pathol* **3**:167–182, 1972.
118. Karvountzis GG, Redeker AG, Peters RL: Long-term follow-up studies of patients surviving fulminant viral hepatitis. *Gastroenterology* **67**:870–877, 1974.
119. Rizzetto M, Verme G, Gerin JL, Purcell RH: Hepatitis delta virus disease, in Popper H, Schaffner F (eds): *Progress in Liver Diseases*, Vol. VIII. New York, Grune & Stratton, 1986, pp. 417–431.
120. Tassopoulos NC, Papaevangelou GJ, Roumeliotou-Karayannis A, et al: Fulminant hepatitis in asymptomatic hepatitis B surface antigen carriers in Greece. *J Med Virol* **20**:371–379, 1986.
121. Govindarajan S, Chin KP, Redeker AG, Peters RL: Fulminant B viral hepatitis: Role of delta agent. *Gastroenterology* **86**:1417–1420, 1984.
122. Govindarajan S, De Cock KM, Peters RL: Morphologic and immunohistochemical features of fulminant delta hepatitis. *Hum Pathol* **16**:262–267, 1985.
123. Bianchi L, De Groote J, Desmet VJ, et al: Morphological criteria in viral hepatitis. *Lancet* **1**:333–337, 1971.
124. Boyer JL: Chronic hepatitis—A perspective on classification and determinants of prognosis. *Gastroenterology* **70**:1161–1171, 1976.
125. Fauerholdt L, Asnaes S, Ranek L, et al: Significance of suspected "chronic aggressive hepatitis" in acute hepatitis. *Gastroenterology* **73**:543–548, 1977.
126. Vanstapel MJ, Van Steenbergen W, De Wolf-Peeters C, et al: Prognostic significance of piecemeal necrosis in acute viral hepatitis. *Liver* **3**:46–57, 1983.

Hepatitis Delta Virus in Acute and Chronic Liver Disease

FERRUCCIO BONINO and MARIO RIZZETTO

BIOLOGY, TRANSMISSION, AND EPIDEMIOLOGY OF HEPATITIS DELTA VIRUS

Biology

Hepatitis delta virus (HDV) is a defective hepatotropic RNA agent that replicates only in hosts who are simultaneously infected with hepatitis B virus (HBV).[1,2] The virion is a spherical 36-nm particle, composed of a lipoprotein envelope. The surface antigen of HBV (HB$_s$Ag) contains delta antigen (HDAg) and an RNA molecule of 1.7 kilobases (kb) (HDV-RNA).[1,2] The detection of HDAg requires treatment with detergents, but nucleocapsidic structures are not seen electron microscopically within the HB$_s$Ag envelope of the particle.[3] HDAg is composed of two major proteins, 24,000–27,000 M_r and 27,000–29,000 M_r molecular weight.[3,4] HDV-RNA is considered the genome of the defective agent. It was reverse transcribed to make complementary DNA (cDNA) that was cloned using appropriate vectors.[5-11] DNA clone fragments of different length, spanning the entire HDV genome, were obtained and sequenced.[5-11] No significant homology was observed between HDV-RNA and HBV-DNA or between HDV-RNA and host DNA. HDV-RNA contains 1679–1683 nucleotides and five open reading frames (ORF) of more than 100 amino acids in both genomic and antigenomic strands.[2,5-11] The largest ORF, present on the antigenomic strand (+) and coding for 214 amino acids, was expressed in bacteria; the resultant fusion protein reacted with human antibodies to HDAg (anti-HD) by Western

FERRUCCIO BONINO and MARIO RIZZETTO • Division of Gastroenterology, San Giovanni Battista Molinette Hospital, 10126 Turin, Italy.

blot analysis.[5] *In vitro* translation of RNA derived from HDV-infected livers using lysates of rabbit reticulocytes produced two major proteins of HDAg that reacted in immunoblot with polyclonal anti-HD antibody and a monoclonal antibody obtained from Epstein–Barr virus (EBV)-transformed human lymphocytes.[5,12] The lack of a 3' poly (A) tract on the virion RNA and its failure to translate HDAg *in vitro* and the presence of HDAg coding sequences on the antigenomic strand of HDV-RNA suggest that HDV is a negatively stranded virus where the complementary strand of the genome (+) serves as messenger RNA (mRNA). HDV particles contain two RNA species that migrated in gel electrophoresis at 1.75 and 2.0 kb, respectively.[5,7] These RNAs reacted only with one of the two strand-specific cDNA probes of HDV-RNA (antigenomic), indicating that they have the same polarity (genomic, +) and possibly that they represent nicked linear and circular forms of the same RNA molecule.[7] These studies and results of HDV-RNA under the electron microscope suggest that HDV contains a single-stranded and covalently closed circular RNA molecule that forms extensive secondary structure. The self-annealing properties and the high GC content (60%) permit the formation of a double-stranded rodlike structure resembling those of a number of different viroidlike RNAs that cause a variety of diseases in plants.[5,13] Different forms of HDV-RNA were found in infected livers, including genomic and antigenomic strands, poly-A RNA, and double-stranded RNA (dsRNA). The dsRNA species could represent replicative forms of HDV-RNA, suggesting a replicative cycle of HDV somewhat similar to that seen in satellites of plant RNA viruses. Satellite RNA of cucumber mosaic virus (CMV) replicate in rolling circle fashion, producing large amounts of double-stranded forms that accumulate in the cell.[14] These forms suppress replication of the helper virus RNA which is produced much less rapidly than satellite RNA[13,14] and thus determines the attenuation of disease symptoms caused by CMV. Occasionally, this apparently defensive mechanism turns out to be deleterious. This happens upon superinfection of a CMV carrier plant with satellites containing a defective necrotizing gene known to cause tremendous epidemics of tomato necrosis.[13,14] Satellite–CMV interference in plants closely resembles that of HDV and HBV in humans and animals. Furthermore, some sequence homology of HDV-RNA with plant virusoids[5] suggests that HDV and these agents may have a common ancestry.

Transmission

Transmission of HDV is linked to that of the helper virus. HDV infection in newborns was documented only in babies born to HB_eAg-positive HDV-infected mothers.[15] Most chronic carriers of HDV have low levels of HBV replication[16]; thus, perinatal transmission of HDV is rare. For the same reason the risk of post-transfusion HBV–HDV infection is negligible ($< 1:3000$) in recipients with negative markers for HBV and HDV.[17] This is conceivable because the presence of HB_sAg in the serum usually prevents the HDV carrier from blood donation. However, the possible inhibition of HB_sAg synthesis to subliminal levels in asymptomatic HDV–HBV carriers indicates a potential risk of transmission.[18-20] The risk becomes dramatically increased when the recipient is also a carrier of HB_sAg, and the amount of HDV to be rescued is infinitessimal because of the persistent and well-established HBV infection. End-point titration of HDV infectivity in chimpanzees have shown that an inoculum, infectious for both HBV and HDV, transmitted HDV infection at a 10^{-11} dilution in HB_sAg-positive animals but only at a 10^{-5} dilution in HB_sAg-negative chimpanzees.[21]

In keeping with the evidence of the high infection rate of HDV in the HB_sAg carrier, anti-HD is usually found in the serum of 30–100% of HB_sAg-carrier hemophiliacs treated with commercial clotting factors prepared from large pools of donors.[17] Anti-HD has a lower prevalence, or it is absent in HB_sAg carriers treated with products prepared from small pools of donors. These results indicate that blood-derived material given to HB_sAg carriers should be obtained from small pools of the safest donors, and it should be carefully checked for all HBV and HDV markers, not only for HB_sAg.

Epidemiology

HDV infection occurs worldwide[1,2] (Table I). The numbers of HB_sAg carriers and the extent of their promiscuity are the major factors determining

TABLE I. Worldwide Prevalence of Anti-HD in the Serum
of HB_sAg Carriers

Continent	Total anti-HD positive %	Highest %	Lowest %
Africa	10	35 (Egypt, Kenya)	<2
America			
North	5	Confined to high-risk groups	
South	10	90 (Amazon Basin)	<2
Asia			
Middle East	20	40 (Kuwait)	5
Far East	2.5	10 (New Guinea)	<2
Australia	20	—	—
Europe	20	60 (Balkan Peninsula)	<2

diffusion of HDV in a given population. In drug addicts and other high-risk populations of HB$_s$Ag carriers (e.g., hemophiliacs, hemodialysis patients, mentally retarded persons)[22-26] HDV is highly endemic independent of its levels in the normal population of the same area. In countries with intermediate or high HBV endemicity (>2%), HDV infection also occurs in normal individuals, after exposure to infectious body fluids during close or intimate contacts. HDV spreads rapidly within the household,[27] and the likelihood of infection increases where persons are crowded together in nonhygienic circumstances. Acupuncture, open skin wounds, and mosquitoes facilitate epidemic diffusion.[23,28] This probably explains why HDV infection is most common in the socially disadvantaged communities of tropical areas.[1,2] The apparent geographic irregularity of HDV prevalence probably reflects variations in serologic testing. Still unexplained is why HDV infection is endemic with severe outbreaks of fulminant hepatitis in South America but rare in the Far East, where the prevalence of HB$_s$Ag carriers is similar.

ACUTE HDV HEPATITIS

HBV and HDV Co-Infection

Experimental transmission of HDV to chimpanzees and epidemiologic studies in humans have shown that HDV infection occurs only in individuals infected with HBV and that immunity against HBV also protects against HDV.[1,2,29] When susceptible individuals are simultaneously exposed to both viruses, the duration of HBV infection is the limiting factor for expression of HDV. Acute HBV infection, even if associated with HDV, rarely reaches chronicity, and HDV cannot persist after clearance of HBV.[30,31] Usually, the acute illness secondary to HBV–HDV co-infection is not clinically different from classic type B hepatitis.[30] The serologic response to HDV is often elusive; it can be totally absent or limited to a transient appearance of IgM anti-HD.[30-33] Occasionally, however, in HBV–HDV co-infection, a strong serologic response to HDV develops; this form predominates in drug addicts and may be associated with severe liver damage.[6,7,15,34] HDAg appears in the serum during the acute phase of infection, followed by rising titers of IgM and IgG anti-HD. A typical clinical course in this case is biphasic hepatitis, in which the acute illness is characterized by two peaks of serum transaminases (ALT).[31,35] When a single inoculum or consecutive injections are highly infectious for both HBV and HDV, massive HBV replication supports the rapid rescue of the defective agent, which, being more efficient than the helper virus, overwhelms and suppresses the synthesis of HBV gene products, thus determining the first elevation of ALT. Subsequently, HBV infection completes its natural course, leading to the second bout of hepatitis. In keeping with this hypothesis, the peak of HD viremia (HDAg) precedes or is associated with the first ALT peak. A strong anti-HD immune response occurs instead at the time of the second ALT elevation where the highest values of HBV replication are usually found. The two necrotic events may represent a higher risk of fulminant hepatitis; however, the outcome of HBV–HDV co-infection is negligible in the great majority of cases and 90% of the patients recover completely with seroconversion to anti-HBs (Table II).[31]

HDV Superinfection of an HB$_s$Ag Carrier

The mechanism and the natural course of HDV infection are different in chronic carriers of HB$_s$Ag superinfected with HDV.[1,2,30,31,36,37] Persistent and well-established HBV infection promotes the florid replication of the defective virus and leads to severe liver damage. This form accounts for a large proportion (30–60%) of fulminant HB$_s$Ag positive hepatitis.[38–40] In HDV superinfection a strong serologic response to HDV develops, characterized by high titers of IgM and IgG anti-HD.[32,33] HDV superinfection has the propensity to become chronic since permanent HBV infection permits the indefinite life of the defective agent (Table II). Transition to chronicity of HDV infection simulates progressive type B hepatitis and poses important diagnostic problems when the HB$_s$Ag carrier status of the patient is unknown. The lack of IgM antibody to HBV "core" antigen in the serum, or persistence of low titers of this antibody during the course of acute HB$_s$Ag positive hepatitis should always raise suspicion of HDV or non-A, non-B superinfection in a previously unrecognized carrier of HB$_s$Ag.[32,33,41] Detection of HDV markers is mandatory also in serum of HB$_s$Ag negative patients with acute hepatitis as the explosive replication of HDV during acute superinfection can suppress the synthesis of HB$_s$Ag to undetectable levels. Since survival of the defective virus depends on the highly efficient use of the same replicative machinery of HBV, HDV may strongly compete with HBV and, being an RNA virus, it may profit by possible reverse transcriptase activity

TABLE II. Outcome of Acute HDV Hepatitis

	HBV–HDV co-infection (%)	HDV superinfection (%)
Benign, self-limiting hepatitis	90	10
Evolution to chronicity	8[a]	85
Fulminant hepatitis	2	5

[a]In drug addicts, up to 20%.

of HBV-DNA polymerase. Obviously, the inhibition exerted by HDV cannot be so intense as to suppress completely the synthesis of HBV, as some degree of replication of this virus is necessary for survival of the defective agent. Occasionally, however, in very rare and fortunate cases, the supervening HDV infection may induce the termination of the HB_sAg carrier state with seroconversion to anti-HB_s and clearance of both HBV and HDV.[42]

The outcome of acute HDV superinfection may depend on whether the carrier of HB_sAg was previously asymptomatic or suffered from an HBV-related illness. In patients with previous HBV-induced liver disease, HDV causes further damage, accelerating the course of chronic hepatitis toward cirrhosis. Unfortunately, however, severe and progressive liver disease develops also in healthy carriers of HB_sAg superinfected with HDV.[30,31] Only a minor proportion experience a self-limited HDV infection, and a very fortunate minority also clear HBV after the acute illness; the great majority of the patients develop chronic liver disease. The evidence that liver damage is invariably present in the liver of both symptomatic and asymptomatic carriers of HDV and the presence of important cytopathic lesions in HDV infected livers (see histopathology) suggested that HDV may be directly pathogenic. However, transmission experiments in animals showed that the first phase in type D hepatitis is the expression of HDAg in the liver cell nuclei, in the absence of cell damage and inflammation. After development of the host's immunologic response (serum anti-HD), immunocomplexes are seen within the hepatocytes, lymphocytes accumulate in portal tracts and sinusoids, and liver necrosis takes place. Therefore available data do not support the hypothesis that HDV has major cytotoxic effects.

CHRONIC HDV HEPATITIS

Clinical, Serologic, and Histologic Features

Chronic HDV hepatitis is not clinically distinguishable from the other forms of viral hepatitis. History of acute hepatitis and splenomegaly are frequently reported in patients chronically infected by HDV (in about 70% of cases) but these cannot be considered specific diagnostic features.[36,43–47]

Autoimmune phenomena such as autoantibodies against microsomal membranes of the liver and kidney, more reactive with human than animal substrates, as well as antibodies to the basal cell layer of rat forestomach and to human tymocytes, were found in 20–65% of the patients with chronic HDV hepatitis, but these autoantibodies were also seen in other forms of liver disease.[48–50] The significance of this association is unknown, but the finding of these reactivities in the absence of HDV infection might suggest the search for a different viral etiology. Morphologists analyzed in detail the liver biopsies of chronically infected patients and animals to identify distinctive features of HDV hepatitis.[34,51-57] A few prevailing characteristics were described: severe lobular damage, eosinophilic and microvesicular (steatosislike) degeneration of liver cells. None of these, however, appeared specific to HDV infection as they were also observed in non-A, non-B hepatitis.

Natural History of Chronic HDV Hepatitis

Chronic HDV hepatitis represents the major cause of cirrhosis in young adults in Italy (Fig. 1).[46] The outcome of this disease was studied in 176 consecutive patients collected in our department from 1972 to 1980.[47] It was rapidly progressive in about 15% of cases with the development of clinical symptoms of cirrhosis within 1 year of the acute illness. It was slowly progressive in most of the patients (70%) with development of clinical cirrhosis in 15–25 years after acute HDV infection and negligible with remission of liver disease only in 15% of cases. The search for predictive markers of unfavorable outcome of HDV infection was extensive; only the persistence of markers of ongoing HDV replication in serum and liver (HDAg and HDV-RNA) and that of florid antibody response to HDAg, of both IgG and IgM type, in serum appear useful. The importance of the original morphologic lesion as a predictor of the course of chronic HDV hepatitis is uncertain. Severe forms of chronic active hepatitis (CAH), seen at admission, may not lead to cirrhosis, while relatively quiescent forms of liver damage may evolve rapidly to liver failure.[34,43,52] Recently we

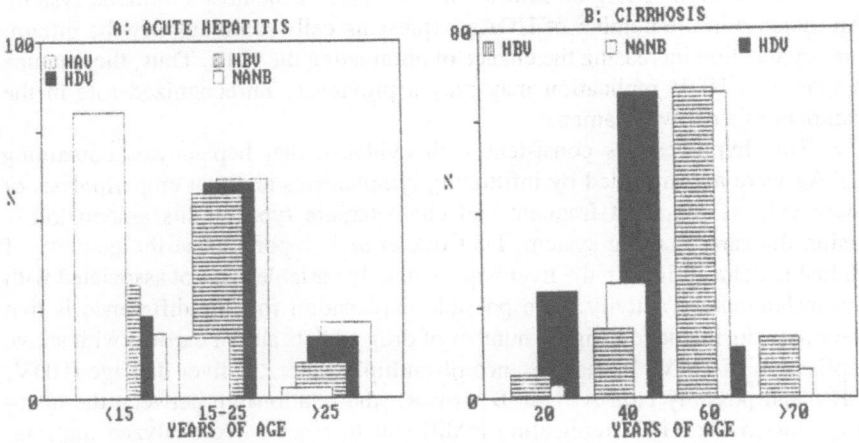

FIGURE 1. Age-specific prevalence of viral hepatitis in Italy. (A) Acute form: 384 total cases. (B) Chronic form: 646 total cases.

studied the expression of intrahepatic delta antigen (HDAg) in relationship to the morphologic features of HDV hepatitis in 101 patients followed for a mean of 12 years. Multiple liver biopsies were available from each patient, and the histologic features were assessed using numerical scores.[34] The prognosis of chronic HDV hepatitis appears unrelated to the original morphologic lesion; piecemeal necrosis, bridging necrosis, or the extent of lobular inflammation were not per se predictive of the course of HDV hepatitis. Cirrhosis was present in the follow-up liver biopsy of 13 of 39 (33%) patients who did not show nodular regeneration in the liver biopsy specimen obtained at admission. Cirrhosis developed in the short follow-up (mean 5 years) both in patients with piecemeal necrosis with and without bridging and in patients with minimal periportal lesions. By contrast, patients with subacute hepatic necrosis and bridging may recover upon remission of viral replication (two cases, in this study). Expression of HDAg in the liver was weakly correlated with the histologic activity index used in our study.[58] Among the four categories composing this index—portal inflammation, periportal necrosis, intralobular necrosis, and fibrosis—a significant positive relationship was observed only between the number of HDAg-positive cells and the extent of portal inflammation (Spearman's rank coefficient: 0.75). The overall level of HDAg and inflammation was twice as high in liver specimens obtained within 10 years of acute HDV hepatitis than afterward. Interestingly, in all the patients who recovered (with disappearance of biochemical signs of liver disease and decrease of serum anti-HD), the biopsy preceding remission showed the highest amount for both inflammatory activity and intrahepatic HDAg. On the contrary, the lowest values were associated with steadiness or progression of disease. These results suggest that the inflammatory response might depend on the recognition of HDAg on infected hepatocytes by the host's immune system. An increase in the number of HDAg-expressing cells could amplify the inflammatory reaction increasing the chance of eliminating the virus. Thus, the immune response to HDV replication may play a previously unrecognized role in the pathogenesis of liver damage.

This hypothesis is consistent with evidence that hepatocytes containing HDAg were accompanied by infiltrating lymphocytes and that emperipolesis of these cells is the most frequent and characteristic type of this association.[59] Using the same scoring system, De Cock et al.[44] reported that the quantity of stainable delta antigen in the liver was extremely variable and not associated with the inflammatory activity. One possible explanation for this difference is that their patients included a higher number of drug addicts and of carriers with active replication of HBV. In the presence of multiple causes of liver damage (HDV, HBV and possibly Non-A, Non-B viruses), the relationship between the histologic lesion and HDV replication is difficult to assess. We analyzed the relationship between intrahepatic expression of HDAg and histologic activity only in patients without a history of drug addiction and without serum and intrahepatic markers of active HBV replication, trying to eliminate the underlying HBV and Non-A, Non-B-induced liver damage.

The number of HDAg-positive cells in the liver appeared to be unrelated to the presence or extent of the degenerative lesions described: acidophilic bodies, eosinophilic or ballooning degeneration.[7,8] The so-called Morula cell degeneration (microsteatosis like lesion of the hepatocyte) was rarely found in our patients suggesting that this lesion is probably peculiar to HDV hepatitis seen in distinct epidemiologic settings, such as the Amazonian basin[11]; environmental factors other than HDV infection might be involved in its pathogenesis.

DIAGNOSIS, THERAPY, AND PROPHYLAXIS

Diagnosis

HDV disease is a multifaceted illness in which clinical and laboratory data as well as liver histology provide useful tools for the evaluation of the extent of liver damage, but specific diagnosis requires detection of markers of HDV infection (Table III). The diagnosis of acute and chronic hepatitis is made by the direct identification of the virus, detecting HDAg and HDV-RNA in serum and liver, or determining the presence of high titers of circulating antibodies of HDAg that represent the host's immune response to HDV infection.

Serum HDAg is detected by sensitive solid-phase radioimmunoassay (RIA) and by enzyme-linked immunosorbent assays (ELISA), or by Western blotting.[3,4,60] Current solid-phase immunoassays do not detect HDAg in the serum of patients with high titers of anti-HD, as the antigen is masked by the homologous antibody after detergent release from virions. In these patients HDAg can

TABLE III. Diagnosis of HDV Hepatitis:
Patterns of HDV Markers[a] in Serum and Liver

Serum HDAg	HDV-RNA	IgM-anti-HD	Anti-HD	Phase	Liver HDAg
Acute HDV hepatitis					
+	+/−	−/+	−	Early	−
+/−	+	+/−	−/+	Clinical	−
−	−	+	−/+	Late	−
Chronic HDV hepatitis					
+/−	+/−	+/−	+	−	+/−

[a]At least two of HDV markers are necessary for the diagnosis.

be detected by Western blotting. Detection of HD antigenemia correlates with expression of HDAg in the liver.

Intrahepatic HDAg is stained by immunohistochemical techniques in frozen or formalin-fixed paraffin-embedded liver specimens using anti-HD labeled with fluorochromes or enzymes. Immunohistology is a sensitive technique for demonstrating active HDV infection and the poor prognosis of HDV infection appears linked to the persistence of intrahepatic HDAg that maintains inflammation. Chronic liver disease, however, may proceed through episodes of recurrent hepatitis with quantitative reduction or disappearance of HDAg from the liver and subsequent new expression of the viral antigen in the hepatocytes.[48,52] These observations indicate the limits of the liver biopsy that offers only a single frame of the moving picture characterizing the evolution of chronic hepatitis. Fortunately, recombinant DNA technology provides useful tools to determine and monitor active HDV replication using simple, noninvasive, serologic methods for the detection of HDV-RNA by molecular hybridization.[5-11] After the introduction of riboprobe-based techniques as a substitute for nick translation in the labeling of HDV-RNA cDNA probes a 90% correspondence was found between detection of intrahepatic HDAg and serum HDV-RNA.[21]

The detection of anti-HD antibodies of IgG and IgM type is currently based on competitive assays for liver or serum derived HDAg[41,60]; in the IgM anti-HD assay, IgM is captured by anti-human IgM antibodies linked to the solid phase. High titers of IgG anti-HD, and particularly of IgM antibodies, reflect continuously active HDV replication.[21,32,41,54] The whole battery of HDV assays together with that of HBV[61] provides the only means of making the diagnosis of HDV hepatitis (see Table III). Acute self-limited hepatitis is characterized by several serologic profiles varying from the early appearance of HDAg followed by seroconversion to IgM anti-HD and IgG anti-HD, to an IgM/IgG response in the absence of detectable HD antigenemia, to the sole and short-lived detection of IgM or IgG anti-HD. Titers of IgM and IgG anti-HD remain relatively low ($<10^4$). Progressive HDV hepatitis is accompanied by the rapid rising of IgM and IgG antibodies to high titers ($>10^4$); their persistence permits diagnosis of chronicity.[32,33] The importance of a correct etiologic diagnosis of liver disease in HB_sAg carriers has important therapeutic implications because of the different response of HBV and HDV disease to treatment.

Therapy

Therapy of chronic HDV hepatitis with corticosteroids, levamisole, and azathioprine was disappointing.[1,2,43] In a randomized study, we observed that therapy with 5 megaunits (MU)/m^2 of recombinant α2-interferon (IFN$_{\alpha2}$), subcutaneously, three times weekly, induced a significant inhibition of HDV replication and a decrement of serum transaminases during treatment in 80% of patients (9 of 12).[62] Unfortunately, the biochemical remission achieved during treatment persisted only in one patient who cleared HDAg and HDV-RNA from serum and intrahepatic HDAg, showing a scarred liver without inflammatory lesions in the liver biopsy obtained 1 year after discontinuation of therapy. No significant changes in HDV replication and in the biochemical signs of liver disease were observed in controls. A temporary inhibition of HDV replication with remission of liver disease was also observed in other studies, which did not include a control group.[63,64] These results of IFN therapy appear less promising than those observed in HB_sAg carriers with type B hepatitis but without HDV superinfection. However, in consideration of the ominous prognosis of HDV disease in untreated patients, the therapeutic potential of interferon suggests a need for further trials of this drug for a longer period, and possibly in association with other untested antiviral drugs.

Recently, Hedin et al.[65,66] reported 75% survival rate in patients with fulminant HBV and HDV co-infection using trisodium phosphonoformate (foscarnet, 20-mg/kg bolus and 0.16 mg/kg per min infusion for 1–14 days), an inhibitor of DNA polymerase. It will take some time before we know how much of this exciting therapeutic potential of these new drugs will become a reality.

Prophylaxis

The use of HBV vaccines may prevent HBV and HDV co-infection; unfortunately, HBV vaccination does not help the estimated 200 million HB_sAg carriers who are at risk of developing HDV superinfection. For these persons, a specific HDV vaccine is required. Employing the subtlest tricks of recombinant DNA it is now possible to manipulate human and virus genes to synthesize drugs and vaccines in vitro. It is our hope that in the near future the blizzard of the genetic revolution will also result in substantial progress both in the therapy and the prophylaxis of HDV hepatitis.

REFERENCES

1. Verme G, Rizzetto M, Bonino F: Viral Hepatitis and Delta Infection. New York, Liss, 1983.
2. Rizzetto M, Gerin JL, Purcell RH: The Hepatitis Delta Virus and Its Infection. New York, Liss, 1987.
3. Bonino F, Hermann KH, Rizzetto M, Gerlich WH: Hepatitis delta virus: Protein composition of delta antigen and its hepatitis B virus derived envelope. J Virol 58:945–950, 1986.
4. Bergman KF, Gerin JL: Antigens of hepatitis delta virus in the liver and serum of humans and animals. J Infect Dis 154:702–706, 1986.

5. Wang KS, Choo QL, Weiner JH, et al: The viroid-like structure of the hepatitis delta genome: Synthesis of a viral antigen in recombinant bacteria. *Proc Clin Biol Res* **234**:71–82, 1987.
6. Kos A, de Reus A, Dubbeld M, et al: Biological and molecular characterization of the hepatitis delta virus. *Proc Clin Biol Res* **234**:83–88, 1987.
7. Baroudy BM, Smedile A, Korba BE, et al: Transcription and replication of hepatitis delta virus. *Proc Clin Biol Res* **234**:89–92, 1987.
8. Taylor J, Chen PJ, Kalpana G, et al: Structure and replication of the genome of hepatitis delta virus. *Proc Clin Biol Res* **234**:93–96, 1987.
9. Denniston KL, Hoyer BH, Smedile A, et al: Cloned fragment of the hepatitis delta virus RNA genome: Sequence and diagnostic application. *Science* **232**:873–875, 1986.
10. Wang KS, Choo QL, Weiner AJ, et al: Structure, sequence and expression of the hepatitis delta virus genome. *Naute* **323**:508–513, 1986.
11. Kos A, Dijkema R, Arnberg AC, et al: The hepatitis delta virus possesses a circular RNA. *Nature (Lond)* **323**:558–560, 1986.
12. Pohl C, Baroudy BM, Bergmann KF, et al: Identification of viral polypeptide and in vitro translation products of the genome of the hepatitis D virus by human monoclonal antibody, in *Abstracts of the 1987 International Symposium on Viral Hepatitis and Liver Disease*, p. 36A.
13. Kaper JM, Tousignant ME: Viral satellites: Parasitic nucleic acids capable of modulating disease expression. *Endeavour* **8**:194–200, 1984.
14. Piazzolla P: Symptom regulation induced by some plant virus-associated satellite-like RNAs. *Proc Clin Biol Res* **234**:19–22, 1987.
15. Zanetti A, Ferroni P, Magliano E, et al: Perinatal transmission of the hepatitis B virus and of the HBV-associated delta agent from mothers to offsprings in northern Italy. *J Med Virol* **9**:139–149, 1982.
16. Bonino F, Negro F, Chiaberge E, et al: Active HBV replication in HBsAg carriers with chronic delta infection. *It J Gastroenterol* **17**:235, 1985.
17. Rosina F, Saracco G, Rizzetto M: Risk of post-transfusion infection with the hepatitis delta virus. A multicenter study. *N Engl J Med* **312**:1488–1491, 1985.
18. Moestrup T, Hannson BG, Widell A, Nordenfelt E: Clinical aspects of delta infection. *Br Med J* **286**:87–90, 1987.
19. De Cock K, Govindarajan S, Redeker AG: Acute delta hepatitis without circulating HBsAg. *Gut* **26**:212–214, 1985.
20. Arico S, Aragona M, Rizzetto M, et al: Clinical significance of antibody to the hepatitis delta virus in symptomless HBsAg carriers. *Lancet* **2**:356–357, 1985.
21. Smedile A, Rizzetto M, Denniston KJ, et al: Type D hepatitis: The clinical significance of HDV RNA in serum as detected by a hybridization-based assay. *Hepatology* **6**:1297–1302, 1986.
22. Gmelin K, Roggendorf M, Schlipkoter U, et al: Delta infection in haemodialyzed patient. *J Infect Dis* **151**:74, 1987.
23. Jacobson IM, Dienstag JL, Werner BG, et al: Epidemiology and clinical impact of hepatitis D virus infection. *Hepatology* **5**:188–191, 1985.
24. Lohiya G, Govindarajan S, Hoefs J, et al: Prevalence of hepatitis B-associated delta agent among mentally retarded carriers of HBsAg. *J Infect Dis* **151**:192–193, 1987.
25. Marinucci G, Valeri L, Di Giacomo C, Morganti D: Spread of delta infection in a group of haemodialysis carriers of HBsAg. *Proc Clin Biol Res* **234**:151–154, 1987.
26. Marinucci G, Di Giacomo C, Morganti D, D'Angelo G: Delta agent diffusion in institutionalized Down's syndrome patients. *It J Gastroenterol* **16**:30–33, 1987.
27. Bonino F, Caporaso N, Dentico P, et al: Familiar clustering and spreading of hepatitis delta virus infection. *J Hepatol* **1**:221–226, 1985.
28. Hadler SC, de Monzon M, Ponzetto A, et al: Delta virus infection and severe hepatitis. *Ann Intern Med* **100**:339–344, 1987.

29. Purcell RH, Gerin JL, Rizzetto M: Experimental transmission of the delta agent in chimpanzees. *Proc Clin Biol Res* **143**:79–90, 1983.
30. Caredda F, Rossi E, D'Arminio Monforte A, et al: Hepatitis B virus-associated coinfection and superinfection with delta agent: Indistinguishable disease with different outcome. *J Infect Dis* **151**:925–928, 1987.
31. Caredda F, Antinori S, Re T, et al: Course and prognosis of acute HDV hepatitis. *Proc Clin Biol Res* **234**:267–276, 1987.
32. Aragona M, Caredda F, Lavarini C, et al: Serological response to the hepatitis delta virus in hepatitis D. *Lancet* **1**:478–480, 1987.
33. Aragona M, Macagno S, Caredda F, et al: IgM anti-HD in acute hepatitis D: Diagnostic and prognostic significance. *Proc Clin Biol Res* **234**:243–248, 1987.
34. Negro F, Baldi M, Bonino F: Chronic HDV hepatitis: Intrahepatic expression of delta antigen, histologic activity and outcome of liver disease. *J Hepatol* **6**:8–14, 1988.
35. Govindarajan S, Valinluck B, Peters RL: Relapse of acute B viral hepatitis—Role of delta agent. *Gut* **27**:19–22, 1986.
36. Hadziyannis SJ, Hatzakis A, Papaionnaou C, et al: Endemic hepatitis delta virus infection in a Greek community. *Prog Clin Biol Res* **234**:209–217, 1987.
37. De Cock KM, Govindarajan S, Chin KP, et al: Delta hepatitis in the Los Angeles Area: A report of 126 cases. *Ann Intern Med* **105**:108–114, 1986.
38. Smedile A, Farci P, Verme G, et al: Influence of delta infection on severity of hepatitis B. *Lancet* **2**:9–15, 1982.
39. Govindarajan S, Chin KP, Redeker AG, et al: Fulminant B viral hepatitis of delta agent. *Gastroenterology* **86**:1417, 1984.
40. De Cock KM, Govindarajan S, Redeker AG, et al: Fulminant delta hepatitis in chronic hepatitis B infection. *JAMA* **252**:2746–2748, 1984.
41. Smedile A, Lavarini C, Crivelli O, et al: Radioimmunoassay detection of IgM antibodies to the HBV associated delta antigen. Clinical significance in delta infection. *J Med Virol* **9**:131–138, 1983.
42. Hansson BG, Norkrans G, Weibull M, et al: Epidemiology of delta infection in Scandinavia. *Prog Clin Biol Res* **143**:155–159, 1983.
43. Rizzetto M, Verme G, Recchia S, et al: Chronic hepatitis in carriers of hepatitis B surface antigen with intrahepatic expression of the delta antigen. An active and progressive disease unresponsive to immunosuppressive treatment. *Ann Intern Med* **98**:437–441, 1983.
44. De Cock KM, Govindarajan S, Redeker AG: Natural course of delta superinfection in chronic hepatitis B virus infected patients. Histopathologic study, in Rizzetto M, Gerin JL, Purcell RH (eds): *The Hepatitis Delta Virus and Its Infection.* New York, Liss, 1987, pp. 167–173.
45. Colombo M, Cambieri R, Rumi MG, et al: Long-term delta superinfection in hepatitis B surface antigen carriers and its relationship to the course of chronic hepatitis. *Gastroenterology* **85**: 235–239, 1983.
46. Brunetto MR, Baldi M, Bonino F: Chronic HDV infection: An important cause of HBsAg positive cirrhosis of young adults. *Proc Clin Biol Res* **234**:209–211, 1987.
47. Bonino F, Negro F, Baldi M, et al: The natural history of chronic delta hepatitis. *Proc Clin Biol Res* **234**:145–152, 1987.
48. Crivelli O, Lavarini C, Chiaberge E, et al: Microsomal autoantibodies in chronic infection with the HBsAg associated delta agent. *Clin Exp Immunol* **54**:232–238, 1983.
49. Lenkei R, Norder H, Biberfeld G, Magnius LO: Autoantibodies to thymic epithelial cells in HDV infection. *J Infect Dis* **152**:232–235, 1987.
50. Zauli D, Fusconi M, Crespi C, et al: Close association between basal cell layer antibodies and hepatitis B virus associated chronic delta infection. *Hepatology* **4**:1103–1106, 1984.

51. Verme G, Amoroso P, Lettieri G, et al: A histological study of hepatitis delta virus liver disease. *Hepatology* **6**:1303–1307, 1986.
52. Verme G, Rocca G, Rizzi R, et al: Histopathology of chronic delta hepatitis. *Prog Clin Biol Res* **143**:169–176, 1983.
53. Popper H, Thung SN, Gerber MA, et al: Histologic studies of severe delta agent infection in Venezuelan Indians. *Hepatology* **3**:906–912, 1983.
54. Andrade ZA, Santos JB, Prata A, Dourado H: Histopatologia da hepatite da Labrea. Revista da *Soc Bras Med Trop* **16**:31–40, 1983.
55. Buitrago B, Poper H, Hadler SC, et al: Specific histologic features of Santa Marta hepatitis: A severe form of hepatitis D virus infection in northern South America. *Hepatology* **6**:1285–1291, 1986.
56. Govindarajan S, De Cock KM, Peters RL: Morphologic and immunohistochemical features of fulminant delta hepatitis. *Hum Pathol* **16**:262–267, 1985.
57. Lok ASF, Lindsay I, Scheuer PJ, Thomas HC: Clinical and histological features of delta infection in chronic hepatitis B virus carriers. *J Clin Pathol* **38**:530–533, 1987.
58. Knodell RG, Ishak KG, Black WC, et al: Formulation and application of a numerical scoring system for assessing histological activity in asymptomatic chronic active hepatitis. *Hepatology* **1**:431–435, 1981.
59. Kojima T, Callea F, Desmyter J: Hepatitis delta antigen (HDAg) in hepatocytes and lymphocyte reaction in immune light and electron microscopic studies in: *Abstracts of the IASL Meeting, Caracas, Venezuela, September 14–17, 1986*, p. 100.
60. Rizzetto M, Shih JW-K, Gerin JL: The hepatitis B virus-associated delta antigen: Isolation from liver, development of solid-phase radioimmunoassays for delta antigen and anti-delta and partial characterization of delta antigen. *J Immunol* **125**:318–324, 1980.
61. Bonino F: The importance of hepatitis B viral DNA in serum and liver. *J Hepatol* **3**:136–141, 1986.
62. Rizzetto M, Rosina F, Saracco G, et al: Treatment of chronic delta hepatitis with alpha-2 recombinant interferon. *J Hepatol* **3**:2295–2335, 1986.
63. Hoofnagle J, Mullen K, Peters M, et al: Treatment of chronic delta hepatitis with recombinant human alpha interferon. *Proc Clin Biol Res* **234**:291–298, 1987.
64. Thomas HC, Farci P, Karayiannis P, et al: Inhibition of hepatitis delta virus replication by lymphoblastoid human alpha interferon. *Proc Clin Biol Res* **234**:277–280, 1987.
65. Hedin G, Weiland O, Ljunggren K, et al: Treatment of fulminant hepatitis B and fulminant hepatitis B and D coinfection with Foscarnet, in *1987 International Symposium on Viral Hepatitis and Liver Disease*, abstract 361, p. 132.
66. Hedin G, Weiland O, Ljunggren K, et al: Treatment of fulminant hepatitis B and fulminant hepatitis B and D coinfection with Foscarnet. *Proc Clin Biol Res* **234**:309–320, 1987.

Non-A, Non-B Hepatitis

VICTOR M. VILLAREJOS

INTRODUCTION

More than a decade has elapsed since the existence of a new type of post-transfusion hepatitis was postulated[1] and confirmed.[2] Provisionally designated non-A, non-B (NANB) hepatitis by exclusion of the two known virus types, a causative agent(s) has not yet been found and the original name is still valid. However, a wealth of information, both positive and negative, has been accumulated and warrants a brief review of the state of the art.

ETIOLOGY

Agent

The causative agent has eluded detection during all these years despite intensive research efforts throughout the world. Among the many etiologic possibilities considered is that NANB is a variant of hepatitis B virus (HBV), a theory repeatedly proposed on both morphologic grounds and observed cross-reactions of NANB sera with hepatitis B core antigen (HB_cAg) and hepatitis B e antigen (HB_eAg).[3] The finding of nucleic acid homology between HBV and NANB viruses has also been reported to prove such a link,[4,5] but other investigators[6,7] did not detect HBV-DNA hybridization in NANB hepatitis sera or liver tissue. Moreover, the substantial serologic data accumulated by etiologic exclusion of HBV would speak against such an association, as well as against NANB being a delta-like incomplete virus, as suggested by Rizzetto et al.[8]

VICTOR M. VILLAREJOS • International Center for Medical Research and Training, Louisiana State University, San Jose, Costa Rica.

A sample of the many viruses that have been described as the causative agent of NANB hepatitis is presented in Table I. The wide spectrum of visualized particles, ranging from 16 to 85 nm in size, gives an idea of the prevailing confusion.

The double-shelled tubular structures described by Jackson et al.[9] in the cytoplasm of hepatocytes of chimpanzees experimentally infected with plasma from NANB hepatitis cases are generally regarded as characteristic of NANB infection in primates. This is the only existing evidence of the presence of the NANB agent, although the viral specificity of these formations remains to be determined. Such cytoplasmic structures seem not to occur in human NANB hepatitis.[10]

Serologic Tests

There have been numerous reports of antigen–antibody systems associated with NANB hepatitis, but none has been confirmed independently,[11] nor could they be reproduced reliably by the same laboratories in unknown sera. In 1981, six selected laboratories, using their own diagnostic systems, failed to identify proven infectious sera in an NIH panel compiled by Alter et al.[12]

Recently, Seto et al.[13] suggested that the NANB virus could be a retrovirus-like agent. These investigators found reverse transcriptase (RT) activity in all of 18 sera from patients with posttransfusion NANB hepatitis and very rarely in control sera. The RT activity was sensitive to RNase and banded at a 1.14-g/m peak in sucrose, which was considered consistent with the agent being a retrovirus; moreover, material from this peak was infectious in chimpanzees. Unfor-

TABLE I. Viral Particles Reported as Associated with Non-A, Non-B Hepatitis

Investigators	Particle	
	Shape	Size (nm)
Cossart et al., 1975[52]	Parvoviruslike	23
Prince et al., 1978[52]	C-type viruslike	60–80
Bradley et al., 1979[52]	Picornaviruslike	25–30
Coursaget et al., 1979[52]	Toga viruslike	60
Woodford et al., 1979[52]	Picornaviruslike	16–25
Diermitzel et al., 1980[52]	With 28- to 40-nm core	36–61
Mori et al., 1980[52]	With 22-nm core	32
Hantz et al., 1980[52]	HBVlike, 22-nm core	35–40
Gmelin et al., 1980[53]	Intranuclear bodies	27
Watanabe et al., 1984[54]	Double-shelled	23
Iwarson et al., 1985[55]	Retroviruslike	60–85

tunately, these exciting results have not yet been confirmed in spite of attempts made by several other investigators. Prince and William[14] reported the isolation of a retroviruslike agent in chimpanzee liver cell cultures inoculated with the Hutchinson strain of NANB virus; the isolate was later recognized as a contaminating chimpanzee spumivirus not causally related to NANB hepatitis. By contrast, a different type of enveloped particle associated with RT activity, described as bunyaviruslike, was found in NANB hepatitis cases,[15] adding confusion to the candidacy of retroviruses.

An innovative approach was followed by Shimitzu et al.,[16] who obtained an antibody from cultured lymphocytes from NANB hepatitis convalescent chimpanzees that would identify a virus-specific antigen. However, the antibody could not be detected free in the serum of either chimpanzees or humans, and was later found to be nonspecific, reacting with human livers infected with HBV or the delta agent and also with alcoholic livers. Since the product identified may be induced by an NANB virus, but probably is not an integral part of the virus, subtractive complementary DNA (cDNA) cloning is being tried to identify it, so far without success.[17]

Thus, up to the present, there is still no specific, reproducible, confirmed, and accepted assay for the identification of either an NANB antigen or an antibody, or both, and the negative characterization of this type of hepatitis as caused by neither type A nor type B viruses remains a nagging admission of our ignorance of the true cause of the infection.

Multiple Agents?

This discouraging situation has led to the alternative suggestion that the disease may be produced by a variety of noninfectious factors. However, there seems to be no doubt that NANB hepatitis is caused by a specific filterable agent(s), as demonstrated by the development of NANB hepatitis after transfusion of blood not known to be otherwise infective and the production of hepatitis in chimpanzees by injection of acute serum from NANB patients or contaminated factor VIII preparations, with subsequent serial transmission of the infection in susceptible animals.[18]

Moreover, the reported occurrence of more than one separate clinical bout of NANB hepatitis[19] suggested the existence of two or more different etiologic agents, as confirmed by cross-challenge studies in chimpanzees using serum and coagulation factor VIII preparations implicated in the transmission of the infection.[20] The production of characteristic cytoplasmic double-shelled structures in the liver of chimpanzees inoculated with sera of some NANB hepatitis cases and the failure of other NANB inocula to produce this effect has also been presented as indirect evidence for the existence of two different agents.[21]

The frustrating failure to detect the virus by serologic means would suggest that either the antiserum employed is too weak, i.e., contains little specific anti-

NANB antibody, or that the concentration of NANB antigen present in the blood is minimal, probably too low for detection by current serologic methods. Moreover, the presence of circulating NANB immune complexes has been reported[22]; these would mask the viral antigen, making it even more difficult to detect. On the other hand, it is possible that the NANB agent belongs to a special, still unknown, class of microorganisms that may give rise to a different kind of response by the infected individual, not necessarily inducing the conventional type of immune reaction. The observed fact that clinical NANB hepatitis frequently develops into chronic liver disease would indicate some failure of the agent to induce an adequate immune response in the infected person, or vice versa.

A diagnostic system associated with NANB hepatitis was recently detected by rheophoresis in our laboratory.[23] This system, which we have called ICMRT NANB antigen and antibody, was translated to third-generation serologic methods, i.e., enzyme-linked immunosorbent assay (ELISA) and radioimmunoassay (RIA), greatly increasing its sensitivity. We have employed this test system widely during the past several years.

CLINICAL COURSE

Acute NANB Hepatitis

Incubation Time

The time elapsed between transfusion of blood and onset of clinical or biochemical signs of hepatitis was observed to range between 2 and 26 weeks, with an average of 8 weeks, which is now the accepted incubation time of post-transfusion NANB hepatitis.[24] Shorter incubation, less than 2 weeks, has been observed, especially after administration of factor VIII to hemophiliacs.[25] For obvious reasons, the incubation time of the sporadic form remains undetermined.

Clinical Characteristics

Approximately two thirds of transfusion-associated NANB hepatitis cases are anicteric and evolve asymptomatically.[12] In the contact-acquired sporadic form, the proportion of inapparent infection is probably higher.

Prodromal symptoms are not usual. Clinical signs and symptoms, even in icteric cases, tend to be mild, and only occasionally does the disease run a more severe course. Initial fever is uncommon. Moderate enlargement of the liver is patent in about one third of cases; less than 20% are found to have abnormal prothrombin time.[26] Serum bilirubin rarely exceeds 3 mg/%, and alanine aminotransferase (ALT) elevations are slight to moderate (mean 514 IU/liter), but usually lower than in type A or B hepatitis[27]; however, some clinically overt cases may show higher biochemical values and run a more severe course. In most instances, immunoglobin M (IgM) levels are only moderately increased (mean 198 U/ml), in contrast with the high values (mean 462 U/ml) seen in type A hepatitis.[28] Nevertheless, clinical and biochemical mildness cannot be used as a differentiating criterion, because of considerable overlapping of values.

Fulminant Hepatitis

Fulminant NANB hepatitis may be relatively frequent. The sporadic form has been found to be the predominant cause of acute liver failure in the English Midlands[29] and was also the most common cause of fulminant hepatitis in Bombay,[30] advanced pregnancy with labor being an important precipitating factor. In the United States, 40% to 50% of fulminant hepatitis cases are attributed to NANB infection.[31] The high relative frequency of NANB fulminant hepatitis was confirmed in a worldwide study by Saracco et al.[32] However, NANB apparently causes fewer fatalities than acute HBV infection in the transfusion setting.[33]

Chronic NANB Hepatitis and Sequelae

The importance of NANB hepatitis lies mainly in its tendency to progress to chronic disease with important sequelae. All studies concur in that at least 50% of acute NANB posttransfusion hepatitis will become chronic; in a recent National Institutes of Health (NIH) series,[34] almost 70% of 75 patients with acute NANB hepatitis had persistent or fluctuating alanine aminotransferase (ALT) elevations for periods up to 3 years, an indication of chronic evolution.

The proportion of acute cases progressing to chronicity varies with the route of acquisition of the infection; it was found highest for posttransfusion and drug addiction hepatitis (58%) and lowest (20%) for sporadic, nonparenterally acquired infections.[35]

After exclusion of noninfectious causes, approximately 50% of chronic hepatitis cases have HBV markers and are probably due to hepatitis B; most of the remainder will have a NANB etiology. In a series of 54 cases of chronic hepatitis with histopathologic changes typical of viral infection, reported by Brenes et al.,[36] HBV markers were present in 25 (46%) cases; of the remaining 29 non-B cases, 19 (66%) were positive for the ICMRT–NANB antigen.

Typically, ALT elevations fluctuate in NANB chronic hepatitis over prolonged periods of time and the pathologic process may persist for years without noticeable symptomatology. Usually, by the time the patient experiences any symptoms, he already has advanced chronic active hepatitis, which then often progresses to postnecrotic cirrhosis. Figure 1 shows an example of the patterns of ALT behavior observed in our patients with chronic NANB hepatitis.

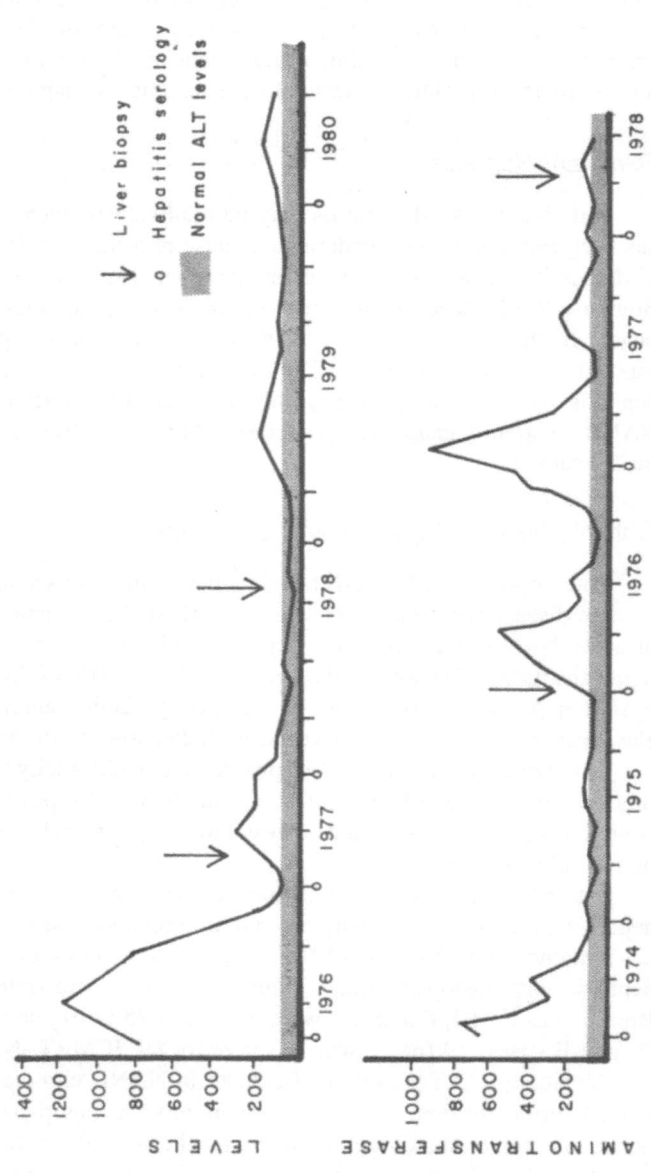

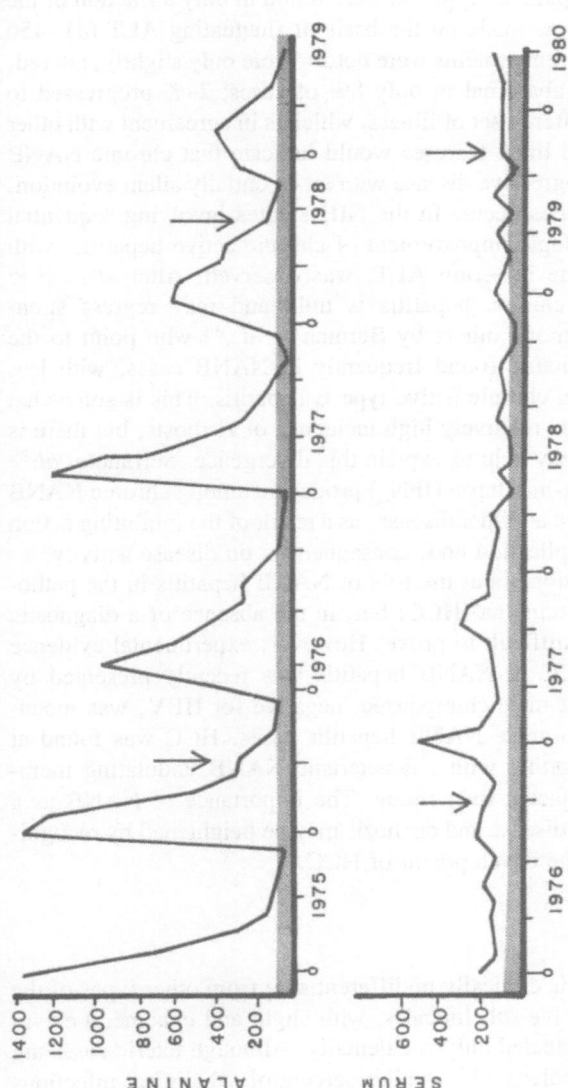

FIGURE 1. Patterns of alanine aminotransferase elevation observed in chronic NANB hepatitis cases. (Courtesy of San Ramon Hospital, Costa Rica.)

In an NIH series of 25 patients with posttransfusion chronic NANB hepatitis,[37] 80% were totally asymptomatic, although mild fatigue was seen in about one half of the cases. None of the patients had jaundice or choluria and bilirubin was essentially normal. Mild degrees of hepatomegaly and splenomegaly, as well as spider angioma and palmar erythema were found in only a fraction of the patients, whose diagnosis was made on the basis of fluctuating ALT (41–456 μ/liter) and liver biopsy. Serum proteins were not, or were only slightly, altered, and prothrombin time was abnormal in only 8% of cases; 24% progressed to cirrhosis within 1–7 years after onset of illness, which is in agreement with other reports in the literature. All these features would indicate that chronic NANB hepatitis is an insidious, progressive disease with an essentially silent evolution.

However, regression does occur. In the NIH studies involving sequential biopsies,[12,34] distinct histologic improvement of chronic active hepatitis, with slow but progressive decline in serum ALT, was observed. Alter et al.[12,24] believe that most NANB chronic hepatitis is mild and may regress spontaneously, a view shared among others by Berman et al.,[38] who point to the moderate histopathologic picture found frequently in NANB cases, with less fibrosis and bridging than in chronic active type B hepatitis. This is somewhat incongruent with the reported relatively high incidence of cirrhosis, but there is an interesting finding that may help to explain this divergence. Serrano et al.[39] reported recently that high α-interferon (IFN$_\alpha$) producers among chronic NANB hepatitis patients tend to have a milder disease, as a result of the inhibiting action of the interferon on viral replication and, consequently, on disease activity.

There is much speculation about the role of NANB hepatitis in the pathogenesis of hepatocellular carcinoma (HCC) but, in the absence of a diagnostic test, such an association is difficult to prove. However, experimental evidence for the development of HCC in NANB hepatitis was recently presented by Muchmore et al.[40] An adult male chimpanzee, negative for HBV, was inoculated with plasma from two acute NANB hepatitis cases. HCC was found at necropsy, 7 years later, together with characteristic NANB undulating membranes in the tumor and adjacent liver tissue. The importance of NANB as a major cause of chronic liver disease and cirrhosis may be heightened by recognition of its possible role in the development of HCC.

Clinical Diagnosis

Acute NANB hepatitis is clinically undifferentiable from other types of the disease. Most infections evolve subclinically, with slight and ephemeral elevations of ALT that may be detected only accidentally. Although icteric cases are more apt to progress to chronicity,[12,34] a high percent of subclinical infections evolve silently toward chronic hepatitis. The lack of symptomatology during most of the evolution makes a clinical diagnosis difficult, if not impossible.

Thus, the presumptive diagnosis of acute or chronic NANB hepatitis relies basically on the finding of ALT elevations and the exclusion of other causes of enzyme alteration, including other hepatotropic viruses. By consensus, the ALT elevation should be at least 2½ times the norm and should be sustained for more than one week in order to be considered suggestive of a viral hepatic process, but ALT levels may fluctuate widely, especially if the disease is progressing toward chronicity.

If either clinical or biochemical signs, or both, of acute hepatitis are present and toxic or other noninfectious causes are excluded, a probable viral diagnosis is made by serologic testing. After initial screening for hepatitis B surface antigen (HB_sAg), IgM class anti-HAV, anti-HB_c, and anti-CMV determinations are the most reliable methods to exclude acute infection by these viruses. If all three tests prove negative, the diagnosis of NANB hepatitis is reasonable. In cases with sustained ALT elevations over 6 months, liver biopsy is indicated to demonstrate an ongoing chronic process.

EPIDEMIOLOGY

NANB hepatitis is not restricted by geographic boundaries and its prevalence is worldwide. At least three distinct modes of transmission have been recognized: parenteral, contact, and waterborne or enteric. The most common vehicle for parenteral infection is transfused blood and blood products, and the use of contaminated syringes by IV drug abusers. Utensils for percutaneous procedures (e.g., tattooing) are also an efficient mechanism of transmission. Sporadic hepatitis may be acquired by a still undisclosed form of personal contact. Enteric infection seems to be responsible for waterborne outbreaks of a disease with characteristics distinct from the other two forms.

NANB Posttransfusion Hepatitis

Since the virtual elimination of HBV from blood banks by HB_sAg screening, NANB accounts for at least 90% of the hepatitis cases still occurring after transfusion. A small proportion is caused by CMV,[12] which seem to have been partly responsible for a surge of posttransfusion hepatitis (PTH) cases in the United States in 1978.

Incidence

In various prospective studies in the United States, the incidence of NANB PTH varied between 7% and 12%. In Europe and Japan, the incidence is essentially similar. The risk of PTH has been shown to be almost eight times higher for recipients of blood from paid donors in the transfusion-transmitted viruses (TTV)[41] and many other studies; hence, the use of only volunteer donors has been the single most effective measure for its control. Obviously, the risk of infection was found to increase with the volume of blood transfused, from two- to sixfold, in recipients of more than 3 units of blood. In the same study, it was noted that elevation of transaminase values in the donor blood was associated with a higher rate of NANB hepatitis.

From the PTH incidence data, it can be inferred that the carrier rate in the general population must be high, at least as high as that of HB_sAg carriers. The tendency to a chronic course of the infection certainly makes this plausible, even though the number of clinical occurrences is relatively low. Consequently, a considerable number of these inapparent infections must result in chronic carriage of the virus.

Detection of Carriers

The real problem being faced now is how to detect those carriers, a feat that has not yet been achieved. None of the numerous assays reported to the present has been able to identify reliably a specific NANB antigen in proven infectious sera. However, there may be a hopeful candidate. In an NIH panel of 60 sera from donors of blood transfused to 10 patients who subsequently developed NANB hepatitis, eight of these donor sera were positive for the ICMRT–NANB antigen. After decoding, it was seen that a unit of positive blood had been transfused to each of 8 of the 10 NANB PTH patients, thus identifying the infecting donor in eight of 10 NANB PTH cases; all 12 control donor sera in the panel were negative. In the same panel, the ICMRT antigen was also found in the sera of 8 (62%) of 13 patients who developed posttransfusion NANB hepatitis, and not in the sera from nine control patients.[41a] Thus, it would seem that this test detects the presence of one agent involved in the transmission of NANB hepatitis. Work to expand these encouraging results to the final goal is hampered' by the scarcity of the specific reagents, which also prevents, for the time being, the evaluation of the method in larger numbers of donor sera.

Surrogate Tests

In the absence of a specific test, blood banks are now resorting to screening of blood with surrogate tests such as determinations of ALT levels and the presence of anti-HB_c for the indirect identification of NANB virus carriers. Because of the high rate of chronic NANB hepatitis with fluctuating ALT, it is to be expected that some carriers with active disease will have elevated ALT values at the time of transfusion. It has been estimated that ALT screening of donors could prevent up to 30% of NANB PTH occurrences.[34] The value of this procedure is still controversial. Elevated ALT, to at least twice the normal value, is very suggestive but not diagnostic of hepatitis; it can occur in other pathologic conditions and is often found in obese persons, or after ingestion of alcohol and other similar transient aggressions to the liver. One is reminded of the popular term "transaminitis" used widely some years ago to depict such conditions.

Testing for anti-HB_c has been proposed on the assumption that, because of the similar modes of transmission people having had hepatitis B would also have had a high risk of exposure to NANB infection. It was indeed found that the rate of NANB hepatitis was higher in anti-HB_c-positive persons than in those negative for the antibody,[42] and it was estimated that a further substantial number of NANB-PTH cases could be prevented by eliminating anti-HB_c-positive donors. The puzzle is that positives in the two surrogate tests do not overlap as was hoped, but apparently belong to different populations.

Foes of the use of these tests point to the loss, by elimination, of many valuable blood units identified as "positive" by both methods, especially when blood donors are scarce, and also to the high economic burden of the testing for blood banks. Nevertheless, ethical considerations would mandate their use, even if only a small percentage of PTH cases could be prevented. Blood banks in the United States are now required to perform both tests by recommendation of the American Association of Blood Banks and various federal agencies.

Currently all donors at the Central Blood Bank in Costa Rica are being screened for HB_sAg and HIV. Recently, determinations of ALT and anti-HB_c, as well as the ICMRT-NANB-associated antigen and antibody, have been added. We hope to be able to evaluate the correlation of the two surrogate tests with the ICMRT-NANB system in the near future.

Sporadic Endemic NANB Hepatitis

Early after the recognition of NANB PTH, it was shown that the infection could also occur endemically in the general population, and that it could be acquired in the absence of blood transfusion or other parenteral means of transmission, presumably by contact.[43] This nontransfusion hepatitis was shown to occur sporadically, but at a much lower level than the two other types, A and B. Initially, only 24 (2.1%) of 1120 hepatitis cases studied in a highly endemic zone of Costa Rica failed to type for either A or B hepatitis by standard serologic methods. Moreover, in the prospective study of families of these cases, transient transaminitis, without serologic hepatitis markers, was observed in 3% of contacts. Retrospective testing of stored sera from these contacts disclosed seven that were positive for the ICMRT antigen. This seems an indication that subclinical NANB is fairly frequent in the general population.

Routine testing of all cases of acute viral hepatitis at the General Hospital in San Jose showed roughly 70% ICMRT-NANB antigen positives among those who were negative for HAV, HBV, and CMV serology. In addition, 21% of the positives for ICMRT-NANB antibody were found in sera from different population groups. Surprisingly, there was not much increase in the prevalence of antibody after 15 years of age, a fact that may suggest evanescence of the antibody.

Sporadic NANB hepatitis has been reported from many other parts of the world, mainly from Europe and the United States, where it represents a high proportion of the total of endemic, nonparenteral hepatitis.[44] The apparent disparity in the incidence of sporadic NANB infection between areas of high and low hepatitis endemicity probably does not reflect a higher frequency of NANB hepatitis but rather a lower incidence of type A hepatitis in industrialized societies, resulting in a higher proportion of NANB hepatitis than in developing countries.

From these data, it would seem that subclinical or inapparent NANB infection is widely present throughout the general population, while clinically overt hepatitis is more or less rare. The ratio of subclinical to clinical infection is probably much higher in NANB hepatitis than in the two other types of hepatitis. A number of sporadic NANB hepatitis cases, especially in children of less developed areas, may be due to primary CMV infection, as reported by Zamora et al.[45]

Epidemic NANB Hepatitis

The NANB nature of waterborne hepatitis epidemics resembling classic type A outbreaks reported from India has been confirmed.[46] It is intriguing that the disease is both epidemic and endemic in the Indian subcontinent, South Central Asia, and the Middle East, is spreading into North and West Africa and seems now to have reached the Western Hemisphere. Two small water-related outbreaks of NANB hepatitis have been reported recently from Mexico.[46a] All evidence indicates that the agent spreads by the fecal–oral route, as does HAV' and all enteroviruses, to the extent that it is now referred to as enteric-transmitted (ET) NANB hepatitis.

The presence of a spherical nonenveloped virus, first identified by Balayan[47] in the feces of infected volunteers, has been confirmed repeatedly. The particles are 27 nm in diameter and band at a buoyant density of 1.34 g/cm^3 in cesium chloride, similar to HAV.[48] Antibodies to these particles were found in the sera of native populations of Central and South East Asia. However, unlike HAV, this virus could not be transmitted to chimpanzees, although it proved infective to tamarins and was serially passaged in cynomolgus monkeys.[49]

Although convalescent patient serum was shown to contain IgM class antibodies that reacted with the particles found in human and primate feces, no reaction could be elicited between human acute and convalescent sera. Viremia or circulating antigen could not be demonstrated, but it is possible that the viremia is very short-lived, as in the case of hepatitis A. The same agent was found in the feces of a few cases of sporadic hepatitis in France,[50] but it is not clear whether the latter infections were acquired in the Orient or locally.

In contrast to hepatitis A, which attacks all ages, especially children under 10 years, and has a negligible mortality rate, ET-NANB occurs predominantly in young adults, with peak incidence in the third and fourth decade of life; it produces moderate to severe disease with elevated mortality, as high as 20%, especially among pregnant women. Unlike the transfusional and sporadic forms, but similar to hepatitis A, the epidemic form apparently does not progress to chronicity.[51] No significant seasonal variation was observed in the incidence of the disease, as opposed to hepatitis A, which shows seasonal peaks of occurrence in endemic areas. All these features, in some respects similar to those of HAV and in other respects different, would suggest that the agent of ET-NANB hepatitis may be a mutant variety of HAV or a related new type of enterovirus.

SUMMARY

After a decade of intensive investigation, much important epidemiologic, clinical, and pathologic information has been accumulated, although the final feat of defining the causative agent or agents of non-A, non-B hepatitis has not yet been achieved. All evidence suggests that the agent of the enterically transmitted epidemic (and endemic) variety has been identified, but those of the parenterally and sporadic forms still elude us, although they are more important to the Western world because of their ominous sequelae.

We hope that more funds can be made available to solve the problems posed by these forms of hepatitis, for they undoubtedly have an important long-term medical impact. Nevertheless, real advances have been made and we should be optimistic and confident of final success.

REFERENCES

1. Prince AM, Grady GF, Hazzi C, et al: Long-incubation post-transfusion hepatitis without serological evidence of exposure to hepatitis B virus. *Lancet* **1**:241–246, 1974.
2. Feinstone SM, Kapikian AZ, Purcell RH, et al: Transfusion-associated hepatitis not due to viral hepatitis type A or B. *N Engl J Med* **292**:767–770, 1975.
3. Trepo CF, Degos L, Vitvitski R, et al: Evidence for a transmissible non-A, non-B agent inextricably linked with hepatitis B virus, in Vyas GN, Dienstag JL, Hoofnagle JH (eds): *Viral Hepatitis and Liver Disease*. Orlando, Florida, Grune & Stratton, 1984, pp. 355–365.
4. Wands JR, Lieberman HM, Muchmore E, et al: Detection and transmission in chimpanzees of

hepatitis B virus related agents formerly designated "non-A, non-B" hepatitis. *Proc Natl Acad Sci USA* **79**:7552–7556, 1982.

5. Charnay P, Brechot C, Vitvitski L, et al: Analysis by hybridization with HBV DNA of hepatocellular DNA from patients with chronic non-A, non-B hepatitis, in Szmuness W, Alter HJ, Maynard JE (eds): *International Symposium on Viral Hepatitis.* Philadelphia, Franklin Institute Press, 1981, pp. 656–657.

6. Fowler MJF, Monjardino J, Weller IV, et al: Failure to detect nucleic acid homology between some non-A, non-B viruses and hepatitis B virus DNA. *J Med Virol* **12**:205–213, 1983.

7. Yap SH, Hellings JA, Rijntjes PJM, et al: Absence of detectable hepatitis B virus DNA in sera and liver of chimpanzees with non-A, non-B hepatitis. *J Med Virol* **15** :343–350, 1985.

8. Rizzetto M, Gerin JL, Purcell RH: Delta antigen: Evidence for a variant of hepatitis B virus or a non-A, non-B hepatitis agent? in *Perspectives on Virology*, Vol. XI. New York, Liss, 1981, pp. 195–217.

9. Jackson D, Tabor E, Gerety RJ: Acute non-A, non-B hepatitis; specific ultrastructural alterations in endoplasmic reticulum of infected hepatocytes. *Lancet* **1**:1249–1250, 1979.

10. Bamber M, Murray A, Lewin J, et al: Ultrastructural features in chronic non-A, non-B (NANB) hepatitis: A controlled blind study. *J Med Virol* **8**:267–275, 1981.

11. Gerety RJ: Virus-like particles and antigen–antibody systems associated with non-A, non-B hepatitis, in Gerety RJ (ed): *Non-A, Non-B Hepatitis.* New York, Academic, 1981, pp. 216–221.

12. Alter HJ, Purcell RH, Feinstone SM, et al: Non-A, non-B hepatitis: Its relationship to cytomegalovirus, to chronic hepatitis and to direct and indirect test methods, in Szmuness W, Alter HJ, Maynard JE (eds): *International Symposium on Viral Hepatitis.* Philadelphia, Franklin Institute Press, 1981, pp. 656–657.

13. Seto B, Iwarson S, Coleman WG, et al: Detection of reverse transcriptase activity in association with the non-A, non-B hepatitis agent(s). *Lancet* **2**:941–943, 1984.

14. Prince AM, William BAA: A spumivirus-like agent isolated from NANB hepatitis: Relation to NANB virus, in *Proceedings of the International Symposium on Viral Hepatitis and AIDS, San Jose, Costa Rica, December 1986.*

15. Herrera MI, Castillo I, and Carreno V: Reverse transcriptase activity and enveloped particles in non-A, non-B hepatitis, in Zuckerman A (ed): *Proceedings of the International Symposium on Viral Hepatitis and Liver Disease, London.* New York, Liss, 1987.

16. Shimitzu YK, OOmura M, Abe K, et al: Production of antibody associated with non-A, non-B hepatitis in a chimpanzee lymphoblastoid cell line established by in vitro transformation with Epstein–Barr virus. *Proc Natl Acad Sci USA* **82**:2138–2142, 1985.

17. Alter HJ: The etiology and clinical spectrum of transfusion-associated NANB hepatitis, in V. M., Villarejos (ed): *Proceedings of the International Symposium on Viral Hepatitis and AIDS, Trejos, San Jose Costa Rica,* pp. 263–272, 1967.

18. Tabor ER, Gerety RJ: The chimpanzee animal model for non-A, non-B hepatitis: New applications, in Szmuness W, Alter HJ, Maynard JE (eds): *International Symposium on Viral Hepatitis.* Philadelphia, Franklin Institute Press, 1981, pp. 305–317.

19. Mosley JW, Redeker AG, Feinstone SM, et al: Multiple hepatitis viruses in multiple attacks of acute viral hepatitis. *N Engl J Med* **296**:75–78, 1977.

20. Hollinger FB, Mosley JW, Szmuness W, et al: Transfusion-transmitted viruses study: Experimental evidence for two non-A, non-B hepatitis agents. *J Infect Dis* **142**:400–407, 1980.

21. Shimitzu YK, Feinstone SM, Purcell RH: Non-A, non-B hepatitis: Ultrastructural evidence for two agents in experimentally infected chimpanzees. *Science* **205**:197–200, 1979.

22. Dienstag JL, Bhan AK, Alter HJ, et al: Circulating immune complexes in non-A, non-B hepatitis: Possible masking of viral antigen. *Lancet* **1**:1265, 1979.

23. Villarejos VM, Visona KA, Serra J: Evaluation of the specificity of an immunoprecipitin test for non-A, non-B hepatitis. *J Infect Dis* **147**:702–710, 1983.

24. Alter HJ, Holland PV, Morrow AG, et al: Clinical and serological analysis of transfusion associated hepatitis. *Lancet* **2**:838–841, 1975.
25. Hruby MA, Schauf V: Transfusion-related short incubation hepatitis in hemophilic patients. *JAMA* **240**:1355, 1978.
26. Blum HE, Vyas GN: Non-A, non-B hepatitis: A contemporary assessment. *Haematologia* **15**:153–173, 1982.
27. Sampliner RE, Woronow DI, Alter HJ, et al: Community acquired non-A, non-B hepatitis: Clinical characteristics and chronicity. *J Med Virol* **13**:125–130, 1984.
28. Mosley JW, Visona KA, Villarejos VM: Immunoglobulin M level in the diagnosis of type A hepatitis. *Am J Clin Pathol* **75**:86–87, 1981.
29. Vickers CS, Hubschen D, Adams R, et al: A predominance of sporadic non-A, non-B hepatitis as a cause of acute liver failure in the Midlands, in Zuckerman A (ed): *Proceedings of the International Symposium on Viral Hepatitis and Liver Disease, London*, 1987. New York, Liss, 1988 (in press).
30. Rath S, Kamat SA, Zuckerman AJ, et al: Fulminant viral hepatitis in Bombay, in Zuckerman A (ed): *Proceedings of the International Symposium on Viral Hepatitis and Liver Disease, London*. New York, Liss, 1988 (in press).
31. Acute Hepatic Failure Study Group: Etiology and prognosis in fulminant hepatitis. *Gastroenterology* **75A**:33, 1979.
32. Saracco C, Papaevangelou G, Govindarajan S, et al: Epidemiology of fulminant HBsAg-positive hepatitis world-wide, in Zuckerman A (ed): *Proceedings of the International Symposium on Viral Hepatitis and Liver Disease, London*. New York, Liss, 1988 (in press).
33. Goldfield M, Black HC, Bill J, et al: The consequences of administering blood pretested for HBsAg by third generation techniques: A progress report. *Am J Med Sci* **270**:335–342, 1975.
34. Alter HJ: Posttransfusion hepatitis: Clinical features, risk and donor testing, in *Infection, Immunity and Blood Transfusion*. New York, Liss, 1985, pp. 47–61.
35. Rakela J, Redeker AG: Chronic liver disease after acute non-A, non-B hepatitis. *Gastroenterology* **77**:1200–1202, 1979.
36. Brenes F, Quirós J, Mora C, et al: Chronic non-B hepatitis and cirrhosis, in Villarejos VM (ed): *Proceedings of the International Symposium on Viral Hepatitis and AIDS, Trejos, San Jose, Costa Rica, 1987*, pp. 285–289.
37. Hoofnagle JH, Alter HJ: Chronic non-A, non-B hepatitis, in *Infection, Immunity and Blood Transfusion*. New York, Liss, 1985, pp. 63–69.
38. Berman M, Alter HJ, Ishak KG, et al: The chronic sequelae of non-A, non-B hepatitis. *Ann Intern Med* **91**:1–6, 1979.
39. Serrano MA, Castilla S, Morte M, et al: Interferon (IFN) production by T cells in chronic non-A, non-B hepatitis (CNANBH) patients: Its relationship with the severity of liver disease, in Zuckerman A (ed): *Proceedings of the International Symposium on Viral Hepatitis and Liver Disease, London*. New York, Liss, 1988 (in press).
40. Muchmore E, Popper H, Linke HK, et al: Non-A, non-B hepatitis related hepatocellular carcinoma in a chimpanzee, in Zuckerman A (ed): *Proceedings of the International Symposium on Viral Hepatitis and Liver Disease, London*. New York, Liss, 1988 (in press).
41. Aach RD, Lander JJ, Sherman LA, et al: Transfusion-transmitted viruses: Interim analysis of hepatitis among transfused and nontransfused patients, in Vyas GN, Cohen SN, and Schmid R (eds): *Proceedings of the Second Symposium on Viral Hepatitis*. Philadelphia, Franklin Institute Press, 1978, pp. 383–396.
41a. Visona KA, Zamora E, Villarejos VM: Evaluation of a serologic test for non-A, non-B hepatitis, in Villarejos VM (ed): *Proceedings of the International Symposium on Viral Hepatitis and AIDS, Trejos, San José, Costa Rica, 1987*, pp. 397–399.
42. Stevens CE, Aach RD, Hollinger FB, et al: Hepatitis B virus antibody in blood donors and the

occurrence of non-A, non-B hepatitis in transfusion recipients: An analysis of the Transfusion-Transmitted Viruses Study. *Ann Intern Med* **101**:733–738, 1984.

43. Villarejos VM, Visona KA, Eduarte CE, et al: Evidence for viral hepatitis other than type A or type B among persons in Costa Rica. *N Engl J Med* **293**:1350–1352, 1975.

44. Dienstag JL, Alaama A, Mosley JW, et al: Etiology of sporadic hepatitis B surface antigen-negative hepatitis. *Ann Intern Med* **87**:1–6, 197.

45. Zamora E, Herrero L, Morales C: Epidemiologic significance of CMV infection, in V. M. Villarejos (ed): *Proceedings of the International Symposium on Viral Hepatitis and AIDS, Trejos, San Jose, Costa Rica, December* pp. 273–278, 1987.

46. Wong DC, Purcell RH, Sreenivasan MA, et al: Epidemic and endemic hepatitis in India: Evidence for non-A, non-B hepatitis virus etiology. *Lancet* **2**:876–878, 1980.

46a. MMWR: Enterically transmitted non-A, non-B hepatitis. **36**:36, 1987.

47. Balayan MS, Andjaparidze AG, Savinskaya SS, et al: Evidence for a virus in non-A, non-B hepatitis transmitted via fecal-oral route. *Intervirology* **20**:23–31, 1983.

48. Balayan MS: Further studies on non-A, non-B transmitted via fecal-oral route, in Zuckerman A (ed): *Proceedings of the International Symposium on Viral Hepatitis and Liver Disease, London.* New York, Liss, 1988 (in press).

49. Bradley DW, Krawczynski K, Cook EH, et al: Enterically transmitted non-A, non-B hepatitis: Serial passage of disease in cynomolgus monkeys and recovery of disease-associated 27–29 nm virus-like particles from infected case and primate stools, in Zuckerman A (ed): *Proceedings of the International Symposium on Viral Hepatitis and Liver Disease, London.* New York, Liss, 1988 (in press).

50. Pillot J, Sharma MD, Grangeot-Keros L, et al: Involvement of the same viral agent in epidemic and sporadic non-A, non-B hepatitis, in Zuckerman A (ed): *Proceedings of the International Symposium on Viral Hepatitis and Liver Disease, London.* New York, Liss, 1988 (in press).

51. Khuroo MS, Saleem M, Telli MR, et al: Failure to detect chronic liver disease after epidemic NANB hepatitis. *Lancet* **1**:97–98, 1980.

52. Gerety RJ (ed): *Non-A, Non-B Hepatitis.* New York, Academic, 1981, pp. 207–215.

53. Gmelin K, Kommerell B, Waldherr R, von Ehrlich B: Intranucleic virus-like particles in a case of sporadic non-A, non-B hepatitis. *J Med Virol* **5**:317–322, 1980.

54. Watanabe S, Reddy KR, Jeffers L, et al: Electron microscopic evidence of non-A, non-B hepatitis markers and virus-like particles in immunocompromised humans. *Hepatology* **4**:628–632, 1984.

55. Iwarson S, Schiff Z, Seto B, et al: Retrovirus-like particles in hepatocytes of patients with transfusion-acquired non-A, non-B hepatitis. *J Med Virol* **16**:37–45, 1985.

Uncommon Forms of Viral Hepatitis

FREDRIC G. REGENSTEIN and
ROBERT P. PERRILLO

INTRODUCTION

Members of the herpesvirus family of viruses are commonly involved in human illness and infection. Herpesviruses are distinguished by the presence of a double-stranded DNA genome, a nucleocapsid composed of 162 capsomeres, and a viral envelope derived from the host nuclear membrane. The size of the complete virion ranges from 120 to 250 nm in diameter, while the nucleocapsid measures 95–100 nm in diameter. Of the approximately 80 herpesviruses characterized, only five agents are responsible for causing infections in humans: herpes simplex virus types 1 and 2 (HSV-1 and HSV-2), varicella–zoster (VZV), cytomegalovirus (CMV), and Epstein–Barr virus (EBV).

The members of the herpesvirus family can be further subdivided according to their host cell range and biologic properties. HSV and VZV are characterized by their fairly rapid growth, ability to replicate in a variety of human and animal cell lines, and ability to cause infections associated with the production of characteristic skin lesions (i.e., vesicles). CMV is distinguished by its slower growth in culture, more restricted ability to replicate in different cell lines, and production of cytomegalic change in infected cells. EBV differs from other members of the family because of its extremely limited host cell range. *In vitro*, EBV is only able to replicate in lymphoblastoid cell lines. Despite these differences, all

FREDRIC G. REGENSTEIN and ROBERT P. PERRILLO • Gastroenterology Section, Veterans Administration Medical Center; and Division of Gastroenterology, Washington University School of Medicine, St. Louis, Missouri 63106.

members of the herpesvirus family are capable of producing latent (i.e., persistent, clinically inapparent) infections. After the primary infection, the viruses can exist in a latent form in neural (HSV, VZV) or lymphoid (CMV, EBV) tissue. Following a variable period of time, unidentified factors can trigger reactivation of infection leading to either clinical illness or asymptomatic viral replication and shedding.

Despite the ubiquitous nature of the herpesviruses, they are infrequently recognized as a cause of clinically significant viral hepatitis. However, because of the prevalence of herpesvirus infections, these agents are in fact responsible for a significant number of hepatitis cases. Unlike the hepatitis viruses (i.e., hepatitis A, hepatitis B, hepatitis D, hepatitis non-A, non-B), the herpesviruses do not exhibit a selective affinity for liver cells (i.e., hepatotropism). Thus, hepatitis occurring secondary to a herpesvirus infection is frequently associated with evidence of a generalized or multisystem infection, with isolated hepatic involvement being the exception. Herpesvirus-related hepatitis may therefore be easily overlooked in cases where the degree of hepatocellular injury is mild or overshadowed by evidence of a generalized infection.

VARICELLA–ZOSTER

Infection with the VZV results in two distinct clinical syndromes, varicella (chickenpox) and zoster (shingles). Varicella is usually a disease of children with only rare cases occurring in adults. It represents the syndrome associated with primary exposure to the VZV. Zoster is a localized infection, usually occurring in elderly or immunocompromised persons, and it represents a reactivation of a latent VZV infection following a prior attack of chickenpox. Both syndromes produce identical skin lesions (i.e., papules, vesicles, and eventually crusted scabs).

Clinical Features

Significant hepatic disease is rare with varicella and zoster infections, and virtually always occurs in the presence of typical skin lesions.[1,2] Herpes zoster is usually localized[3,4]; therefore, if hepatitis occurs, it must be preceded by an episode of viral dissemination. Isolated liver involvement in herpes zoster infection is extremely unusual.[5] Varicella–zoster infection appears to play a role in the development of Reye's syndrome. While the pathogenesis of Reye's syndrome remains obscure, preceding VZV infection occurs in approximately 20% of cases.[6]

Diagnosis

Infection with VZV produces a syndrome associated with typical skin lesions occurring in a characteristic distribution that is unlikely to be confused with other entities. Vesicular lesions may be scraped and stained, in a Tzanck preparation, exhibiting the characteristic multinucleated giant cells and intranuclear inclusions. In rare cases, disseminated herpes simplex may resemble VZV infection. Distinction between the two can be made on the basis of viral culture or by direct identification of viral antigens or DNA from the involved tissue. Serologic tests are available but are rarely helpful in establishing a diagnosis in the acute setting.

Liver Histology

A variety of histologic lesions have been reported with VZV infection.[1,2,5] Focal necrosis appears to be the most common histologic finding, but granulomas and submassive necrosis can also occur.

HERPES SIMPLEX

The two serotypes, HSV-1 and HSV-2, share many features, but the primary clinical distinction between the two is the predilection for primary HSV-1 infection to result in mucocutaneous lesions involving the oral cavity, while HSV-2 infections usually involve the genitalia. HSV-1 and HSV-2 are both capable of producing latent and recurrent infections as a consequence of their ability to reside in sensory nerve ganglia.

Herpes simplex infections are extremely common in humans. Poor hygiene and overcrowding appear to promote the spread of HSV. Seroepidemiologic studies indicate that antibodies to HSV can be detected in nearly 100% of adults from underdeveloped areas and lower socioeconomic groups, while substantially lower seropositive rates, 40–50%, are reported for persons from upper socioeconomic classes.[7]

Clinical Features

First episodes of HSV infections are deemed primary infections. Many primary infections are subclinical, and seropositive persons often give no history of having had a primary infection.[8] Symptomatic primary infections with HSV-1 typically cause constitutional symptoms, gingivostomatitis, pharyngitis, and cervical lymphadenopathy. Reactivated HSV-1 is often accompanied by the occurrence of fever blisters (herpes labialis); however, many reactivations are asymptomatic. In immunosuppressed persons, reactivation infections are more likely to be severe and can serve as a source for a disseminated infection. Primary genital HSV-2 infections are characterized by constitutional symptoms and typical vesicular lesions in the genital area. Local symptoms such as pain, itching, dysuria, vaginal or urethral discharge, and inguinal adenopathy are also common. As with HSV-1, reactivation of HSV-2 is often asymptomatic but can be associated with any of the symptoms present in primary genital HSV-2 infections.

Herpes simplex hepatitis can be caused by either HSV-1 or HSV-2. Infection of the liver occurs following viremia and can occur with either primary or reactivated infections. In addition to the liver, multiple organs are usually involved once the infection has disseminated. As a group, neonates have the highest frequency of disseminated infection; however, visceral HSV infections occur in adults as well. Most cases of HSV-associated hepatitis have been reported in immunocompromised persons. Cases occurring in patients with cancer or receiving chemotherapy or corticosteroids,[9–12] in transplant recipients,[13–17] in burn victims,[18] and in pregnant women, especially those in the third trimester,[19–21] have all been described. Occasional episodes of herpes hepatitis have been reported in apparently normal hosts, although detailed assessments of immunologic function were not performed in most of these cases.[22–27]

In adults, herpes hepatitis usually presents with the acute onset of a severe hepatitis associated with fever. Constitutional symptoms may precede the onset of hepatitis by several days, but are nonspecific and of little help in suggesting the correct diagnosis. Evidence of herpetic lesions elsewhere (e.g., fever blisters, herpes genitalis, herpes esophagitis) may be found, but their presence is not a universal feature. The liver may be enlarged and tender, while splenomegaly is unusual.

Laboratory Features

Marked aminotransferase elevations associated with mild bilirubin and alkaline phosphatase elevations are typical. Aminotransferase values of 1000–5000 U/liter are common, while bilirubin levels rarely exceed 5.0 mg/dl and are usually normal or minimally elevated until the terminal phase of the disease. Leukopenia, thrombocytopenia, and disseminated intravascular coagulation (DIC) are commonly seen.

Diagnosis

A high index of suspicion is required if the diagnosis is to be made early enough for treatment to be successful. Onset of an acute illness associated with fever, severe hepatocellular injury, and coagulopathy, especially in an immunocompromised host (Table I), should raise suspicion enough to begin empiric therapy for presumed herpes hepatitis. Definitive diagnosis is based on the isolation of HSV in tissue culture, but this usually requires 24–96 hr. More rapid diagnosis can be made by identifying viral antigens in infected cells using immunofluorescence, enzyme-linked immunosorbent assay (ELISA), or DNA-hybridization techniques. Serologic tests for antibodies against HSV are available, but are rarely helpful in establishing the diagnosis of herpes hepatitis.

Liver Histology

Evidence of infection with HSV is readily identified in biopsy specimens from infected tissue. The histologic features of herpes hepatitis are quite characteristic. Areas of coagulative necrosis are a major histologic feature, with hepatocytes adjacent to the areas of necrosis exhibiting intranuclear inclusions. Inclusions surrounded by a clear halo between the inclusion and the marginated chromatin at the nuclear membrane are designated Cowdry's type A inclusions. Nuclei may also exhibit a homogeneous "ground glass" appearance, and multinucleated cells forming a syncytium may be seen (Fig. 1). Cytoplasmic changes are less apparent but occasionally, degenerating cells resembling acidophil bodies can be seen. Both microvesicular and macrovesicular fat may also be present. Hepatocytes surviving in areas surrounding the involved parenchyma often demonstrate reactive and regenerative changes.

TABLE I. Summary of Key Diagnostic Features
in Herpesvirus-Related Hepatitis

Agent	Diagnostic feature
Herpes simplex	Mucocutaneous herpes simplex lesion
	Fever
	Aminotransferases >1000 U/liter, normal bilirubin
	Disseminated intravascular coagulation
Cytomegalovirus	Fever, fatigue, malaise, anorexia
	Atypical lymphocytosis
	Heterophile-antibody negative
Epstein–Barr virus	Fever, fatigue, malaise, anorexia
	Lymphadenopathy, pharyngitis
	Atypical lymphocytosis
	Heterophile-antibody positive
Varicella–zoster	Characteristic skin lesions

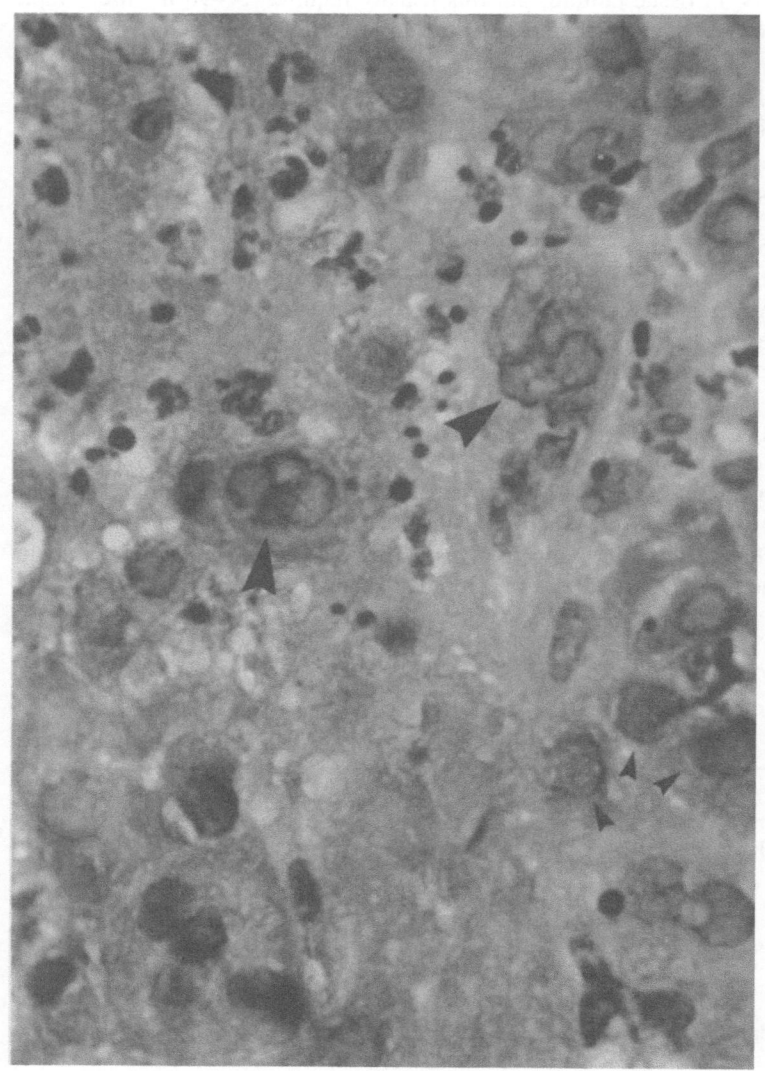

FIGURE 1. Multinucleated syncytial cells (large arrows) and nuclei with ground-glass changes (small arrows) are seen adjacent to an area of necrosis in a patient with herpes simplex hepatitis. (Photograph courtesy of Dr. Elizabeth Brunt.)

Treatment

Few data and no controlled trials are available on the effects of therapy in patients with HSV hepatitis.[21,27] Both vidarabine (ara-A) and acyclovir have demonstrable activity against HSV.[28] Acyclovir is much less toxic and is the preferred agent.[29]

Outcome

Death due to fulminant hepatic failure or disseminated HSV infection is a frequent occurrence in patients with hepatitis secondary to HSV. Prompt initiation of therapy in suspected cases may reduce the extremely high mortality rate seen with this disease.

CYTOMEGALOVIRUS

Cytomegalovirus infections are extremely common. Infected persons shed virus in their secretions, and the infection is disseminated by close personal contact. Poor sanitary conditions and overcrowding promote the spread of infection. Most primary and reactivated CMV infections are asymptomatic. In some cases, a mononucleosislike illness or hepatitis occurs. Both primary and reactivated CMV infections are associated with asymptomatic viral shedding. The asymptomatic excretion of virus in saliva and urine represents an important means of transmitting CMV infection to susceptible persons.

Clinical and Laboratory Features

Neonatal Infection

In the perinatal setting, CMV infection can occur as a consequence of transplacental passage of the virus, resulting in a congenital infection, or as a neonatal infection, occurring during or shortly after the birth process. The latter can occur as a result of either blood transfusion, breast milk transmission, or close contact with someone who sheds the virus. In the mother, the source of the CMV infection can be either a primary or reactivated infection. Intrauterine infection appears to occur more often following a primary maternal infection. Congenital CMV infection occurs in approximately 0.2–2.0% of live births, but only about 10% of these cases are associated with clinical sequelae.[30] The typical features of congenital CMV, petechiae, hepatosplenomegaly, jaundice, microcephaly, chorioretinitis, and thrombocytopenia are only seen in 2–

5% of affected cases. The most common laboratory abnormalities associated with congenital CMV are elevated aspartate aminotransferase and direct bilirubin, atypical lymphocytosis, and an increased cord IgM level.

The clinical course is variable, and the hepatitis usually resolves during the first year of life. In some cases, progression to chronic liver disease may occur.[31,32] The role, if any, played by CMV in the pathogenesis of biliary atresia remains to be determined.[33]

Infection in Nonimmunocompromised Hosts

In normal hosts, primary episodes of CMV are occasionally symptomatic and are associated with an illness suggestive of infectious mononucleosis. Fatigue, fever, and myalgias are often present. Pharyngitis and lymphadenopathy are less common with CMV than with EBV infection, but atypical lymphocytes are present in both disorders.

In most cases of symptomatic CMV infection in normal hosts, the mononucleosislike illness predominates, and the associated hepatic dysfunction is mild.[34,35] Typically, aminotransferases, alkaline phosphatase, and bilirubin are elevated less than threefold.[36-38] Icteric hepatitis is unusual, but occasional cases present with predominant liver involvement, or marked cholestasis.[39,40] Persistent fever and an atypical lymphocytosis are frequently present and should provide a clue to the correct diagnosis (Table I). Fulminant CMV hepatitis has only been reported on rare occasions.[41]

Cytomegalovirus hepatitis can also occur following blood transfusion. In the posttransfusion setting, CMV can occur as either a primary or recurrent infection. In primary infections, the host is presumably CMV seronegative and receives blood from a seropositive donor resulting in CMV transmission. In recurrent infections, the seropositive host either reactivates a latent CMV infection, through yet-to-be identified mechanisms, or a new infection occurs due to exposure to a different viral strain. Most cases of posttransfusion CMV are asymptomatic and appear to be due to reactivation of a latent infection. In symptomatic cases, an infectious mononucleosislike illness is typically present. If hepatocellular injury occurs, it is generally mild.

During the late 1960s and early 1970s, posttransfusion CMV infection occurred frequently in patients undergoing cardiac surgery. Subsequently, CMV infections following transfusion have occurred less often.[42] Factors that may help explain the lower frequency of posttransfusion CMV infections in recent years include the use of less blood during cardiac surgery, increasing reliance on banked donor blood instead of fresh blood, and greater usage of blood from volunteer donors.

Infection in Immunocompromised Hosts

Cytomegalovirus infections represent a major problem and a significant cause of morbidity in immunocompromised individuals.[43,44] CMV infections are especially troublesome when they occur in the transplant setting. In organ transplant recipients, CMV can be transmitted to the seronegative recipient via the donor organ or as a result of a transfusion. Alternatively, in seropositive recipients, CMV can reactivate during immunosuppressive therapy.

Both primary and recurrent CMV infections are more likely to be symptomatic in immunosuppressed than in normal hosts. Symptomatic patients generally experience a febrile illness associated with varying degrees of constitutional symptoms. In immunosuppressed patients with CMV infection, viral excretion may persist for prolonged intervals. If liver involvement occurs, it is generally mild and associated with minimal elevations of aminotransferases and alkaline phosphatase.[45] In severe cases, evidence of hepatic involvement may be the predominant disease manifestation. These patients may present with jaundice and marked elevations in liver function tests. Even in severe cases, however, the hepatic involvement is usually overshadowed by evidence of disseminated infection. Persistent fever, leukopenia, thrombocytopenia, and pneumonitis are typical findings in disseminated infections. Severe CMV infections often occur in close relation to the administration of immunosuppressive therapy used to control episodes of organ rejection.

Cytomegalovirus alone is an infrequent cause of hepatitis in patients with acquired immune deficiency syndrome (AIDS), but the virus is often isolated from these patients as a consequence of persistent viral shedding. In most AIDS cases, several pathogens may be present, and multiple etiologies for liver dysfunction can be identified.[46]

A clinical picture resembling sclerosing cholangitis and papillary stenosis has recently been described in patients with AIDS. Biliary tract infection with CMV has been implicated in the pathogenesis of this syndrome.[46a]

Diagnosis

The diagnosis of congenital CMV is best established by isolating the virus in cell culture, and the organism can usually be cultured from urine, blood, or saliva. When CMV hepatitis is suspected, the diagnosis can be confirmed by isolating the virus from a liver biopsy specimen. When sensitive techniques become widely available, detection of IgM antibody against CMV in cord sera may be helpful in rapidly establishing the diagnosis of congenital CMV infection.

In acquired CMV infection isolation of the virus from blood, rather than from urine or saliva, correlates best with the presence of disseminated infection. The diagnosis of CMV by culture techniques is limited by the 4-week or more delay that may be required before the virus can be isolated. Serologic tests for IgG antibody to the CMV agent are useful in diagnosing primary CMV infections (Table II). A fourfold rise in IgG antibody titer is indicative of an acute infection. The major limitations of the IgG antibody test is its difficulty in establishing the diagnosis of recurrent infections in normal hosts, unpredictability in diagnosing primary or recurrent CMV infection in immunosuppressed persons, and the 2- to 3-week delay necessary in order to demonstrate a rising antibody titer. Recently described techniques for detecting IgM antibodies against CMV appear to be very useful in diagnosing primary CMV infections in normal hosts.[47] The value of IgM antibody testing to diagnose recurrent infections or infections in immunocompromised hosts remains to be determined.[48,49] Newer techniques using monoclonal antibodies directed against CMV proteins and DNA-hybridization probes[50–52] hold future promise for making the diagnosis of CMV infection easier and more quickly than current culture techniques.

Liver Histology

Histologic features of CMV hepatitis in immunocompromised hosts appear to differ from those found in normal individuals. In normal hosts, the major findings consist of a mononuclear infiltrate in the sinusoids and portal tracts, mild hepatocellular necrosis, granuloma formation, damaged bile duct epithelium, and rare CMV nuclear inclusions. Immunoperoxidase stains detecting CMV antigens in liver tissue are often negative in normal hosts.[53] By contrast, immunosuppressed persons tend to have more extensive liver cell necrosis, less inflammatory infiltrates, and greater numbers of intracellular viral inclusions than do normal hosts (Fig. 2). Immunoperoxidase stains for CMV antigens are usually positive in these people.[53,54] The differing histologic features between normal and immunocompromised hosts are most likely related to the difference in the immunologic response in the respective groups. In the immunocompromised

TABLE II. Interpretation of
Cytomegalovirus Serologic Markers

CMV antibody present		
IgM	IgG	Interpretation
+	+	Primary CMV infection
+/−	+	Reactivated CMV infection
−	+	Remote CMV infection

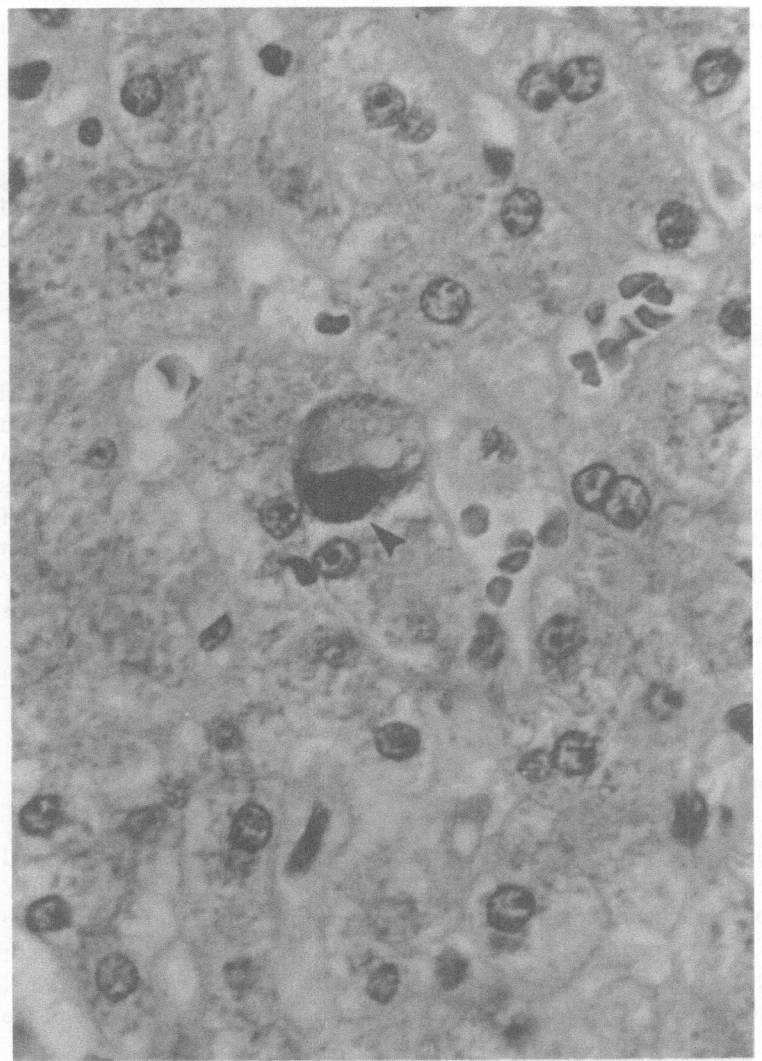

FIGURE 2. Intranuclear inclusion (arrow) in an immunosuppressed patient with cytomegalovirus hepatitis. (Photograph courtesy of Dr. Elizabeth Brunt.)

host, viral replication proceeds without an effective cell-mediated immune response, leading to viral proliferation and greater intracellular expression of viral proteins. Eventually cell death probably occurs as a result of viral-mediated cytolysis. In normal hosts, the cellular immune response to CMV results in lymphocyte-mediated destruction of CMV-infected cells limiting the expression of complete CMV virions.[54]

Treatment

Gangciclovin, 9-(1,3-dihydroxy-2-propoxymethyl)guanine is an analog with activity against CMV.[55] There are no controlled trials; however, anecdotal experience with gongciclovin appears very favorable. The agent appears to be primarily limited by its bone-marrow toxicity.

Outcome

Most cases of mild CMV hepatitis are self-limited and are not associated with long-term sequelae. In severe cases, mortality can be high, and death usually occurs as a result of multiorgan CMV infection. Death due to fulminant liver failure is unusual. The role of CMV infection in chronic hepatitis remains unclear. In several series, patients with chronic liver dysfunction and evidence of active CMV infections were presumed to have chronic CMV hepatitis.[56] Most cases of chronic hepatitis associated with positive CMV cultures or rising CMV antibody titers are probably due to underlying chronic non-A, non-B hepatitis and a superimposed recurrent CMV infection. Until a reliable marker for non-A, non-B hepatitis becomes available, the role of CMV in this setting will remain unsettled.

EPSTEIN–BARR VIRUS

The Epstein–Barr virus is the herpesvirus responsible for the classic clinical syndrome of infectious mononucleosis. As with the other herpesviruses, EBV appears to establish a lifelong latent infection following primary infection. Aside from its ability to establish latent infection in B lymphocytes, EBV is capable of producing the indefinite proliferation of B lymphocytes *in vitro*. Crowding, lower socioeconomic status, and poor sanitary conditions promote spread of the virus and lead to acquisition of infection at an early age.

Clinical Features

Most primary EBV infections occur in young children and are asymptomatic or associated with a nonspecific virallike illness. The clinical syndrome of infectious mononucleosis typically occurs in older children, adolescents, or young adults. Older patients tend to have a more severe illness and are more likely to present in an unusual fashion.[57-61]

Typical infectious mononucleosis is characterized by malaise, fatigue, sore throat, fever, and lymphadenopathy. Less often, headache, myalgias, anorexia, nausea, and vomiting may be present. Clinical signs suggestive of infectious mononucleosis include an evanescent rash, periorbital edema, severe pharyngitis with tonsillar exudate, hepatosplenomegaly, palatal petechiae, and occasionally thrombocytopenia or hemolytic anemia.

Most cases of EBV-related infectious mononucleosis are associated with hepatic dysfunction, but clinically detectable jaundice is present in only 4–17% of cases.[62-64] Hepatitis associated with fever, pharyngitis, or lymphadenopathy should lead one to consider the diagnosis of EBV infection. In addition, clinically significant hepatitis occurs more often in elderly patients than in younger persons.[58,65]

Laboratory Features

In patients undergoing serial blood testing, elevations in aspartate aminotransferase and alkaline phosphatase can be demonstrated in more than 80% of cases.[37] Aminotransferase levels are usually elevated less than fivefold, while serum alkaline phosphatase levels are typically less than threefold increased. In occasional cases, markedly elevated levels of aminotransferases can be seen; however, values in excess of 1000 U/liter are very rare. Marked serum alkaline phosphatase elevations can also occur and often are associated with normal or near-normal levels of serum bilirubin.[66]

Diagnosis

Infection with CMV can cause a similar illness and needs to be excluded in patients presenting with an infectious mononucleosislike illness (Table I). The diagnosis of an EBV infection is easy to establish when atypical lymphocytosis and the Paul–Bunnell heterophile antibody are present. Additional studies may be necessary when the Paul–Bunnell heterophile antibody test is negative. Detection of antibodies directed against various EBV-related antigens (Table III) can be used to establish the diagnosis of EBV in atypical or unusual cases.[67] Newer methods employing monoclonal antibodies and DNA-hybridization techniques are available in research settings and can be used to detect viral antigens or EBV-associated DNA in infected tissues.[67]

In primary EBV infections, antibodies against the viral capsid antigen (anti-VCA) develop early, and levels peak at 3–4 weeks following the acquisition of an infection. Anti-VCA of the IgM class are usually detectable for up to 12 weeks following infection, while levels of IgG anti-VCA remain detectable

TABLE III. Interpretation of Epstein–Barr Virus
Serologic Markers

Antibody present				
Anti-viral capsid antigen		Anti-early antigen	Anti-nuclear antigen	Interpretation
IgM	IgG			
+	+	+	−	Acute EBV infection
−	+	−	+	Remote EBV infection
+/−	+	+	+	Reactivated EBV infection
+/−	+	+/−	+/−	Chronic EBV infection

indefinitely after an infection. The presence of IgM anti-VCA, therefore, is quite specific for acute infection. Very high levels of IgG anti-VCA are usually indicative of an acute infection, although in some cases, high levels may persist long after the initial infection. Antibodies against EBV-related early antigens (anti-EA) can also be identified. Like IgM anti-VCA, anti-EA levels are usually present for up to 12 weeks after a primary infection; however, in a variety of immunodeficiency states, anti-EA levels may remain elevated for prolonged periods. Antibodies against the EBV nuclear antigen (anti-EBNA) usually develop 2 to 3 months following a primary infection. Anti-EBNA persists indefinitely, and its presence indicates that EBV infection is not recent.

Liver Histology

In most cases, a liver biopsy is neither required nor necessary to establish the diagnosis. In unusual or atypical cases, biopsy may be useful in order to exclude other causes of liver disease. The biopsy typically demonstrates preservation of the hepatic architecture and infiltration of the sinusoids and portal tracts with a pleomorphic cellular infiltrate.[68–72] The infiltrate usually consists of large atypical lymphocytes, smaller lymphocytes, plasma cells, and granulocytes. Kupffer cell hyperplasia, fatty change, and evidence of regenerative activity may be present, but, extensive liver cell necrosis is very rare. The relatively normal-appearing hepatocytes and the minimal amounts of focal necrosis help distinguish EBV infection from typical viral hepatitis.

Treatment

No specific therapy is available for EBV infection. Corticosteroids are occasionally administered in cases associated with thrombocytopenia, hemolytic anemia, or massive lymphadenopathy that result in airway compromise or inability to swallow. In a case report, acyclovir was associated with temporary clinical improvement in a patient with EBV-induced lymphoproliferation.[73] In a controlled trial, acyclovir appeared to decrease EBV excretion; however, no apparent clinical benefit could be demonstrated from this antiviral effect.[74]

Outcome

In young adults with symptomatic disease, constitutional symptoms usually resolve within 3 weeks. Recrudescence of constitutional symptoms, especially fatigue and occasionally fever, can occur. In addition to having a more severe illness, older persons tend to recover more slowly. Irrespective of age, aminotransferase and alkaline phosphatase levels usually return to normal range within 3 months. Currently, there is no convincing evidence to implicate EBV infection as a causative agent in either chronic hepatitis or cirrhosis.[75]

Fulminant hepatic failure secondary to EBV infection has been described and appears to be rare.[76,77] Fatal cases may be more apt to occur in persons with underlying immune deficiencies.[78] In these situations, severe hepatic dysfunction due to massive tissue infiltration with EBV-infected B lymphocytes can occur.

Recently, a syndrome presumed to be secondary to chronic EBV disease has been described.[79,80] Most patients complain of chronic fatigue and of intermittent episodes of low-grade fever, pharyngitis, lymphadenopathy, depression, musculoskeletal pains, and headache. Hepatosplenomegaly and elevated aminotransferases are occasionally present. The heterophile antibody is usually absent, but other EBV markers (i.e., anti-VCA, anti-EA) are typically positive. The relationship of this clinical syndrome to a chronic EBV infection has been questioned.[81] However, in patients with extremely high titers of anti-VCA and anti-EA and in people whose illness follows an acute episode of EBV mononucleosis, chronic EBV infection seems likely.[82]

REFERENCES

1. Eschar J, Reif L, Waron M, et al: Hepatic lesion in chickenpox. A case report. *Gastroenterology* **64:**462–466, 1973.
2. Keene JK, Lowe DK, Grosfeld JL, et al: Disseminated varicella complicating ulcerative colitis. *JAMA* **239:**45–46, 1978.
3. Burgoon LF, Burgoon JS, Baldridge CD: The natural history of herpes zoster. *JAMA* **164:**265–270, 1957.
4. Mazur MH, Dolin R: Herpes zoster at the NIH: A 20 year experience. *Am J Med* **65:**738–744, 1978.
5. Ross JS, Fanning WL, Beautyman W, et al: Fatal massive hepatic necrosis from varicella-zoster hepatitis. *Am J Gastroenterol* **74:**423–427, 1980.

6. Centers for Disease Control: Follow-up on Reye's syndrome—United States. *MMWR* **29**:1–3, 1980.
7. Rooney JF: Epidemiology of herpes simplex. Herpes simplex virus infection: Biology, treatment, prevention. *Ann Intern Med* **103**:404–419, 1985.
8. Corey L, Spear PG: Infection with herpes simplex viruses. *N Engl J Med* **314**:686–691, 749–757, 1986.
9. Lee JC, Fortuny IE: Adult herpes simplex hepatitis. *Hum Pathol* **3**:277–281, 1972.
10. Orenstein JM, Castadot MF, Wylens SL: Fatal herpes hepatitis associated with pemphigus vulgaris and steroids in an adult. *Hum Pathol* **5**:489–493, 1974.
11. Keane JT, Malkindon FD, Bryant J, et al: Herpes virus hominis hepatitis and disseminated intravascular coagulation: Occurrence in an adult with pemphigus vulgaris. *Arch Intern Med* **136**:1312–1317, 1976.
12. Williams TL, Morgan JR, Denzler TB: Fulminant herpes simplex hepatitis following coronary bypass and postcardiotomy syndrome. *Am Heart J* **110**:679–680, 1985.
13. Anuras S, Summers R: Fulminant herpes simplex hepatitis in an adult: Report of a case in renal transplant recipient. *Gastroenterology* **70**:425–428, 1976.
14. Moses MF, Ascher NL, Balfour HH, et al: Jaundice after renal transplantation. *Ann Surg* **188**:783–790, 1978.
15. Elliot WC, Houghton DC, Bryant RE, et al: Herpes simplex type 1 hepatitis in renal transplantation. *Arch Intern Med* **140**:1656–1660, 1980.
16. Walker DP, Langson M, Lawler W, et al: Disseminated herpes simplex virus infection with hepatitis in an adult renal transplant recipient. *J Clin Pathol* **34**:1044–1046, 1981.
17. Taylor RJ, Saul SH, Dowling JN, et al: Primary disseminated herpes simplex infection with fulminant hepatitis following transplantation. *Arch Intern Med* **141**:1519–1521, 1981.
18. Foley FD, Greenawald KA, Nash G, et al: Herpes virus infection in burned patients. *N Engl J Med* **282**:652–656, 1970.
19. Flewitt TH, Parker RGF, Philip WM: Acute hepatitis due to herpes simplex virus in an adult. *J Clin Pathol* **22**:60–66, 1969.
20. Young EJ, Killam AP, Greene JF: Disseminated herpesvirus infection in pregnancy. Association with primary genital herpes in pregnancy. *JAMA* **235**:2731–2733, 1976.
21. Lagrew DC, Furlow TG, Hager WD, et al: Disseminated herpes simplex virus infection in pregnancy. Successful treatment with acyclovir. *JAMA* **252**:2058–2059, 1984.
22. Francis TI, Osunyokun BO, Kemp GE: Fulminant hepatitis due to herpes hominis in an adult human. *Am J Gastroenterol* **57**:329–332, 1972.
23. Eron L, Kosininski K, Hitsch MS: Hepatitis in an adult caused by herpes simplex virus type 1. *Gastroenterology* **71**:500–504, 1976.
24. Connor RW, Lorts G, Gilbert DN: Lethal herpes simplex virus type 1 hepatitis in a normal adult. *Gastroenterology* **76**:590–594, 1979.
25. Rubin MH, Ward DM, Painter J: Fulminant hepatic failure caused by genital herpes in a healthy person. *JAMA* **253**:1299–1301, 1985.
26. Goodman ZD, Ishak KG, and Sesterhenn IA: Herpes simplex hepatitis in apparently immunocompetent adults. *Am J Clin Pathol* **85**:694–699, 1986.
27. Baxter RP, Phillips LE, Faro S, et al: Hepatitis due to herpes simplex virus in a nonpregnant patient. Treatment with acyclovir. *Sex Transm Dis* **13**:174–176, 1986.
28. Hirsch MS, Schooley RT: Treatment of herpesvirus infections. *N Engl J Med* **309**:963–970; 1034–1039, 1983.
29. Whitley RJ, Alford CA, Hirsch MS, et al: Vidarabine versus acyclovir therapy in herpes simplex encephalitis. *N Engl J Med* **314**:144–149, 1986.
30. Stagno S, Whitley RJ: Herpesvirus infections of pregnancy. Part 1. Cytomegalovirus and Epstein–Barr virus infections. *N Engl J Med* **313**:1270–1274, 1985.

31. Dresler S, Linder D: Noncirrhotic portal fibrosis following neonatal cytomegalic inclusion disease. *J Pediatr* **93**:887–888, 1978.
32. Zuppan CW, Bui HD, Grill BG: Diffuse hepatic fibrosis in congenital cytomegalovirus infection. *J Pediatr Gastroenterol Nutr* **5**:489–491, 1986.
33. Oppenheimer EH, Esterly JR: Cytomegalovirus infection: A possible cause of biliary atresia. *Am J Pathol* **13**:2a, 1973.
34. Bonkowsky HL, Lee RV, Klatskin G: Acute granulomatous hepatitis. Occurrence in cytomegalovirus mononucleosis. *JAMA* **233**:1284–1288, 1975.
35. Clarke J, Craig RM, Saffro R, et al: Cytomegalovirus granulomatous hepatitis. *Am J Med* **66**:264–269, 1979.
36. Horwitz CA, Henle W, Hemle G, et al: Heterophile-negative infectious mononucleosis and mononucleosis-like illnesses. Laboratory confirmation of 43 cases. *Am J Med* **63**:947–957, 1977.
37. Horwitz CA, Burke MD, Grimes P, et al: Hepatic function in mononucleosis induced by Epstein–Barr virus and cytomegalovirus. *Clin Chem* **26**:243–246, 1980.
38. Cohen JI, Corey GR: Cytomegalovirus infection in the normal host. *Medicine (Baltimore)* **64**:100–114, 1985.
39. Lamb SG, Stern H: Cytomegalovirus mononucleosis with jaundice as presenting sign. *Lancet* **2**:1003–1006, 1966.
40. Toghill PJ, Bailey ME, Williams R, et al: Cytomegalovirus hepatitis in the adult. *Lancet* **1**:1351–1354, 1967.
41. Shusterman NH, Frauenhoffer C, Kinsey MD: Fatal hepatic necrosis in cytomegalovirus mononucleosis. *Ann Intern Med* **88**:810–812, 1978.
42. Tegtmeier GE: Cytomegalovirus infection as a complication of blood transfusion. *Semin Liver Dis* **6**:82–95, 1986.
43. Rubin RH, Cosimi AB, Tolkoff-Rubin NE, et al: Infectious disease syndromes attributable to cytomegalovirus and their significance among renal transplant recipients. *Transplantation* **24**:458–464, 1977.
44. Peterson PK, Balfour HH, Marker SC, et al: Cytomegalovirus disease in renal allograft recipients: A prospective study of the clinical features, risk factors, and impact on transplantation. *Medicine (Baltimore)* **59**:283–300, 1980.
45. Aldrete JS, Sterling WA, Hathaway BH, et al: Gastrointestinal and hepatic complications affecting patients with renal allografts. *Am J Surg* **129**:115–124, 1975.
46. Lebovics E, Thung SW, Schaffner F: The liver in acquired immunodeficiency syndrome: A clinical and histologic study. *Hepatology* **5**:293–299, 1985.
46a. Schneiderman DJ, Cello JP, Laing FC: Papillary Stenosis and Sclerosing Cholangitis in the Acquired Immunodeficiency Syndrome. *Ann Intern Med* **106**:546–549, 1987.
47. Griffiths PD: Diagnostic techniques for cytomegalovirus infection. *Clin Hematol* **13**:631–644, 1984.
48. Rasmussen L, Kelsall D, Nelson R et al: Virus-specific IgG and IgM antibodies in normal and immunocompromised subjects infected with cytomegalovirus. *J Infect Dis* **145**:191–199, 1982.
49. Pass RF, Griffiths PD, August A: Antibody response to cytomegalovirus after renal transplantation: Comparison of patients with primary and recurrent infection. *J Infect Dis* **147**:40–46, 1983.
50. Chou S, Merigan TC: Rapid detection and quantitation of human cytomegalovirus in urine through DNA hybridization. *N Engl J Med* **308**:921–925, 1983.
51. Shuster EA, Beneke JS, Tegtmeier GE, et al: Monoclonal antibody for rapid laboratory detection of cytomegalovirus infections: Characterization and diagnostic application. *Mayo Clin Proc* **60**:577–558, 1985.
52. Unger ER, Budgeon LR, Myerson D, et al: Viral diagnosis by in situ hybridization. Description of a rapid simplified colorimetric method. *Am J Surg Pathol* **10**:1–8, 1986.

53. Snover DC, Horwitz CA: Liver disease in cytomegalovirus mononucleosis: A light micro-scopical and immunoperoxidase study of six cases. *Hepatology* **4:**408–412, 1984.
54. Ten Napel CHH, Houthoff HJ, The TH: Cytomegalovirus hepatitis in normal and immune compromised hosts. *Liver* **4:**184–194, 1984.
55. Jacobson MA, Mills J: Serious cytomegalovirus disease in the Acquired Immunodeficiency Syndrome: Clinical findings, diagnosis, and treatment **108:**585–594, 1988.
56. Ware AJ, Luby JP, Hollinger B, et al: Etiology of liver disease in renal-transplant patients. *Ann Intern Med* **91:**364–371, 1979.
57. Ansari A, Grotte, M: Acute hepatitis as a primary manifestation of infectious mononucleosis in a 53-year-old man. *Am J Gastroenterol* **79:**471–473, 1984.
58. Horwitz CA, Henle W, Henle G, et al: Clinical and laboratory evaluation of elderly patients with heterophile antibody positive infectious mononucleosis. Report of 7 patients ages 40–78. *Am J Med* **6:**333–339, 1976.
59. Carter JW, Edson RS, Kennedy CC: Infectious mononucleosis in the older patient. *Mayo Clin Proc* **53:**146–150, 1978.
60. McKendrick MW, Gesses AM, Edwards J: Atypical infectious mononucleosis in the elderly. *Br Med J* **2:**970, 1979.
61. Pickens S, McMurdoch CJ: Infectious mononucleosis in the elderly. *Age Aging* **8:**93–95, 1979.
62. Hoagland RJ, McClusky RT: Hepatitis in mononucleosis. *Ann Intern Med* **43:**1019–1036, 1955.
63. Hoagland RJ: The clinical manifestations of infectious mononucleosis. A report of 200 cases. *Am J Med Sci* **240:**21–29, 1960.
64. Baron DN, Bell JL, Dunnet WN: Biochemical studies on hepatic involvement in infectious mononucleosis. *J Clin Pathol* **18:**209–211, 1965.
65. Horwitz CA, Henle W, Henle G, et al: Infectious mononucleosis in patients aged 40–72 years. Report of 27 cases including 3 without heterophile antibody responses. *Medicine (Baltimore)* **62:**256–262, 1983.
66. Shuster F, Ognibene AI: Dissociation of serum bilirubin and alkaline phosphatase in infectious mononucleosis. *JAMA* **209:**267–268, 1969.
67. Sumaya CV: Epstein–Barr virus serologic testing: Diagnostic indications and interpretations. *Pediatr Infect Dis* **5:**337–342, 1986.
68. Nelson RS, Darragh JH: Infectious mononucleosis hepatitis. *Am J Med* **21:**26–33, 1950.
69. Wadsworth RC, Keil PG: Biopsy of the liver in infectious mononucleosis. *Am J Pathol* **28:**1003–1026, 1952.
70. Kilpatrick ZM: Structural and functional abnormalities of liver in infectious mononucleosis. *Arch Intern Med* **117:**47–53, 1966.
71. White NJ, Juel-Jensen BE: Infectious mononucleosis hepatitis. *Semin Liver Dis* **4:**301–306, 1984.
72. Lloyd-Still JD, Scott JP, Crussi F: The spectrum of Epstein–Barr virus hepatitis in children. *Pediatr Pathol* **5:**337–351, 1986.
73. Hanto DW, Frizzer G, Gajl-Peczalska KJ, et al: Epstein–Barr virus induced B-cell lymphoma after renal transplantation: Acyclovir therapy and transition from polyclonal to monoclonal B-cell proliferation. *N Engl J Med* **306:**913–918, 1982.
74. Andersson J, Skoldenberg B, Ernberg I, et al: Acyclovir treatment in primary Epstein–Barr virus infection. A double-blind placebo controlled study. *Scand J Infect Dis (Suppl)* **47:**107–111, 1985.
75. Tanaka K, Shimada M, Sasahara A, et al: Chronic hepatitis associated with Epstein–Barr virus infection in an infant. *J Pediatr Gastroenterol Nutr* **5:**467–471, 1986.
76. Pelletier LL, Bores DM, Roning DA, et al: Disseminated intravascular coagulation and hepatic necrosis. Complications of infectious mononucleosis. *JAMA* **235:**1144–1146, 1976.
77. Davies MH, Morgan Capner P, Portman B, et al: A fatal case of Epstein–Barr virus infection with jaundice and renal failure. *Postgrad Med J* **56:**794–795, 1980.

78. Crawford DH, Epstein MA, Achong BG, et al: Virological and immunological studies on a fatal case of infectious mononucleosis. *J Infect* 1:37–48, 1979.
79. Jones JF, Ray CG, Minnich LL, et al: Evidence for active Epstein–Barr virus infection in patients with persistent, unexplained illness: Elevated anti-early antigen antibodies. *Ann Intern Med* 102:1–6, 1985.
80. Straus SE, Tosato G, Armstrong G, et al: Persisting illness and fatigue in adults with evidence of Epstein–Barr virus infection. *Ann Intern Med* 102:7–16, 1985.
81. Merlin TL: Chronic mononucleosis: Pitfalls in the laboratory diagnosis. *Hum Pathol* 17:2–8, 1986.
82. Tobi M, Straus SE: Chronic Epstein–Barr virus disease: A workshop held by the National Institute of Allergy and Infectious Diseases. *Ann Intern Med* 103:951–953, 1985.

Acute Viral Hepatitis
Treatment

JACK PEICHER and EUGENE R. SCHIFF

INTRODUCTION

Most people with acute viral hepatitis are anicteric and asymptomatic and infrequently seek medical attention. The physician therefore is more likely to see the patient with more severe disease that is clinically apparent. A safe and effective antiviral agent is not available although putative agents are being tested. Management of patients with viral hepatitis can be subdivided into several categories: acute uncomplicated viral hepatitis, cholestatic hepatitis, subacute fulminant hepatitis, and fulminant hepatitis.

UNCOMPLICATED VIRAL HEPATITIS

Most patients with acute viral A and B hepatitis will have an uncomplicated course and will eventually completely resolve the infection. Older patients with posttransfusion non-A, non-B hepatitis have a disproportionately greater likelihood of developing chronic hepatitis.

Hospitalization

Patients with uncomplicated viral hepatitis should be hospitalized if they are vomiting and are unable to eat, or if the prothrombin time is prolonged and

JACK PEICHER • Department of Gastroenterology, University of Southern California, Los Angeles, California 90033.   EUGENE R. SCHIFF • Division of Hepatology, University of Miami School of Medicine, and Hepatology Section, Veterans Administration Medical Center, Miami, Florida 33125.

fulminant hepatitis may be evolving. Older and chronically ill patients should probably be hospitalized because they are more susceptible to complications. Unreliable patients or those who are unable to care for themselves should also be hospitalized.

Isolation

Most patients with viral hepatitis are unlikely to transmit the infection to another patient in a hospital setting. However, from a practical standpoint, it is preferable to put these patients in a private room, to prevent undue stress to susceptible roommates and avoid medicolegal consequences. Exceptions are patients with type A hepatitis who are fecally incontinent or small children who are likely to transmit the infection via toys soiled with feces.[1]

Hepatitis B, delta and posttransfusion non-A, non-B are not transmitted by the fecal–oral route; therefore, these patients do not require a private room. Needle precautions should be instituted for all patients regardless of a diagnosis of viral hepatitis.

Household contacts of patients who stay at home should be given immune serum globulin (0.02 ml/kg IM) if the patient has hepatitis A. Sexually active spouses of patients with hepatitis B should receive hepatitis B immune globulin 0.06 ml/kg IM as soon as possible following exposure (preferably within 7 days). If active vaccination that provides long-term immunity is not elected hepatitis B immune globulin (HBIG) in the same dose should be repeated 1 month later. It is recommended that spouses of patients with acute non-A, non-B hepatitis receive a single dose of immune serum globulin (0.06 ml/kg IM) if they are sexually active.

Restriction of Activity

Patients with acute viral hepatitis feel tired and initially will want to rest. However, if they feel well enough to move around, they should be permitted to be mobile. The policy of prolonged and strict bed rest until normalization of liver tests was based on an early experience in the Mediterranean theater during World War II.[2,3] Patients with hepatitis were permitted early ambulation and this seemed to increase the frequency of relapse. It was postulated that the upright posture decreased blood flow to the liver and further compromised liver function. The average duration of bed rest for soldiers was extended from 30 days in 1943 to 89 days in 1951.[4] Subsequently, many other studies have shown that even vigorous physical exercise during acute hepatitis has no untoward effects.[5,6]

Forced bed rest should be discouraged and may lead to a posthepatitis syndrome characterized by prolonged fatigue in the absence of abnormal liver chemistries. Patients prescribed strict rest are also predisposed to deep vein thrombosis and pulmonary emboli. Thus, during the acute illness, the patient should be encouraged to use the bathroom and gradually progress to full ambulation. The decision to allow the patient to return to work should be tailored to the specific circumstances. In general the patient should be able to physically tolerate the work and the icterus should be mild or absent. Although jaundice is not necessarily detrimental, it may create fears among co-workers.

Diet

Most patients with acute hepatitis are anorectic and nauseous. The anorexia is in part due to disordered gustatory acuity.[7] Adequate nutrition may necessitate supplements with high caloric junk food. The diet should include at least 4 g glucose per kilogram of body weight. Candy, soft drinks, and juices are usually well tolerated; if not, IV glucose should be used. Infusion of at least 10% glucose solution is mandatory if the patient has severe liver necrosis and hypoglycemia. The safety and efficacy of amino acid supplements in acute viral hepatitis have not been well determined.

As the patient starts to eat more, frequent small feedings (six per day instead of three per day) are better tolerated. Nausea tends to worsen throughout the day, therefore breakfast should be the largest meal. Fatty foods are often avoided but may be ingested if tolerated.

Vitamin supplements are not necessary in well-nourished patients. If the prothrombin time is prolonged, vitamin K injected SC in a dosage of 10 mg/day for 3 days should be tried. Improvement is more likely to occur if cholestasis is prominent. In the patient with persistent vomiting, IV fluid and electrolyte replacement will be necessary.

Specific Therapy

No agent has been shown to decrease mortality or evolution into a chronic state, even though multiple trials have been conducted. Corticosteroids have no role in the treatment of uncomplicated viral hepatitis. Early studies showed that treatment with adrenocorticotropic hormone (ACTH) decreased bilirubin levels rapidly but recovery was slower and relapses more common.[8] Later studies comparing prednisone to placebo showed no differences in the duration of illness.[9]

Also, corticosteroids potentially might convert a self-limited acute hepatitis B to chronic active hepatitis by impairing viral clearance. There are no data that justify the use of corticosteroids in the treatment of acute viral hepatitis, with the possible exception of cholestatic hepatitis A.

Numerous antiviral forms of therapy have been studied. Ribavirin inhibits synthesis of viral nucleic acid. In one study, it was shown to decrease the serum bilirubin and aminotransferases, but no other clinical data are described.[10]

The free radical acceptor, (+)-cyanidanol-3, was used in a double-blind trial on 124 randomized patients with acute viral hepatitis: 58 were given 3 g of (+)-cyanidanol-3 per day and 66 were given placebo. The serum bilirubin and aminotransferases were checked every 5 days. For the total group of patients, the aminotransferases were lower in the cyanidanol group than in the control group from the thirtieth to the fiftieth day of treatment, but the duration of hospitalization was the same for both groups.[11] Acyclovir given IV in a dosage of 10 or 15 mg/kg every 8 hr (q8h) was shown to inhibit production of complete hepatitis B virus particles in two patients,[12] but further studies are required.

α-Interferon (IFN_α) was given to five patients with acute hepatitis with rapid activation of their interferon systems (which was shown to be depressed prior to treatment), and three of them had a rapid and uncomplicated recovery. Levin and Hahn[13] suggested that interferon be studied in the early treatment for severe viral hepatitis. Immune globulin and even hyperimmune serum globulin have been found to be ineffective in acute hepatitis.[14] None of the drugs tested can be recommended as routine treatment for acute viral hepatitis.

Supportive Measures

Nausea is usually short-lived, but it can be treated with metoclopramide, 10 mg IV or IM prior to meals. It is the drug of choice because it promotes gastric emptying and has few hepatic side effects. Phenothiazines may be effective but are not preferred because of potential cholestatic side effects.

Pruritus can be a major problem, and the antihistamine of choice is hydroxyzine 50 mg q6h. It also has antiemetic properties. Cholestyramine should be used if hydroxyzine does not work, but it usually takes 2 or 3 days to have an effect and constipation is a common side effect. The usual dose is 4 g before each meal and at bedtime, but it may be increased to 6 g four times daily.

Abdominal pain is usually not a problem in hepatitis, but with stretching of Glisson's capsule severe pain may occur and may require narcotics, e.g., meperidine. If further treatment with narcotics is necessary, the patient should be carefully monitored for evidence of encephalopathy. In the patient who is symptomatic from a high fever, acetaminophen in doses totaling less than 2.5 g/day may be used. Sedation should be avoided but, if absolutely necessary, oxazepam is preferred, since it is excreted at a normal rate by patients with hepatitis.[15]

Use of Other Medications

In general, all unnecessary medications should be stopped, particularly narcotics and tranquilizers, but drugs such as oral contraceptives may be continued unless no longer needed. Obviously sexual intercourse should be discouraged to prevent transmission of the infection. In a retrospective study of women with acute hepatitis, no adverse effect was seen with oral contraceptive use.[16]

Alcohol

It is prudent for patients with acute hepatitis to abstain from alcohol intake. A study conducted in 1949 demonstrated adverse effects of alcohol in patients with hepatitis.[17] However, a more recent study showed that one dose of 80 mg ethanol per kilogram of body weight, given IV during acute hepatitis, had no effect on aminotransferases.[18] Alcohol ingestion has not been shown to be more harmful in patients 6–12 months after recovery from viral hepatitis than in the general population.[17] Nevertheless, if underlying alcoholism is suspected, abstinence should be sustained indefinitely.

Elective Surgery

Elective surgery should be postponed until acute hepatitis has resolved. Even though evidence is meager, one study showed that among 42 patients with acute viral hepatitis undergoing surgery, 4 died and 5 others had major complications.[19]

CHOLESTATIC HEPATITIS

Cholestatic hepatitis is a rare presentation of acute hepatitis characterized by pruritus and persistent jaundice. These patients usually present with a prolonged prothrombin time that improves with vitamin K administration. In a recent paper, cholestatic type A hepatitis responded to oral prednisone, 40 mg/day for 4 days followed by tapering off the medication over weeks.[20] Prednisone resulted in symptomatic relief and a rapid initial drop in serum bilirubin levels, followed by a slower fall. In cholestatic hepatitis B and non-A, non-B, steroids should not be used because of the potential for promoting chronicity of the hepatitis.

SUBACUTE FULMINANT HEPATITIS

This type of viral hepatitis is quite severe but is more prolonged than fulminant hepatitis; it usually evolves into chronic liver disease or is fatal. It is characterized clinically by ascites, edema, encephalopathy, high serum bilirubin levels, and a course that can last months. Corticosteroid use does not enhance survival and may even be detrimental.

Corticosteroids were first used during the early 1950s.[21] Even though the studies were uncontrolled, the therapy seemed to work; however, in 1976, a controlled trial of steroid therapy in severe hepatitis showed that this form of treatment could be detrimental.[22] Patients with severe viral hepatitis were randomly assigned to methyl prednisolone or placebo treatment groups. These patients had at least one of the following features: bilirubin >25 mg/dl; prothrombin time <50% of normal; serum albumin <2.5 g/dl; ascites; encephalopathy; edema; and/or bridging necrosis, and the duration of illness was less than 3 months. Nine of the 29 patients died during the study. Seven received steroids (methylprednisolone 48 mg in divided doses), and two received placebo. All nine patients had bridging necrosis or bridging fibrosis. Two of the steroid-treated patients had pulmonary candidiasis, one had systemic aspergillosis, and another one died of complications of peptic ulcer disease. Ascites should be treated with diuretics, watching carefully for electrolyte imbalances. Encephalopathy is treated with lactulose or neomycin (500 mg PO q8h), or both. If the patient develops cerebral edema, he or she should be treated as in fulminant hepatitis.

FULMINANT HEPATITIS

Fulminant hepatitis is the clinical syndrome associated with massive necrosis of the liver. It is characterized by liver failure associated with impairment of consciousness within 8 weeks of the onset of the illness.[23] Mortality rates as high as 95% are not unusual. There is no specific therapy for this form of liver disease; only supportive measures. Complications include cerebral edema, gastrointestinal (GI) bleeding, renal failure, electrolyte imbalances, respiratory insufficiency, hypoglycemia, sepsis, seizures, disseminated intravascular coagulation (DIC), hypotension, and death. Patients with fulminant hepatitis should be transferred to an intensive care setting where they can be watched carefully.

Cerebral edema is usually treated with IV mannitol, 1 g/kg q4–6h, while monitoring the serum osmolarity carefully. If it exceeds 320 mOsmole/liter, mannitol should be stopped and restarted when osmolarity returns to normal.[24] Routine use of intracranial pressure monitoring is not indicated. Dexamethasone[24] and high-frequency ventilation[25] have no effect on survival. Gastrointestinal bleeding has been shown to be reduced in patients treated with IV cimetidine, 300 mg q6h or as a continuous drip at 50 mg/hr.[26]

Electrolyte imbalance can be caused by the excessive use of lactulose resulting in hypernatremia secondary to diarrhea. Lactulose will only control hyperammonemia, and the dosage should be adjusted to produce two to three bowel movements daily.

Hypoglycemia should be recognized and treated aggressively with 10–25% glucose solutions. However, hyperalimentation with amino acid solutions or lipids has no role in fulminant hepatitis and potentially can be deleterious. Fresh-frozen plasma should only be used if the patient is actively bleeding, or if an invasive procedure such as endotracheal intubation or central vein cannulation is planned. Patients with fulminant hepatic failure can become combative and must be restrained. Small doses of intravenous lorazepam can be used. If the patient develops seizures, diazepam is the drug of choice.

Several forms of therapy have been found to be useless. Hyperimmune globulin therapy was ineffective in the treatment of patients with fulminant hepatitis B.[14] Glucagon-insulin therapy has been used to stimulate hepatic regeneration in mice[27] but has not proved efficacious in human subjects.

High doses of corticosteroids have been assessed in the treatment of fulminant hepatic failure. In 1979 the Acute Hepatic Failure Study Group conducted a double-blind study regimen.[28] High (800 mg/day) and low (400 mg/day) doses of hydrocortisone were compared with placebo. Most of the patients had hepatitis types B and non-A, non-B. Overall survival was 33% for fulminant B and 13% for fulminant non-A, non-B hepatitis. Neither high-dose nor low-dose hydrocortisone therapy had any beneficial effect.

Exchange transfusions,[29] cross-circulation with animals, perfusion of pig and baboon livers, and total body washout were heroic measures used in the past, which have been abandoned because of failure to improve survival as compared with conservative therapy. There have been attempts to create forms of artificial hepatic support: charcoal hemoperfusion and hemoperfusion using a polyacrylonitrite membrane has been shown by some investigators to increase survival in patients with grade III coma,[30] but most of these patients had drug-induced hepatitis. Although survival may not be improved, encephalopathy is lessened, and there may be a place for hemoperfusion in the preparation of a patient for liver transplantation. There is a need for controlled trials assessing the safety and efficacy of charcoal hemoperfusion in fulminant hepatic failure.

Liver transplantation is being evaluated in fulminant hepatitis. In 1985, the Pittsburgh group reported a 50% survival in 10 patients transplanted, but overall survival was only 19% for all patients referred to the institution.[31]

There are multiple practical problems in preparing these patients for transplantation. Time is limited and a donor may not be available. The decision to transplant can be difficult. The physician must differentiate the patient who will recover spontaneously from the patient who will fail to regenerate sufficient hepatic parenchyma in time to survive. The timing of transplantation is critical. The presence of cerebral edema and waiting for stage IV encephalopathy makes the risk for surgery increasingly high.

REFERENCES

1. Favero MS, Maynard JE, Leger RT, et al: Guidelines for the care of patients hospitalized with viral hepatitis. *Ann Intern Med* **91:**872–876, 1979.
2. Capps RB, Barker MH: The management of infectious hepatitis. *Ann Intern Med* **26:**405–416, 1947.

3. Havens WP Jr: Infectious hepatitis in the Middle East: A clinical review of 200 cases seen in a military hospital. *JAMA* **126**:17–23, 1944.
4. Havens WP Jr: Infectious hepatitis. *Medicine (Baltimore)* **27**:279–326, 1948.
5. Nelson RS, Sprinz H, Colbert JW, et al: Effect of physical activity on recovery from hepatitis. *Am J Med* **16**:780–789, 1954.
6. Nefger MD, Chalmers TC: The treatment of acute infectious hepatitis: Ten-year follow-up study of the effects of diet and rest. *Am J Med* **35**:299–309, 1963.
7. Smith FR, Henkin RK, Dell RB: Disordered gustatory activity in liver disease. *Gastroenterology* **70**:568–571, 1976.
8. Evans AS, Spring H, Nelson RS: Adrenal hormone therapy in viral hepatitis. I. The effect of ACTH in the acute disease. II. The effect of cortisone in the acute disease. *Ann Intern Med* **38**:1115–1133, 1953.
9. DeRitis F, Giusti G, Malluci L, et al: Negative results of prednisone therapy in viral hepatitis. *Lancet* **1**:533–534, 1964.
10. Ayrosa-Galvao PA, Castro IO: The effect of 1-β-D-ribofuranosyl-1,2,4,-triazole-3-carboxamide on acute viral hepatitis. *Ann NY Acad Sci* **284**:278–283, 1977.
11. Piazza M, Guadagnino V, Picciotto L, et al: Effect of (+)-cyanidanol-3 in acute HAV, HBV, and non-A, non-B viral hepatitis. *Hepatology* **3**:45–49, 1983.
12. Weller IVD, Carreno V, Fowler MJF, et al: Acyclovir inhibits hepatitis B virus replication in man. *Lancet* **1**:273, 1982.
13. Levin S, Hahn T: Interferon system in acute viral hepatitis. *Lancet* **1**:592–594, 1982.
14. Acute Hepatic Failure Study Group: Failure of specific immunotherapy in fulminant type B hepatitis. *Ann Intern Med* **86**:272–277, 1977.
15. Shull H Jr, Wilkinson GR, Johnson R, et al: Normal disposition of oxazepam in acute viral hepatitis and cirrhosis. *Ann Intern Med* **84**:420–425, 1976.
16. Schweitzer IL, Weiner JM, McPeak CM, et al: Oral contraceptives in acute viral hepatitis. *JAMA* **233**:979–980, 1975.
17. Gardner HT, Rovelstad RA, Moore DJ, et al: Hepatitis among American occupational troops in Germany: A follow-up study with particular reference to interim alcohol and physical activity. *Ann Intern Med* **30**:1009–1019, 1949.
18. Galambos JT, Asada M, Shanks JZ: The effect of intravenous ethanol on serum enzymes in patients with normal or diseased liver. *Gastroenterology* **44**:267–274, 1963.
19. Harville DD, Summerskill WHJ: Surgery in acute hepatitis: Cause and effects. *JAMA* **184**:257–261, 1963.
20. Gordon SC, Reddy KR, Schiff L, et al: Prolonged intrahepatic cholestasis secondary to acute hepatitis A. *Ann Intern Med* **101**:635–637, 1984.
21. Ducci H, Katz R: Cortisone, ACTH and antibiotics in fulminant hepatitis. *Gastroenterology* **21**:357–374, 1952.
22. Gregory PB, Knaver CM, Kempson RL, et al: Steroid therapy in severe viral hepatitis. A double-blind, randomized trial of methyl-prednisolone versus placebo. *N Engl J Med* **294**:681–687, 1976.
23. Trey C, Davidson CS: The management of fulminant hepatic liver failure. *Prog Liver Dis* **3**:282–298, 1970.
24. Canalese J, Gimson AES, Davis C, et al: Controlled trial of dexamethesone and mannitol for the cerebral oedema of fulminant hepatic failure. *Gut* **23**:625–629, 1982.
25. Ede RJ, Gimson AES, Bihari D, et al: Controlled hyperventilation in the prevention of cerebral oedema in fulminant hepatic failure. *J Hepatol* **2**:43–51, 1986.
26. MacDougall BRD, Williams R: H₂ receptor antagonist in the prevention of acute upper gastrointestinal hemorrhage in fulminant hepatic failure: A controlled trial. *Gastroenterology* **74**:464–465, 1978.

27. Farivar M, Wands JR, Isselbacher KJ, et al: Effect of insulin and glucagon on fulminant murine hepatitis. *N Engl J Med* **295:**1517–1519, 1976.
28. Acute Hepatic Failure Study Group: Etiology and prognosis in fulminant hepatitis. *Gastroenterology* **77:**A33, 1979.
29. Redeker AG, Yamahiro HS: Controlled trial of exchange-transfusion therapy in fulminant hepatitis. *Lancet* **1:**3–6, 1973.
30. Gimson AES, Braude S, Mellon PJ, et al: Earlier charcoal haemoperfusion in fulminant hepatic failure. *Lancet* **2:**681–683, 1982.
31. Peleman RR, Gavaler JS, Van Thiel DH, et al: Liver transplantation for acute and subacute hepatic failure. *Hepatology* **5:**1045, 1985.

Prognosis of Acute Viral Hepatitis

Now You Got It, Now You Don't (Or Do You?)

RONALD L. KORETZ

*Prognosis—a forecast or forecasting; esp., a
prediction of the probable course of a disease
in an individual and the chance of recovery.*
Webster's New World Dictionary, 1974

Acute viral hepatitis (AVH) results in only a limited number of outcomes. The patient may or may not recover from the infection and get rid of the virus (while having either a symptomatic or an asymptomatic illness). The "may not" occurs if the patient dies during the acute phase (in particular, from fulminant hepatitis) or if the patient develops a chronic infection.

This seemingly simple concept is not always so readily translatable in clinical practice. For example, suppose the clinician sees a patient with an acute icteric disease (with biochemical evidence of hepatitis) and hepatitis B surface antigen (HB_sAg) demonstrated in the blood. Although it would be tempting to call this illness acute hepatitis B, the clinician may be seeing a previously asymptomatic HB_sAg chronic carrier who now has a superimposed non-B (and perhaps even nonviral) hepatitis. By contrast, suppose a routine chemistry panel has been obtained for an asymptomatic patient and the alanine aminotransferase (ALT) level is high. Is this an acute or chronic process? Certainly just because

---

RONALD L. KORETZ • Division of Gastroenterology, Olive View Medical Center, Sylmar, California 91342; and Department of Medicine, University of California School of Medicine, Los Angeles, California 90024.

the abnormality has been found on that day, it cannot be assumed that it began at that time. (Australia was the largest island in the world even before it was discovered.)

When the medical literature is reviewed to find out the prognosis of AVH, two problems become immediately apparent. These problems are due to the way most of these data are collected; patients with symptomatic disease are arbitrarily assumed to have acute hepatitis, and their course is then described from the time of presentation. How can we be sure that some of these patients did not have "acute-on-chronic" processes rather than true AVH? How can we define prognosis in patients who have initially asymptomatic infections? (These latter patients are usually not seen at the time of infection.)

A third limitation of the available data is the inability to identify specific viral infections prior to the late 1960s. Thus, most of the information presented in this chapter are from more recent publications.

This chapter reviews the information available in the literature and attempts to provide some insight into the shortcomings of these data, where they exist. In spite of these problems, we can glean some understanding of what happens to people when they are infected with hepatitis viruses. For our purposes, we employ the following definitions:

Viral hepatitis (VH): An inflammatory condition in the liver presumed due to a viral infection and manifested by an increased ACT or aspartate aminotransferase (AST) level. (This definition does not make any restriction concerning the length of time for which the process has been going on, the presence or absence of associated clinical symptoms, or even the underlying histologic appearance.)

Acute viral hepatitis (AVH): Hepatitis that has been recognized for less than 6 months and/or a process in which a liver biopsy has demonstrated the typical appearance of acute disease (intralobular necrosis rather than predominantly portal tract disease).

Chronic viral hepatitis (CVH): Hepatitis that has been documented to persist for at least 6 months and/or a process in which a liver biopsy has demonstrated one of the typical inflammatory patterns of chronic disease (predominantly portal tract inflammation with or without associated cirrhosis).

Chronic viral carrier state: A condition in which one or more hepatitis viruses are known or presumed to be in the bloodstream for at least 6 months. (This definition does not require the presence of concomitant hepatic inflammation, i.e., a chronic carrier may have normal ALT and AST levels.)

PROGNOSIS OF ACUTE HEPATITIS A

Several lines of evidence support the concept that chronic liver disease does not result from hepatitis A infection. Serologic evaluations of patients with chronic liver disease or cirrhosis or both have failed to find an increased frequency of markers for hepatitis A infection.[1-4] Examinations of patients many years after their episode of infectious hepatitis have failed to indicate any greater than expected frequency of chronic liver disease.[5-8] Long-term follow-up studies of patients with AVHA have invariably found that the IgM-specific antibody resolves, fecal excretion of virus ceases, and enzyme levels become normal.[9-13] No patient has ever been reported to develop true chronic liver disease from hepatitis A (no reference available).

The fact that the disease ultimately resolves does not mean that it always does so within 6 months; this is one of the problems with arbitrary definitions such as those I made above. Protracted courses of AVHA, with enzyme abnormalities persisting for months, can occur[9-11,14-22]; the duration of the "illness" may be more than 1 year.[14,15,22] These long courses may be polyphasic (i.e., rises and falls in aminotransferase levels with the rise often associated with symptomatic exacerbations).[10,11,14,15,18-21] Gocke[22] estimated that as many as 10% of patients with hepatitis A may pursue this polyphasic course.

Table I displays the data from three prospective studies of patients with AVHA, indicating the likelihood of abnormal aminotransferases persisting over time; whereas 10–20% of patients may still have abnormal tests after 6 months, only a very small number will still be abnormal after 1 year. It should be stressed that, even when patients have long periods of enzyme abnormalities, they are usually asymptomatic. Even the symptomatic exacerbations, when they occur, are not as severe as the initial episode.[16,18] However, during polyphasic relapses, hepatitis A virus may be present in the stool.[23]

An unusual manifestation of AVHA is cholestasis.[16,17] In this situation, patients develop pruritus, higher bilirubin levels, and more dramatic elevations

TABLE I. Aminotransferase Resolution in Hepatitis A over Time

No. of patients	Percentage of patients with abnormal enzymes at			Reference
	3 months	6 months	12 months	
60	62	10	0	Bamber et al.[10]
377	3		<3	Boughton et al.[11]
69		19	6	Caredda et al.[15]

of the alkaline phosphatase. This condition also resolves, but it is obviously easily confused with obstructive jaundice.

Finally, with regard to the chronicity of hepatitis A, there is one report, in 1954, of a child with (presumed) hepatitis A who was demonstrated to have infective stools 67 weeks after the onset of his illness.[24] At the time, a chronic carrier state for hepatitis A was postulated. Recently the investigator found in his freezer a small amount of serum from this patient; it was positive for HB_sAg.[25]

The other issue of prognosis in AVHA is the development of fulminant hepatitis. How often does this occur? This is an impossible question to answer, since most hepatitis A infections go unnoticed. It is certainly an unusual course for AVHA to pursue, occurring in far less than 1% of infections. However, among patients with fulminant hepatitis, hepatitis A is a common cause. In three large series, hepatitis A infection was present in 3%, 25%, and 32% of the cases.[26-28] (The 3% figure is probably not representative, since many of the hepatitis B cases were specifically referred for a treatment trial, inflating the number of B patients and proportionately reducing the other etiologic categories.)

PROGNOSIS OF ACUTE HEPATITIS B

The ability of the hepatitis B virus (HBV) to establish chronic infections is the reason for the ultimate discovery of HB_sAg in Australian aborigines. The chronic infection may not necessarily be associated with clinical, or even biochemical, evidence of disease; in fact, chronic HB_sAg carriers with normal aminotransferase levels are very unlikely to have significant (i.e., chronic active hepatitis or cirrhosis, or both) liver disease.[29] By contrast, when chronic hepatitis is present, hepatitis B appears to be a common cause.[30-34]

It is often stated that 10% of patients with AVHB develop chronic disease. This figure comes from a 1971 Copenhagen study, in which 11 of 112 patients who were hospitalized with acute hepatitis B (a diagnosis made on clinical, biochemical, histologic, and serologic grounds) had persisting HB_sAg positivity and subsequent biopsy evidence of chronic disease.[35] Several problems are inherent in this observation. Even with the biopsy-proven documentation of AVH, how can we be sure that the acute disease was not a non-B process superimposed on a chronic HB_sAg carrier (e.g., delta infection[36])? Also, the long-term course of an asymptomatic infection (or at least one not resulting in hospitalization) is undefined in this type of study. Finally, in 1971, the techniques employed for HB_sAg detection were substantially less sensitive than they are currently.

Certainly the best way to answer this question is to identify and follow patients from a time before they are infected; if the hypothetical patient in the introductory comments had been known to be HB_sAg-negative a few weeks or months earlier, the diagnosis of AVHB could be made with great confidence. A few prospective studies have been performed in which the baseline serologic states of the participants was established; these data are summarized in Table II.[37–40] The drawback in these reports is that only a defined group of people is followed, and we have to assume that the data can be extrapolated to the general population. However, at least in male homosexuals and Eskimos the 10% frequency of chronicity may be a reasonable expectation. It appears to be lower in Taiwanese college students.

Why is the virus cleared by most people, but not by the rest? We assume that the factors responsible reside in the host and relate to immunologic responsiveness. Although the precise details are unknown, we have a few clues. Males are more likely than females to become chronic carriers.[41,42] Neonates of mothers who are hepatitis B e antigen (HB_eAg)-positive HB_sAg chronic carriers are at high risk of becoming chronically infected themselves.[42,43] Patients with Downs' syndrome have a propensity to develop the carrier state, a phenomenon ascribed to some (undefined) genetic defect in viral clearance.[44] With respect to genetic factors in the general population, however, no consistent association has been found between HLA subtypes and chronic hepatitis B infection in a large number of studies.[45–53]

Acquired factors are also important in some people. Patients with chronic renal failure (CRF) and lepromatous leprosy, diseases causing immunosuppression, seem less able to clear hepatitis B infections.[54] This same propensity for chronicity has been reported in acquired immune deficiency syndrome (AIDS), but the data to date are scarce.[55] Concomitant delta virus infection in (presumed) AVHB has not appeared to result in a higher rate of chronicity, although these studies suffer from many of the design defects we have already discussed.[56–60]

What is the likelihood of AVHB pursuing a fulminant course? In patients hospitalized with presumptive AVHB, this problem is uncommon; in two large

TABLE II. Frequency of Development of Chronic Hepatitis
from Documented Acute Hepatitis B Infections

Study population	No. of patients with AVHB	No. (%) developing chronic infections	Reference
Taiwanese college students	39	1 (3%)	Beasley et al.[37]
Homosexuals[a]	66	4 (6%)	Shah et al.[38]
Homosexuals[a]	127	10 (8%)	Szmuness et al.[39]
Eskimos	188	25 (13%)	McMahon et al.[40]

[a]Placebo recipients in vaccine trials.

series of such patients, the mortality rate (reflecting the occurrence of fulminant disease) was 0% [61] and 0.5%.[62] As was seen for hepatitis A, HB_sAg positivity is commonly found in series of patients with fulminant disease; the previously cited series attributed the process to the HBV in 62%, 50%, and 25% of the cases.[26–28] Many of these patients may have had concomitant hepatitis B and delta virus infection, or even been chronic carriers with superimposed delta (or possibly other non-A, non-B) infection.[63,64]

PROGNOSIS OF ACUTE NON-A, NON-B HEPATITIS

When it became possible to identify both hepatitis A and B serologically, it became apparent that there were yet other hepatitis viruses. In fact, since patients were seen with two episodes of non-A, non-B (NANB) disease, it was suspected that multiple such agents existed.[65] Most chimpanzees, when exposed to hepatitis viruses, become immune; by using such animals (immune to one NANB agent), it has been demonstrated that at least two such agents exist.[66–68] By challenging unexposed chimpanzees with serum specimens obtained years apart from the same patient, the chronic carrier state for NANB disease was also demonstrated,[69] and chronic infection can occur.

The major problem in defining the course of NANB disease is obviously the inability to identify the viruses. In practice, NANB hepatitis is defined when a person develops a disease clinically consistent with hepatitis that is epidemiologically compatible with a viral infection and serologically negative for hepatitis A and B. This definition cannot distinguish the different NANB agents, and the marker for ongoing infection is an abnormal aminotransferase level.

NANB infections appear to be particularly prone to produce chronic disease (persistently abnormal aminotransferases). This phenomenon has been especially appreciated in the posttransfusion hepatitis situation. Several prospective studies have followed patients from the time of transfusion; as such, these people are known not to have underlying chronic hepatitis. Furthermore, asymptomatic people are identified, since the enzyme levels are serially determined in all participants. These data may not be extrapolatable to the general population for a number of reasons. The virus(es) may not be the same as the one(s) seen in nontransfusion disease. The dose of virus contained in a unit of blood is likely much greater than that seen in the usual hepatitis exposure. Patients receiving units of blood have some underlying disease and may be receiving medications; both factors could have an impact on the course of infection.

Keeping these reservations in mind, the frequency of chronicity in NANB posttransfusion hepatitis is displayed on Table III, and the number ranges from 16% to 68%.[70–74] In a recent review, Alter[74] estimated that this rate would be at least 50%. Although most of these patients have asymptomatic CVH (i.e., they

TABLE III. Frequency of Chronicity in NANB PTH[a]

Underlying disease	No. of patients with NANB PTH	No. (%) patients developing CVH	Reference
Various	62	40[b] (65%)	Koretz et al.[70]
Cardiac surgery	26[c]	12 (46%)	Berman et al.[71]
Cardiac surgery	44	10[b] (23%)	Knodell et al.[72]
Various surgeries	116	19 (16%)	Tateda et al.[73]
Cardiac surgery	75	51 (68%)	Alter[74]

[a]PTH, Posttransfusion hepatitis; CVH, chronic viral hepatitis (aminotransferase abnormalities persisting for more than 6 months).
[b]Aminotransferase abnormalities persisting more than 1 year.
[c]Some of these patients may be included in ref. 74.

do not have jaundice, fatigue, or the other clinical manifestations of inflammatory liver disease), 10–20% will develop histologic evidence of cirrhosis over the next decade.[70–72,74]

The rates of development of CVH in the nontransfusion situation are less well defined. These data are derived from following patients identified with presumed AVH and thus are subject to the same limitations as we have previously described. In these studies, chronicity appears to occur more often than in hepatitis B similarly identified,[75,76] with estimates ranging as high as 50%.[77]

Fulminant hepatitis is an occasional outcome of NANB AVH. Furthermore, its mortality appears to be higher.[26–28] However, these data must be interpreted from the perspective that, in single cases, we will not be absolutely certain that a viral infection is the cause until specific serologic tests become available.

A separate form of NANB hepatitis has been recognized in less-developed areas of the world. The illness appears to be waterborne and is analogous to hepatitis A.[78] This disease does not result in chronic hepatitis,[79] although there may be an increased incidence of fulminant disease in pregnant women.[80,81]

PROGNOSTICATION OF PROGNOSIS

Can one foretell which patients will develop CVH? Although not absolutely reliable as predictive markers, there are tendencies for CVHB to occur in males, neonates (especially if the mother is an HB_eAg-positive carrier), and the immunosuppressed.

It has been often claimed that patients in whom chronic disease develops are more likely to have had asymptomatic infections. Certainly, if one interviews known chronic carriers, they usually fail to identify a preceding acute episode.[42]

It is believed that the intensity of the initial illness is a reflection of the host-immune response and that those with impaired ability to clear the virus are more prone to anicteric, or even asymptomatic, initial infections; at the other extreme, it has been stated that patients with fulminant disease rarely become chronic carriers.[42,82]

This tempting concept (relating active disease, viral clearance, and immune status) seems logical. The actual observations, however, at least those made in apparently immunologically intact individuals, are based on faulty data. These studies are usually retrospective and cannot identify all the individuals infected by the hepatitis agents. For example, although most HB_sAg chronic carriers do not have histories of icteric hepatitis, neither do most people who have convalescent antibodies[83]; these latter people did manage to clear the virus without large-scale destruction of their hepatocytes.

Does an acute infection manifested by an icteric illness result in a lower frequency of CVH? The best way to answer this question is to identify all cases of hepatitis prospectively and then ascertain what percentages of icteric and anicteric cases progress. This is difficult to do in practice, as we have seen; asymptomatic people do not report their "illnesses." A few prospective studies have looked at this question. In one study following the placebo recipients in a vaccine trial, no clinical feature of the AVHB identified homosexuals whose disease progressed to CVHB.[38] The data from two prospective studies of NANB posttransfusion hepatitis are summarized in Table IV[71,84]; although the incidence of chronic disease was arithmetically higher in those with anicteric AVH, the differences were not statistically significant and a sizable proportion of those with icteric AVH did develop CVH. From a practical perspective, the occurrence of jaundice in the AVH phase cannot rule out the subsequent development of CVH.

Two groups have reported that patients with NANB hepatitis who demonstrate polyphasic patterns of aminotransferase abnormalities are more likely to develop CVH.[85,86] This is a self-fulfilling prophesy, of course, since, by definition, monophasic disease requires the stepwise reduction in the elevated value with ultimate normalization. It is also of little clinical value, since the patient

TABLE IV. Frequency of NANB CVH in Icteric
and Anicteric Disease

Incidence chronicity		
Icteric hepatitis	Anicteric hepatitis	Reference
7/14 (50%)	22/23 (67%)	Koretz et al.[84]
3/8 (38%)	9/18 (50%)	Berman et al.[71]

must still be followed until the enzyme values become normal or CVH becomes obvious.

For this same reason, monitoring HB_eAg, DNA polymerase, HBV DNA, or IgM-specific anti-HB_c has no clinical utility. Persistence of these markers has been associated with the development of CVHB.[87-90] However, their positive and negative predictiveness is not always 100% compared with the gold standard—HB_sAg clearance and subsequent development of antibody (anti-HB_s) along with aminotransferase normalization. These gold standard tests are not only routinely available, they are usually less expensive.

Liver biopsies are rarely indicated in AVH, as the diagnosis is established clinically and there is no effective intervention to alter the natural history. Some investigators have retrospectively identified an association between the presence of bridging necrosis on liver biopsies obtained during the acute phase and the subsequent development of CVH.[91,92] However, patients with this histologic finding usually have more severe disease; when these clinical parameters are also taken into account in the comparison, bridging necrosis loses its predictive capacity.[93] Thus, it does not seem reasonable to advocate liver biopsy during the acute phase for prognostic purposes.

One might wonder why the early identification of patients who are going to pursue a chronic course should even be an issue? By (my) definition, this question will be answered in 6 months. The same laboratory tests will be obtained in the interim (liver tests and serology). There is no way to stop it, one way or the other. Thus, in the day-to-day management of patients with presumed AVH, one need only monitor those tests that will prove whether or not the inflammation has resolved (aminotransferase levels) and whether the virus has been cleared [up to now, an issue only in AVHB, where HB_sAg should disappear and the convalescent antibody (anti-HB_s) appear].

CONCLUSIONS

Since this chapter is in the acute hepatitis section, we can bring it to an end. The important concepts to remember are the following:

1. Hepatitis A very occasionally results in death from fulminant hepatic failure, but everyone else recovers without chronic sequelae.
2. Hepatitis B progresses to chronic disease in a small percentage of apparently acute patients (perhaps up to 10%), and to fulminant disease in an occasional person (<1%).
3. NANB hepatitis has a remarkable tendency to cause CVH; like the other viral agents, it causes fulminant hepatitis in only a very rare individual.
4. The waterborne type of NANB hepatitis, analogous to hepatitis A, does

not cause chronic disease but may produce fulminant hepatitis in pregnant women at a higher rate than do other hepatitis viruses.

5. Any patient with presumed AVH needs to be followed until the inflammatory process resolves and the viral agent disappears; this latter goal can, at this time, only be realized for hepatitis B.

Got it?

REFERENCES

1. Boyer JL: Chronic hepatitis—a perspective on classification and determinants of prognosis. *Gastroenterology* **70**:1161–1171, 1976.
2. Rakela J, Radeker AG, Edwards VM, et al: Hepatitis A virus infection in fulminant hepatitis and chronic active hepatitis. *Gastroenterology* **74**:879–882, 1978.
3. Mathiesen LR, Hardt F, Dietrichson O, et al: The role of acute hepatitis type A, B, and non-A, non-B in the development of chronic active liver disease. *Scand J Gastroenterol* **15**:49–54, 1980.
4. Agarwal S, Lahori UC, Mehta SK, et al: Hepatitis A and Indian childhood cirrhosis. *Arch Dis Child* **54**:901–903, 1979.
5. Zieve L, Hill E, Nesbitt S, et al: The incidence of residuals of viral hepatitis. *Gastroenterology* **25**:495–531, 1953.
6. Neefe JR, Bambescia JM, Kurtz CH, et al: Prevalence and nature of hepatic disturbance following acute viral hepatitis with jaundice. *Ann Intern Med* **43**:1–32, 1955.
7. Cullinan ER, King RC, Rivers JS: The prognosis of infective hepatitis. *Br Med J* **1**:1315–1317, 1958.
8. Sorenson TIA, Skinhoj P, Aldershvile J, et al: Mortality after acute hepatitis type A,B, and non-A, non-B in 981 patients followed for up to 10 years. *Scand J Gastroenterol* **17**:193–198, 1982.
9. Dienstag JL: Viral hepatitis type A: Virology and course. *Clin Gastroenterol* **9**:135–154, 1980.
10. Bamber M, Thomas HC, Bannister B, et al: Acute type A, B, and non-A, non-B hepatitis in a hospital population in London: Clinical and epidemiological features. *Gut* **24**:561–564, 1983.
11. Boughton CR, Hawkes RA, Schroeter DR, et al: A four-year hospital and general-practice study in Sydney. *Med J. Aust* **1**:113–119, 1982.
12. Routenberg JA, Dienstag JL, Harrison WO, et al: Foodborne outbreak of hepatitis A: Clinical and laboratory features of acute and protracted illness. *Am J Med Sci* **278**:123–137, 1979.
13. Muller R: Hepatitis A virus infection: Clinical disease, absence of chronicity and long-term prognosis. *Infection* **7**:206, 1979.
14. Cornu C, Lamy ME, Geubel A, et al: Persistence of immunoglobulin M antibody to hepatitis A virus and relapse of hepatitis A infection. *Eur J Clin Microbiol* **3**:45–46, 1984.
15. Caredda F, d'Arminio Monforte A, Rossi E, et al: Prolonged course and relapses of acute type A separarl hepatitis. *Bull Ist Sieroter Milan* **63**:34–36, 1984.
16. Jacobson IM, Nath BJ, Dienstag JL: Relapsing viral hepatitis type A. *J Med Virol* **16**:163–169, 1985.
17. Gordon SC, Reddy R, Schiff L, et al: Prolonged intrahepatic cholestasis secondary to acute hepatitis A. *Ann Intern Med* **101**:635–637, 1984.
18. Raimondo G, Longo G, Caredda F, et al: Prolonged, polyphasic infection with hepatitis A. (Letter.) *J Infect Dis* **153**:172–173, 1986.
19. Chiriaco' P, Guadalupi C, Armigliato M, et al: Polyphasic course of hepatitis type A in children. (Letter.) *J Infect Dis* **153**:378–379, 1986.

20. Cobden I, James OFW: A biphasic illness associated with acute hepatitis A virus infection. *J Hepatol* **2**:19–23, 1986.
21. Gruer LD, McKendrick MW, Beeching NJ, et al: Relapsing hepatitis associated with hepatitis A virus. (Letter.) *Lancet* **2**:163, 1982.
22. Gocke DJ: Hepatitis A revisited. (Editorial.) *Ann Intern Med* **105**:960–961, 1986.
23. Sjogren MH, Tanno, H, Fay O, et al: Hepatitis A virus in stool during clinical relapse. *Ann Intern Med* **106**:221–226, 1987.
24. Stokes J, Berk JE, Malamut LL, et al: The carrier state in viral hepatitis. *JAMA* **154**:1059–1065, 1954.
25. Holmes AW: Chronic hepatitis A. *J Med Virol* **15**:101–110, 1985.
26. Rakela J: Etiology and prognosis in fulminant hepatitis. *Gastroenterology* **77**:A33, 1979 (abst). 1986.
27. Mathiesen LR, Skinhoj P, Nielson JO, et al: Hepatitis type A, B, and non-A, non-B in fulminant hepatitis. *Gut* **21**:72–77, 1980.
28. Gimson AES, White YS, Eddleston ALWF, et al: Clinical and prognostic differences in fulminant hepatitis type A, B, and non-A, non-B. *Gut* **24**:1194–1198, 1983.
29. Koretz RL, Lewin KH, Rebhun DJ, et al: Hepatitis B surface antigen carriers: To biopsy or not to biopsy. *Gastroenterology* **75**:860–863, 1978.
30. Wewalka F, Hadziyannis JM, Pesendorfer FX, et al: OMGE-Study on prevalence of hepatitis B surface antigen in different liver diseases. *Scand J Gastroenterol* **14**(suppl 56):55–68, 1979.
31. Borhanmesh F, Behforouz N, Sanadizadeh M, et al: Hepatitis-associated antigen in patients with liver diseases and in rural population of Iran. *Acta Hepatogastroenterol* **26**:358–363, 1979.
32. Po JY, Park CI. Lee YB: Prevalence of the hepatitis B surface antigen in various liver diseases among Koreans demonstrated by orcein staining of 614 biopsies. *Yonsei Med J* **19**:56–69, 1978.
33. Nakamura S, Takezawa Y, Sato T, et al: Hepatitis B antigens and antibodies in asymptomatic carriers and in chronic liver diseases. *Tohoku J Exp Med* **128**:81–87, 1979.
34. Tanno H, Fay O, Findor J, et al: The role of hepatitis B virus infection in patients with chronic hepatitis in Argentina. *J Med Virol* **3**:119–123, 1978.
35. Nielsen JO, Dietrichson O, Elling P, et al: Incidence and meaning of persistence of Australia antigen in patients with acute viral hepatitis: Development of chronic hepatitis. *N Engl J Med* **285**:1157–1160, 1971.
36. Smedile A, Dentico P, Zanetti A, et al: Infection with the delta (δ) agent in chronic HBsAg carriers. *Gastroenterology* **81**:992–997, 1981.
37. Beasley P, Hwang L-Y, Lin C-C, et al: Incidence of hepatitis among students at a university in Taiwan. *Am J Epidemiol* **117**:213–222, 1983.
38. Shah N, Ostrow D, Altman N, et al: Evolution of acute hepatitis B in homosexual men to chronic hepatitis B. *Arch Intern Med* **145**:881–882, 1985.
39. Szmuness W, Stevens CE, Zang EA, et al: A controlled clinical trial of the efficacy of the hepatitis B vaccine (Heptavax B): A final report. *Hepatology* **1**:377–385, 1981.
40. McMahon BJ, Alward WLM, Hall DB, et al: Acute hepatitis B virus infection: Relation of age to the clinical expression of disease and subsequent development of the carrier state. *J Infect Dis* **151**:599–603, 1985.
41. Szmuness W: On the role of certain socio-demographic factors in the epidemiology of hepatitis B. *Infection* **7**:210, 1979.
42. Ganem D: Persistent infection of humans with hepatitis B virus: Mechanisms and consequences. *Rev Infect Dis* **4**:1026–1047, 1982.
43. Koretz RL: Hepatitis: same time, same station, in Gitnick GL (ed): *Current Hepatology*, Vol. 3. New York, Wiley, 1983, pp. 1–47.
44. Koretz RL: Hepatitis: Problems and promises, in Gitnick GL (ed): *Current Hepatology*, Vol. 1. Boston, Houghton-Mifflin, 1980, pp. 1–39.
45. Eddleston ALWF, Williams R: HLA and liver disease. *Br Med Bull* **34**:295–300, 1978.

46. Giani G, Chiramonte M, Pasini CV, et al: Hepatitis B surface antigenemia and HLA antigens. (Letter.) *N Engl J Med* **300**:1056, 1979.
47. Majsky A, Horejsi J, Cerhova M, et al: Independent HBs antigen occurrence on HLA system. *Tissue Antigens* **13**:170–171, 1979.
48. Kew MC, Gear AJ, Baumgarten I, et al: Histocompatibility antigens in patients with hepatocellular carcinoma and their relationship to chronic hepatitis B virus infection in these patients. *Gastroenterology* **77**:537–539, 1979.
49. Par A, Bajtai G, Goydi E, et al: HLA antigens in chronic active hepatitis. *Acta Med Acad Sci Hung* **37**:17–24, 1980.
50. Chan SH, Wee GB, Srinivasan N, et al: HLA and Chinese HBsAg carriers. *Singapore Med J* **20**:339–349, 1979.
51. Van Hattum J, Schreuder GMT, Schalm SW: HLA antigens in patients with various courses after hepatitis B virus infection. *Hepatology* **7**:11–14, 1987.
52. Black FL, Pandey JP, Capper RA: Hepatitis B epidemiology and its relation to immunogenetic traits in South American Indians. *Am J Epidemiol* **123**:336–343, 1986.
53. Forzani B, Actis GC, Verme G, et al: HLA-DR antigens in HBsAg-positive chronic active liver disease with and without associated delta infection. *Hepatology* **4**:1107–1110, 1984.
54. Koretz RL: Hepatitis: Acute and chronic and Arthur Conan, in Gitnick GL (ed): *Current Hepatology*, Vol. 4. New York, Wiley, 1984, pp. 1–42.
55. Underhill GS, Jeffries DJ, Forsten GE, et al: Correlation between fulminant form of viral hepatitis and retrovirus infection associated with AIDS. (Letter.) *Br Med J* **292**:1080–1081, 1986.
56. Moestrup T, Hansson BG, Widell A, et al: Clinical aspects of delta infection. *Br Med J* **286**:87–90, 1983.
57. Hansson BG, Moestrup T, Widell A, et al: Infection with delta agent in Sweden: Introduction of a new hepatitis agent. *J Infect Dis* **146**:472–478, 1982.
58. Shattock AG, Morgan BM, Peutherer J, et al: High incidence of delta antigen in serum. *Lancet* **2**:104–105, 1983.
59. Shattock AG, Fielding JF: Exacerbation of chronic liver disease due to hepatitis B surface antigen after delta infection. *Br Med J* **286**:1279–1280, 1983.
60. Farci P, Smedile A, Lavarini C, et al: Delta hepatitis in inapparent carriers of hepatitis B surface antigen. *Gastroenterology* **85**:669–673, 1983.
61. McCaughan GW, Gallagher ND, Parsons L: Acute hepatitis B in a metropolitan population. *Med J Aust* **2**:333–335, 1979.
62. Norkrans G, Hermodsson S, Lundin P, et al: The long-term outcome of hepatitis B. *Infection* **4**:70–72, 1976.
63. Smedile A, Farci P, Verme G, et al: Influence of delta infection on severity of hepatitis B. *Lancet* **2**:945–947, 1981.
64. Koretz RL: Hepatitis: serious papers, funny papers, in Gitnick GL (ed): *Current Hepatology*, Vol. 7. Chicago, Year Book Medical, 1986, pp. 1–63.
65. Mosley JW, Redeker AG, Feinstone SM, et al: Multiple hepatitis viruses in multiple attacks of acute viral hepatitis. *N Engl J Med* **296**:75–78, 1977.
66. Hollinger FB, Mosley JW, Szmuness W, et al: Transfusion-transmitted viruses study: Experimental evidence for two non-A, non-B hepatitis agents. *J Infect Dis* **142**:400–407, 1980.
67. Bradley DW, Maynard JE, Cook EH, et al: Non-A, non-B hepatitis in experimentally infected chimpanzees: Cross-challenge and electron microscopic studies. *J Med Virol* **6**:185–201, 1980.
68. Yoshizawa H, Itoh Y, Iwakiri S, et al: Demonstration of two different types of non-A, non-B hepatitis by reinjection and cross-challenge studies in chimpanzees. *Gastroenterology* **81**:107–113, 1981.
69. Hollinger FB, Gitnick GL, Aach RD, et al: Non-A, non-B hepatitis transmission in chimpanzees: A project of the transfusion-transmitted viruses study group. *Intervirology* **10**:60–68, 1978.

70. Koretz RL, Stone O, Mousa M, et al: Non-A, non-B post-transfusion hepatitis—A decade later. *Gastroenterology* **88**:1251–1254, 1985.
71. Berman M, Alter HJ, Ishak KG, et al: The chronic sequelae of non-A, non-B hepatitis. *Ann Intern Med* **91**:1–6, 1979.
72. Knodell RG, Conrad ME, Ishak KG: Development of chronic liver disease after acute non-A, non-B post-transfusion hepatitis: Role of γ-globulin prophylaxis in its prevention. *Gastroenterology* **72**:902–909, 1977.
73. Tateda A, Kikuchi K, Numazaki Y, et al: Non-B hepatitis in Japanese recipients of blood transfusions: Clinical and serologic studies after introduction of laboratory screening of donor blood for hepatitis B surface antigen. *J Infect Dis* **139**:511–518, 1979.
74. Alter HJ: Post-transfusion hepatitis: Clinical features, risk, and donor testing, in Dodd RY, Barker LF (eds): *Infection, Immunity, and Blood Transfusion*. New York, Liss, 1985, pp. 47–61.
75. Nagata A, Kiyosawa K, Koike Y, et al: Epidemiology of sporadic acute non-A, non-B hepatitis in Japan: A comparison with hepatitis A and B. *Am J Gastroenterol* **80**:298–302, 1985.
76. Hyodo I, Yamada G, Nishihara T, et al: Clinical and histological features of sporadic non-A, non-B hepatiis. *Acta Med Okayama* **38**:389–401, 1984.
77. Sampliner RE, Woronow DI, Alter MJ, et al: Community-acquired non-A, non-B hepatitis. *J Med Virol* **13**:125–130, 1984.
78. Khuroo MS: Study of an epidemic of non-A, non-B hepatitis. *Am J Med* **68**:818–824, 1980.
79. Khuroo MS, Saleem M, Teli MS, et al: Failure to detect chronic liver disease after epidemic non-A, non-B hepatitis. *Lancet* **2**:97–98, 1980.
80. Kane MA, Bradley DW, Shrestha SM, et al: Epidemic non-A, non-B hepatitis. *JAMA* **252**:3140–3145, 1984.
81. Belabbes E, Boughuermouth A, Benatallah A, et al: Epidemic non-A, non-B hepatitis in Algeria. *J Med Virol* **16**:257–263, 1985.
82. Sherlock S: Predicting progression of acute type-B hepatitis to chronicity. *Lancet* **2**:354–356, 1976.
83. Tedder RS, Cameron CH, Barbara JAJ, et al: Viral hepatitis markers in blood donors with history of jaundice. (Letter.) *Lancet* **1**:595–596, 1980.
84. Koretz RL, Suffin SC, Gitnick GL: Post-transfusion chronic liver disease. *Gastroenterology* **71**:797–803, 1976.
85. Barcena R, Suarez-Garcia E, Gil LA, et al: Post-transfusion non-A, non-B hepatitis: A prospective study. *Liver* **5**:71–76, 1985.
86. Pastore G, Monno L, Santantonio T, et al: Monophasic and polyphasic pattern of alanineaminotransferase in acute non-A, non-B hepatitis: Clinical and prognostic implications. *Hepatogastroenterology* **32**:155–158, 1985.
87. Schulman AN, Fagen ND, Brezina M, et al: HBe-antigen in the course and prognosis of hepatitis B infection: A prospective study. *Gastroenterology* **78**:253–258, 1980.
88. Alberti A, Diana S, Eddleston ALWF, et al: Changes in hepatitis B virus DNA polymerase in relation to the outcome of acute hepatitis type B. *Gut* **20**:190–195, 1979.
89. Pontisso P, Bartolotti F, Schiavon E, et al: Serum hepatitis B virus DNA in acute hepatitis type B. *Digestion* **34**: 46–50, 1986.
90. Cappel R, Van Beers D, Maes F, et al: Significance of persisting IgM anti-Hbc antibodies in hepatitis B virus infection. *J Med Virol* **8**:201–205, 1981.
91. Boyer JL, Klatskin G: Pattern of necrosis in acute viral hepatitis. *N Engl J Med* **283**:1063–1071, 1970.
92. Tandon BN, Nayak NC, Tandon HD, et al: Acute viral hepatitis with bridging necrosis. Collaborative study on chronic hepatitis. *Liver* **3**:140–146, 1983.
93. Ware AJ, Cuthbert JA, Shorey J, et al: A prospective trial of steroid therapy in severe viral hepatitis. *Gastroenterology* **80**:219–224, 1981.

Hepatitis Prophylaxis

BARBARA G. WERNER and GEORGE F. GRADY

INTRODUCTION

Prophylaxis is discussed traditionally in terms of preexposure and postexposure situations. In the case of preexposure prophylaxis, the practitioner must commit to a current action of uncertain necessity that carries a specific risk of adverse reactions. For postexposure prophylaxis, the need to deal with a present danger is clear but there is a reduced efficacy of the late-starting immunoprophylaxis. Intervention may be by either passive or active immunization. In passive immunization, the patient receives short-term protection from antibody present in immune globulins (IG), whereas an active response to vaccine is expected to produce endogenous antibody and long-term immunity. In some situations, a combined passive–active immunization may result from IG that attenuates infection without inhibiting antibody production.

IMMUNOGLOBULIN FOR PASSIVE IMMUNIZATION

Immunoglobulin G (IgG) fraction of human plasma contains antibodies against a wide array of bacterial and viral antigens. Studies describing their use for the prevention of viral hepatitis extend back to the 1940s.[1,2] Today intravenous (IV) as well as intramuscular (IM) formulations exist for prevention or attenuation of a variety of diseases. The IM formulation of IG is the only practical mode for office practice. With this formulation, however, the volume injected at each site must be limited to no more than 2–3 ml because swelling and pain can result from the hypertonicity of U.S.-manufactured preparations, which are usually 16% protein. Some of the European products are less concentrated. The

BARBARA G. WERNER and GEORGE F. GRADY • Massachusetts Center for Disease Control, Department of Public Health, and Department of Medicine, Tufts University School of Medicine, Boston, Massachusetts 02130.

intramuscular formulation in the United States has remained unchanged since the earliest licensure studies showed that small volumes are efficacious and stable at high concentrations. Intravenous formulations are an alternative if large volumes are indicated; however, higher cost and delivery logistics must be considered.

Protection in passive immunization is limited by the continuously declining levels of exogenous antibody and by the impracticality of spacing doses too closely. The lower the likelihood that hepatitis would occur in the absence of prophylaxis, the more one must keep the possibility of adverse reactions in mind. Possible side effects include anaphylaxis (rarely), angioneurotic edema or rash, bleeding or soreness at the injection site, and misplaced injections (e.g., into the sciatic nerve, intradermally, or intravenously—possibly one of the causes of rare anaphylactic reactions). Minor reactions occur with a frequency of about 2–3%, whereas the more serious ones occur in about 1 : 1000 injections.

The gluteal region normally provides the necessary muscle bed for the recommended deep IM injection, hence is the preferred site. Smaller amounts, e.g., a single dose of ≤2 ml, are sometimes given in the deltoid for reasons of convenience or the modesty of some patients (see Table I for usage).

HEPATITIS A

Immunoglobulin Usage

An immunoglobulin dose on a body-weight basis of 0.02 ml/kg or 0.01 ml/lb is usually protective against short-term exposure to hepatitis A.[3] No potency standard exists for hepatitis A antibody in IG, but Federal Drug Administration (FDA) studies have shown that all commercial IG preparations contain an amount presumed to be adequate.[3,4] International travelers to developing countries are a major target for preexposure prophylaxis of hepatitis A. For such travelers, a single IG dose of 0.02 ml/kg is recommended if travel is for less than 2 months. If extended travel is anticipated, 0.06 ml/kg should be given every 5 months.[3]

Children and staff in day-care centers are another group at increased risk of hepatitis A infection. Although continuously repeating IG injections is of limited practicality and may increase the risk of adverse reaction, a series of two or three doses of IG may cover an initial period of risk or attenuate natural infection and result in passive–active immunization.

If the typical incubation period of hepatitis A is assumed to be about 30 days, globulin given before exposure or during the first 10 days of the incubation period can be expected to be about 80–90% protective. If given during the second 10 days, it is only about 50% effective, and if delayed beyond 20 days it is of only marginal value. Protection refers to attenuation or modification of the infection such that clinical disease does not develop. Globulin given early may abort infection so completely that virus shedding in the stool is also prevented.

Appropriate postexposure prophylaxis may require serologic testing to determine the type of hepatitis and the immune status of those involved. Hepatitis A is transmitted primarily by person-to-person contact or by infected food or water, generally through inadvertent fecal contamination. If hepatitis A is suspected, serologic confirmation of the index case is recommended before prophylaxis of contacts. The diagnosis of acute hepatitis A is confirmed by finding IgM-class anti-HAV in serum collected during the acute or early convalescent phase of disease. In the index case, IgG-class anti-HAV in the absence of IgM is inconsistent with current hepatitis A infection; rather, it indicates immunity against disease following infection at some undetermined time in the past. IgG antibody in the contacts of a hepatitis A case indicates immunity and the lack of need for IG. In actual practice, however, the redundancy of IG administration to antibody-positive contacts is accepted to make sure of early administration to those who truly need IG, and because cost-efficiency considerations argue against routine testing to identify susceptible patients.

Because the index case of hepatitis A does not present continuous exposure to contacts, i.e., there is no long-term carrier state, a single IM dose of 0.02 ml/kg IG is recommended for postexposure prophylaxis unless there is subsequent evidence of a multigenerational outbreak.[3] For simplicity, an alternative dosage can be employed: 2.0 ml for adults, 1.0 ml for children weighing 50–100 lb, and 0.5 ml for smaller children. IG is generally available in 2-, 5-, or 10-ml vials.

Postexposure prophylaxis of hepatitis A using IG is indicated for all household and sexual contacts of persons with hepatitis A as well as for staff and attendees of day-care centers in which hepatitis A cases are seen. Workers at day-care centers with children in diapers should be especially aware of the possibility of transmission of hepatitis A in this setting. Since casual contact in nonhousehold settings does not result in virus transmission, routine IG administration is not indicated for the usual school, office, factory, or hospital settings. If epidemiologic studies indicate that transmission is occurring, prophylaxis may, however, be indicated for contacts in these settings.[3]

A foodhandler with diagnosed hepatitis A represents a special case since common source transmission occurs occasionally. Co-workers in the food service establishment should be given IG as soon as possible, unless prior evidence of immunity exists. If the index case handles foods that are served without cooking without gloves, and if patrons can be identified and treated within 2 weeks of exposure, IG should be considered for them as well.

Hepatitis A Vaccines

Live attentuated and killed vaccines against hepatitis A are under evaluation and have proved to be immunogenic in animal studies.[5–7] Live attentuated vaccine candidates must induce a protective antibody response without causing

TABLE I. Pre- and Postexposure Prophylaxis Recommendations[a]

Group	Preexposure				Postexposure			
	Hepatitis A	Hepatitis B	Hepatitis NANB (enteric)	Hepatitis NANB (bloodborne)	Hepatitis A	Hepatitis B	Hepatitis NANB (enteric)	Hepatitis NANB (bloodborne)
Children								
Universal	[V]?				IG	HBIG or HBIG, V[c]	IG?	IG
Day care								
Routine	[V]				IG	HBIG	IG?	IG
High risk	IG, [V]	V?			IG	HBIG, V	IG?	IG
Immigrants from endemic areas	[V]?	V[b]			IG	HBIG, V	IG?	IG
Institutionalized (developmentally disabled)	IG, [V]	V			IG	HBIG, V	IG?	IG
Born to infected mother			IG?	IG?	IG	HBIG, V	IG?	IG

Adults					
Sexual exposures					
Homosexual males	IG?	V		HBIG, V	IG?	IG
Prostitutes		V		HBIG, V	IG?	IG
Multiple partners		V?		HBIG, V	IG?	IG
Spouses		V		HBIG, or HBIG, V[c]	IG?	IG
IV drug abusers		V	IG?	HBIG, V	IG?	IG
Health care workers						
Laboratory		V		HBIG, V	IG?	IG
Medical/surgical		V		HBIG, V	IG?	IG
Institutional		V		HBIG, V	IG?	IG
First responder		V	IG?	HBIG, V	IG?	IG
Traveler (international)	IG	V[b]	IG?	HBIG, or HBIG, V	IG?	IG[b]
Transfusion recipients	IG			HBIG	IG?	IG

[a] IG, immune globulin; HBIG, hepatitis B immune globulin; V, vaccine; [V], vaccine pending future availability.
[b] See ref. 3.
[c] Vaccine if continued exposure likely.

even mild hepatitis. Formalin-inactivated vaccines are not accompanied by the worry of causing hepatitis but may need to be given in multiple doses to elicit effective antibody. Even though some candidate vaccines have undergone limited trials in human volunteers,[5,8,9] licensed products probably will not be available for several years.

Prime targets will be children and staff of day-care centers and institutions for the developmentally disabled. Consideration might also be given to routine immunization of all children in the future, after initial experience establishes safety and efficacy in higher-risk groups (see Table I).

HEPATITIS B

Immunoglobulin Usage

Passive immunization is recommended for sexual exposure to hepatitis B virus (HBV) if additional exposure is not anticipated[3]; (Table II). Infectivity of the source person is indicated by the presence of hepatitis B surface antigen (HB_sAg). In situations for which globulin is indicated, hepatitis B immune globulin (HBIG) is preferred to IG in spite of higher cost. The titer of specific anti-HB_s in HBIG is approximately 1000 times that in IG, but IG may be used to provide some protection if HBIG is unobtainable. Current recommendations for pre-exposure and postexposure generally call for use of vaccine (active immu-

TABLE II. Hepatitis B Virus Postexposure Recommendations[a]

	HBIG		Vaccine[b]	
	Dose	Recommended timing	Dose	Recommended timing
Perinatal exposure	0.5 ml IM	Within 12 hours	0.5 ml (10 μg) IM (plasma derived) 0.5 ml (5 μg) IM (recombinant)	Within 12 hours of birth[c]; repeat at 1 and 6 months
Sexual exposure	0.06 ml/kg IM	Single dose within 14 days of sexual contact		

[a]Adapted from ref. 3.
[b]Vaccine is recommended for homosexual men and for regular sexual contacts of hepatitis B virus carriers. It is optional in initial treatment of heterosexual contacts of persons with acute hepatitis B but may be given if slow resolution of infection presents continued risk.
[c]The first dose can be given at the same time as the dose of hepatitis B immune globulin (HBIG) but at a different site. IM = intramuscular.

TABLE III. Recommendations for Hepatitis B Prophylaxis
after Percutaneous Exposure[a]

HB$_s$Ag status of source	Exposed person	
	Unvaccinated	Vaccinated
HB$_s$Ag positive	One dose of HBIG[b] immediately Initiate HB vaccine series	Confirm that exposed person has anti-HBs (>10 sample ratio units by RIA, or positive by EIA) If not, give one dose of HBIG[b] immediately plus HB vaccine booster dose
High probability HB$_s$Ag positive	Initiate HB vaccine series Test source for HB$_s$Ag; if positive, give HBIG[b]	If exposed person is vaccine non-responder and if source is HB$_s$Ag positive, give one dose of HBIG[b] immediately plus HB vaccine booster dose
Low probability HB$_s$Ag positive	Initiate HB vaccine series	Nothing required
Unknown source	Initiate HB vaccine series; IG optional	Nothing required; IG optional

[a]Adapted from ref. 3.
[b]One dose of hepatitis B immune globulin (HBIG) is 0.06 ml/kg body weight, intramuscularly. HB$_s$Ag, hepatitis B surface antigen; RIA, radioimmunoassay; EIA, enzyme immunoassay; anti-HB$_s$, antibody to HBsAg.
[c]Hepatitis B vaccine series using plasma-derived vaccine, e.g., Heptavax B, is 20 μg intramuscularly for adults, 10 μg intramuscularly for infants or children under 10 years of age; the series using recombinant vaccine, e.g., Recombivax, is 10 μg IM for adults and 5 μg for children. The first dose is given within 1 week of exposure, and the second and third doses, 1 and 6 months later, respectively.

nization) or for globulin in conjunction with vaccine (another type of passive–active immunization). HBIG alone is partially effective in preventing the chronic carrier state following perinatal transmission[10] and will reduce the amount of hepatitis B following accidental needlestick inoculation[11,12] (Tables I and III).

Hepatitis B Vaccines

Two U.S.-manufactured vaccines are currently licensed: a vaccine derived from human plasma (Heptavax-B; Merck Sharp & Dohme) available since mid-1982, and a recombinant vaccine (Recombivax HB; Merck Sharp & Dohme) on the market since early 1987 (Table IV). The plasma-derived vaccine consists of purified noninfectious 22-nm HB$_s$Ag particles that induce the protective anti-HB$_s$ in recipients.[13] Antibodies to other viral components, hepatitis B core and e antigens (HB$_c$Ag and HB$_e$Ag) are not produced. The recombinant vaccine is produced by the yeast, *Saccharomyces cerevisiae*, into which a plasmid

TABLE IV. Characteristics of U.S. Licensed Hepatitis B Vaccines

	Plasma derived	Yeast derived
Antigen source	Plasma from human hepatitis B carriers	Yeast carrying a plasmid with gene for HB_sAg
Purification	Ammonium sulfate Isopycnic banding Rate zonal sedimentation	Cell disruption Chromatography: hydrophobic interaction, size exclusion
Treatment	Urea, pepsin, formaldehyde	Formaldehyde
HB_sAg particle	22 nm	17–25 nm
Subtype	ad	ad
Adjuvant	Aluminum hydroxide	Aluminum hydroxide
Preservative	Thimerosal	Thimerosal
Protective efficacy (chimpanzees)	adr, ayw subtypes	adr, ayw subtypes
Name	Heptavax—B	Recombivax HB
Dose		
Adults	20 μg	10 μg
Children	10 μg	5 μg
Schedule	0, 1, 6 months	0, 1, 6 months
Immunogenicity	>90% seroconversion	>90% seroconversion Titers <Heptavax
Protection duration	5–7 yr	?
Tolerance	Good	Good

containing the gene for HB_sAg has been inserted.[14] The purified recombinant HB_sAg particles are 17–25 nm in diameter and are similar in appearance to human plasma-derived HB_sAg. Both vaccines are safe, immunogenic, efficacious, and equally costly. A superior immunogenicity of the plasma-derived vaccine was seen in most studies.[15–17] Because higher titers of antibody increase the duration of detectable antibody, fewer or less frequent booster doses may be needed.[18] The long-term duration of immunity induced by the plasma-derived vaccine is not known, but it appears to be at least 5–7 years.[19,20] No formal recommendations for timing of booster doses currently exist.[20]

Testing after vaccination is not routinely recommended because more than 90% of healthy persons are expected to respond adequately. Selected persons, such as dialysis patients whose response may be expected to be suboptimal, should be tested to confirm an immune response. In addition, some healthy persons at risk of hepatitis B infections may choose, for personal reassurance, to have postimmunization tests for anti-HB_s.

Subunit polypeptide vaccines[21–23] or chemically synthesized polypeptide vaccines[24] and vaccines produced using other recombinant viruses[25,26] are currently in the research and development stage, and may someday replace the currently available vaccines as alternative means of immunoprophylaxis.

Vaccine can be used effectively in combination with HBIG for postexposure prophylaxis. Studies of plasma-derived and recombinant vaccine indicate that the exogenously administered anti-HB$_s$ from the IG does not interfere with a recipient's ability to respond to vaccine given in separate sites.[17,27] This passive–active immunization approach is recommended for prophylaxis in infants born to HBV carrier mothers, in recipients of accidental needlesticks, and in those who may experience repeated sexual contact with chronic carriers or individuals at high risk for hepatitis B infection.[3,20] Current dosage recommendations are shown in Tables II and III.

Some people may not respond even to two full series (six doses) of the plasma-derived vaccine; insufficient information is available to indicate whether nonresponders will respond to revaccination with the recombinant vaccine. Interestingly, the nonresponders do not necessarily become chronic carriers if infected with HBV after failing to respond.[13] Failure to respond is not fully understood; one study found certain HLA haplotypes to be associated with failure to respond.[28] We also know that a lower response rate is associated with increased age and body weight of vaccine recipients. Site of injection is important; reduced response is seen with buttock injection.[29] The plasma-derived or recombinant HB vaccine should be given to older children and adults in the deltoid muscle and to neonates and infants in the anterolateral thigh muscle.[20] A reduced response rate has been reported among dialysis patients in some studies[30] and, at this time, only the plasma-derived vaccine is recommended for these patients.[20] Because both licensed vaccines lose potency if frozen, proper storage is essential to maximize immunogenicity. The vaccines should be stored at 2–6°C (36–43°F).

DELTA HEPATITIS

Hepatitis delta virus (HDV) is a defective virus dependent on the presence of HB$_s$Ag for its expression. HDV infection can occur as a co-infection with HBV or by superinfection of HBV chronic carriers. No specific prophylaxis for HDV infection exists at present but, because HDV is so uniquely dependent on HBV, prevention is achievable incidental to immunization against hepatitis B unless the individual already is a HB$_s$Ag carrier. Therefore, the preexposure and postexposure recommendations are the same as for HB; the prevention of HBV infection will prevent HDV infection.[3]

NON-A, NON-B (NANB) HEPATITIS

NANB hepatitis appears to be caused by multiple viruses that fall into two major categories. One category seen in developed countries consists of at least

TABLE V. Prophylaxis of Posttransfusion NANB Hepatitis[a]

Study	Mean units of blood	IG dosage schedule	Incidence of icteric NANB hepatitis	
			Immunoglobulin	Placebo
Seeff et al.[38]	3	Dose 1: 0–4 days	9/1094 (0.8%)	20/1110 (1.8%)
		Dose 2: 28 days		
Knodell et al.[39]	12	Dose 1: before transfusion	1/93 (1.1%)	7/94 (7.4%)[b]
Kuhns et al.[40]	18	Dose 1: 3–10 days	6/93 (6.5%)	8/102 (7.8%)
		Dose 2: 30 days		

[a]Adapted from ref. 2.
[b]$p < 0.05$; also reduced incidence of chronic NANB.

two distinct agents that seem to be responsible for a parenterally transmitted form epidemiologically similar to hepatitis B.[31–33] The other category contains a fecally transmitted NANB, more like hepatitis A, that is endemic to the Indian subcontinent, Southeast Asia, and Africa.[33–35] Epidemic transmission of this enterically transmitted form (ET-NANB) has only recently been reported in the Americas, in two villages in Mexico.[36] Limited data suggest that pooled IG from Mexico was not effective in preventing subsequent cases of ET-NANB hepatitis. The enteric or epidemic form of NANB has been identified in the United States in only a few people whose probable exposure was in endemic areas.[37] Therefore, IG prepared in the United States may lack specific antibody and is of uncertain value for passive immunoprophylaxis of this type of NANB hepatitis.

Although specific prophylaxis, passive or active, is not possible without clear identification of the viral agents involved, there is limited evidence to suggest that IG may be beneficial in modification of posttransfusion NANB (Table V). From these posttransfusion studies as well as experimental studies in chimpanzees, it seems reasonable to administer IG 0.06 ml/kg as soon as possible to persons with percutaneous exposure to blood from a NANB hepatitis patient.

STERILIZATION OR DISINFECTION OF INSTRUMENTS AND WORK AREAS

The human hepatitis viruses (A, B, and NANB) are susceptible to common methods of sterilization and disinfection, but disposable equipment should be used when possible to minimize any risk of cross-contamination. Sharp items that may be contaminated with blood or other infectious body fluids should be handled and disposed of with special care to prevent accidental injuries. Environmental surfaces and nondisposable instruments or devices should be thoroughly washed before terminal disinfection or sterilization. Precleaning of surfaces with detergent washes away excess contaminants and provides access for disinfecting agents. In addition to disinfectants ordinarily used by health care facilities, a fresh solution of 5000 ppm sodium hypochlorite (household bleach at a 1 : 10 dilution) is an inexpensive and effective germicide.[41] Additional safety recommendations, including selection of methods for sterilization, appear in the cited reviews.[42,43]

FEAR OF AIDS

Concerns about the safety of IG preparations and the plasma-derived hepatitis B vaccine with respect to human immunodeficiency virus (HIV) infections have proved to be unfounded. Mandatory screening of all donor blood for antibody to human immunodeficiency virus (anti-HIV) is the major method for excluding HIV. Viral inactivation and partitioning during alcohol fractionation of plasma in the preparation of IG also help ensure safety.[44] No well-documented cases of acquired immune deficiency syndrome (AIDS) attributable to administration of IGs have been seen.

No human or animal plasma is used in the preparation of recombinant HB vaccine; the manufacturing process for plasma-derived HB vaccine includes multiple purification steps that inactivate known infectious agents, including retroviruses such as HIV.[45] AIDS has not occurred among vaccine recipients who did not have a history of risk factors. Furthermore, no seroconversion to anti-HIV was observed among a group of health care workers tested after receiving the plasma-derived vaccine.[46] Persons at risk of hepatitis should not procrastinate about following the recommendations for prophylaxis.[3,20]

REFERENCES

1. Maynard JE: Passive and active immunization in the control of viral hepatitis, in Szmuness W, Alter HJ, Maynard JE (eds): *Viral Hepatitis*. Philadelphia, The Franklin Institute Press, 1982, pp. 379–384.
2. Grady GF: Prevention of hepatitis by passive immunization, in Dienhardt F, Dienhardt J (eds): *Viral Hepatitis: Laboratory and Clinical Science*. New York, Dekker, 1983, pp. 241–256.
3. ACIP: Recommendations for protection against viral hepatitis. *MMWR* **34:**313–324, 329–335, 1985.
4. Smallwood LA, Tabor E, Finlayson JS, Gerety RJ: Antibodies to hepatitis A virus in immune serum globulin. *J Med Virol* **7:**21–27, 1981.
5. McLean AA: Development of vaccines against hepatitis A and hepatitis B. *Rev Infect Dis* **8:**591–598, 1986.
6. Provost PJ, Emini EA: Progress towards the development of a hepatitis A vaccine, in *International Symposium on Viral Hepatitis and Liver Disease, London, 1987*, p. 24 (abst).
7. Binn LN, Bancroft WH, Eckels KH, et al: Inactivated hepatitis A virus vaccine produced in

human diploid MRC-5 cells, in: *International Symposium on Viral Hepatitis and Liver Disease, London, 1987*, p. 25 (abst).

8. Sjogren MH, Eckels KH, Binn LN, et al: Safety and immunogenicity of an inactivated hepatitis A vaccine in volunteers, in: *International Symposium on Viral Hepatitis and Liver Disease, London, 1987*, p. 25 (abst).

9. Flemmig B, Haage A, Heinricy V, Pfisterer M. Immunogenicity of a hepatitis A vaccine, in: *International Symposium on Viral Hepatitis and Liver Disease, London, 1987*, p. 25 (abst).

10. Stevens CE, Beasley RP, Lin C-C, et al: Perinatal hepatitis B virus infection: Use of hepatitis B immune globulin, in: Szmuness W, Alter HJ, Maynard JE (eds): *Viral Hepatitis*. Philadelphia, Franklin Institute Press, 1982, pp. 527–535.

11. Seeff LB, Wright EC, Zimmerman HJ, et al: Type B hepatitis after needle-stick exposure: Prevention with hepatitis B immune globulin: Final report of the VA Cooperative Study. *Ann Intern Med* **88:**285–293, 1978.

12. Grady GF, Lee VA, Prince AM, et al: Hepatitis B immune globulin for accidental exposures among medical personnel: Final report of a multi-center controlled trial. *J Infect Dis* **138:**626–638, 1978.

13. Szmuness W, Stevens CE, Harley EJ, et al: Hepatitis B vaccine: Demonstration of efficacy in a controlled clinical trial in a high-risk population in the United States. *N Engl J Med* **303:**833–841, 1980.

14. McAleer WJ, Buynak EB, Maigetter RZ, et al: Human hepatitis B vaccine from recombinant yeast. *Nature (Lond)* **307:**178–180, 1984.

15. Davidson M, Krugman S: Recombinant yeast hepatitis B vaccine compared with plasma derived vaccine: Immunogenicity and effect of a booster dose. *J Infect* **13**(suppl A):31–38, 1986.

16. Hollinger FB, Troisi CL, Pepe PE: Anti-HBs responses to vaccination with a human hepatitis B vaccine made by recombinant DNA technology in yeast. *J Infect Dis* **153:**156–159, 1986.

17. Stevens CE, Taylor PE, Tong MJ, et al: Yeast-recombinant hepatitis B vaccine: Efficacy with hepatitis B immune globulin in prevention of perinatal hepatitis B virus transmission. *JAMA* **257:**2612–2616, 1987.

18. Hollinger FB: Hepatitis B vaccines—to switch or not to switch. (Editorial.) *JAMA* **257:**2634–2636, 1987.

19. Krugman S, Davidson M: Hepatitis B vaccine: Prospects for duration of immunity. *Yale J Biol Med* **60:**333–338, 1987.

20. ACIP: Update on hepatitis B prevention. *MMWR* **36:**353–360, 366, 1987.

21. Tabor E, Howard CR, Skelly J, et al: Immunogenicity in chimpanzees of experimental hepatitis B vaccines made from intact hepatitis B virus, purified polypeptides or polypeptides in micelles. *J Med Virol* **10:**65–74, 1982.

22. Sanchez Y, Ionescu-Matiu I, Melnick JL, et al: Comparative studies of the immunogenic activity of hepatitis B surface antigen (HBsAg) and HBsAg polypeptides. *J Med Virol* **11:**115–124, 1983.

23. Howard CR, Young P, Steward MW, et al: Development of novel hepatitis B vaccines. *Dev Biol Std* **59:**89–98, 1985.

24. Brown SE, Howard CR, Zuckerman AJ, et al: Affinity of antibody responses in man to hepatitis B vaccine determined with synthetic peptides. *Lancet* **2:**184–187, 1984.

25. Moss B, Smith GL, Gerin JL, et al: Live recombinant vaccinia virus protects chimpanzees against hepatitis B. *Nature (Lond)* **311:**67–69, 1984.

26. Paoletti E, Lipinskas BR, Samsonoff C, et al: Construction of live vaccines using genetically engineered poxviruses: Biological activity of vaccinia virus recombinants expressing the hepatitis B surface antigen and the herpes simplex virus glycoprotein D. *Proc Natl Acad Sci USA* **81:**193–197, 1984.

27. Beasley RP, Hwang LY, Lee GC, et al: Prevention of perinatally transmitted hepatitis B

infections with hepatitis B immune globulin and hepatitis B vaccine. *Lancet* **2:**1099–1102, 1983.

28. Craven DE, Awdeh ZL, Kunches LM, et al: Nonresponsiveness to hepatitis B vaccine in health care workers. *Ann Intern Med* **105:**356–360, 1986.

29. Centers for Disease Control: Suboptimal response to hepatitis B vaccine given by injection into the buttock. *MMWR* **34:**105–109, 1985.

30. Stevens CE, Alter HJ, Taylor PE, et al: Hepatitis B vaccine in patients receiving hemodialysis: Immunogenicity and efficacy. *N Engl J Med* **311:**496–501, 1984.

31. Aach RD, Szmuness W, Mosley JW, et al: Serum alanine aminotransferase of donors in relation to the risk of non-A, non-B hepatitis in recipients. *N Engl J Med* **304:**989–994, 1981.

32. Hollinger FB, Alter HJ, Holland PV, Aach RD: Non-A, non-B posttransfusion hepatitis in the United States, in Gerety RJ (ed): *Non-A, Non-B Hepatitis*. New York, Academic, 1981, pp. 49–70.

33. Bradley DW, Maynard JE: Etiology and natural history of post-transfusion and enterically-transmitted non-A, non-B hepatitis. *Semin Liver Dis* **6:**56–66, 1986.

34. Wong DC, Purcell RH, Sreenivasan MA, et al: Epidemic and endemic hepatitis in India: Evidence for a non-A, non-B hepatitis virus aetiology. *Lancet* **2:**876–879, 1980.

35. Khuroo MS: Study of an epidemic of non-A, non-B hepatitis: Possibility of another type of human hepatitis virus distinct from post-transfusion non-A, non-B type. *Am J Med* **68:**818–824, 1980.

36. Center for Disease Control: Enterically transmitted non-A, non-B hepatitis—Mexico. *MMWR* **36:**597–602, 1987.

37. DeCock KM, Bradley DW, Sandford NL, et al: Epidemic non-A, non-B hepatitis in patients from Pakistan. *Ann Intern Med* **106:**227–230, 1987.

38. Seeff LB, Zimmerman HJ, Wright EC, and the Veterans Administration Cooperative Study Group: A randomized, double-blind controlled trial of the efficacy of immune serum globulin for the prevention of post-transfusion hepatitis. *Gastroenterology* **72:**111–121, 1977.

39. Knodell RG, Conrad ME, Ginsberg AL, et al: Efficacy of prophylactic gammaglobulin in preventing non-A, non-B post-transfusion hepatitis. *Lancet* **1:**557–561, 1976.

40. Kuhns WJ, Prince AM, Brotman B, et al: A clinical and laboratory evaluation of immune serum globulin from donors with a history of hepatitis: Attempted prevention of post-transfusion hepatitis. *Am J Med Sci* **272:**255–261, 1977.

41. Bond WW, Petersen NJ, Favero MS: Viral hepatitis B: Aspects of environmental control. *Health Lab Sci* **14:**235–252, 1977.

42. Favero MS: Sterilization, disinfection, and antisepsis in the hospital, in: *Manual of Clinical Microbiology*, 4th Ed. Washington, DC, American Society for Microbiology, 1985, pp. 129–137.

43. Garner JS, Favero MS: *Guideline for Handwashing and Hospital Environmental Control, 1985*. Publication No. 99-1117. Atlanta: Centers for Disease Control, 1985.

44. Wells M, Wittek A, Epstein J, et al: Inactivation and partitioning of human T-cell lymphotropic virus, type III, during ethanol fractionation of plasma. *Transfusion* **26:**210–213, 1986.

45. Francis DP, Feorino PM, McDougal S, et al: The safety of hepatitis B vaccine: Inactivation of the AIDS virus during routine vaccine manufacture. *JAMA* **256:**869–872, 1986.

46. Dienstag JL, Werner BG, McLane MF, et al: Absence of antibodies to human T cell leukemia virus, type III in health workers after hepatitis B vaccination. *JAMA* **254:**1064–1066, 1985.

Toxic and Drug-Induced Hepatitis

ANDREW STOLZ

INTRODUCTION

The liver is the major site for the biotransformation of drugs and toxins. The formation of reactive metabolites during this process of biotransformation places the liver at risk for the development of hepatic injury. This chapter reviews the basic principles and classifications of drug-induced hepatic injury, with emphasis on hepatocellular damage. In addition, recent advances are presented in a select number of drugs that may cause hepatitis.

CLASSIFICATION OF DRUG-INDUCED LIVER INJURY

Various systems for the classification of drug-induced liver injury exist based on clinical presentation, histopathology, and mechanisms of toxicity. Drugs or toxins can be broadly separated into two groups: predictable and non-predictable hepatotoxins. A predictable hepatotoxin is one in which toxicity occurs in a dose-related fashion and is often reproducible in a laboratory animal model. In most of these cases, the parent drug is metabolized in a predictable fashion to form a toxic metabolite. This metabolite may overwhelm the liver's normal mechanism for detoxification allowing for this reactive species to disable critical proteins or membrane structures required for normal hepatocellular function. Eventually, a critical number of targets are affected, and cell death occurs. The exact mechanism for cell death is still unknown and is an area of active

ANDREW STOLZ • Department of Medicine, UCLA School of Medicine, Los Angeles, California 90024; and Wadsworth Veterans Administration Medical Center, Los Angeles, California 90073.

investigation. The prime examples of predictable hepatotoxins are the analgesic agent, acetaminophen, and the organic solvent, carbon tetrachloride. Although the mechanisms of toxicity are best understood for these classes of hepatotoxins, these drugs clinically account for only a small percentage of the overall drug-induced hepatocellular injury.

Most drugs are unpredictable hepatotoxins that occur in only a small percentage of patients.[1] Toxicity with these drugs may occur during varying length of treatment or after previous exposure to the agent. Often, no reliable animal model exists for these toxins. Unpredictable toxins may be classified into two categories, depending on the presence or absence of immunological features associated with the hepatotoxicity. Those patients with immune-mediated disease may present with fever, rash, and eosinophilia and have a history of prior exposure to the therapeutic agent. Sensitization of lymphocytes to newly generated epitopes on hepatic plasma membranes is thought to be one of the bases for this hepatotoxicity. These new epitopes may be generated by reactive metabolites of the parent drug interacting with plasma membranes creating neoantigens. Patients may be susceptible to idiosyncratic, non-immune-mediated drug toxicity because of multiple factors. These factors include genetic variations in the biotransformation capacity, environment factors, such as concomitant drugs or alcohol use, decreased detoxification capacity, or a combination of all three. Previous studies have identified genetic variability in content and properties of the mixed-function oxidase enzymes that participate in phase I hydroxylation reactions. A concomitant drug may compete for the same biotransformation enzyme or lead to the induction of the cytochrome P450 resulting in an increased production of a toxic metabolite. Pharmacokinetic effects such as delayed excretion of the drug may also influence the development of hepatotoxicity. Thus, the development of unpredictable, non-immune-mediated hepatotoxicity may have multifactorial causes with various interactions between environmental and genetic factors.

BIOTRANSFORMATION OF DRUGS

The liver is remarkably designed to biotransform a host of endogenous and exogenous compounds. Typically, the liver transforms a lipophilic poorly water-soluble compound into a hydrophilic compound that then may be eliminated by excretion into urine or bile. Usually, this process sequentially proceeds by two distinct steps, referred to as phases I and II of biotransformation. Phase I consists of oxidation of the drug by the mixed-function oxidases, the cytochrome P450 system. During the formation of this hydroxylated compound, reactive metabolites can be generated that may react with macromolecules, including the cytochrome P450 components themselves. The newly positioned hydroxyl group on the drug is now available for conjugation with either glucuronide, sulfate, amino acids, or glutathione. Conjugation with these compounds enhances the polarity of the parent compound, leading to its ultimate excretion. Occasionally, phase II conjugation may occur before phase I. Compounds possessing a hydroxyl group may undergo conjugation directly by phase II enzymes.

MECHANISM OF DIRECT-ACTING TOXINS

Reactive metabolites generated by the cytochrome P450 system may be divided into two groups: electrophiles and free radicals. Electrophiles are produced as intermediates during the oxidation of the drug. These electrophile intermediates seek nucleophiles to covalently bind to, which stabilizes these reactive intermediates. The predominant nucleophile within hepatocytes is thiol groups of cysteine which are present in proteins and in the tripeptide, gamma-glutamylcysteinylglycine, glutathione. One of the important routes for the detoxification of electrophilic intermediates of drug metabolism is via conjugation to glutathione (GSH). This conjugation may proceed chemically but is most often catalyzed by the glutathione S-transferases, a family of cytosolic enzymes involved in detoxification of a wide variety of electrophiles. In the case of acetaminophen and the toxin bromobenzene, the generation of electrophilic metabolites may overwhelm the hepatic GSH allowing for electrophiles to interact with other thiol groups present in proteins. Covalent binding to these thiols can result in inactivation of the protein (enzyme), leading to cell death. Acetaminophen and bromobenzene exhibit a distinct GSH concentration below which cell necrosis routinely occurs. This GSH threshold is not typical for other electrophilic toxins.

The other major class of reactive metabolites are free radicals that contain an unpaired electron.[2] These free radicals may be produced by either reduction or oxidation by the cytochrome P450 system. In low oxygen concentrations, the cytochrome P450 system may transfer only one electron to the drug, yielding a free radical metabolite. Oxygen concentration therefore may influence the route of metabolism of a drug. This free radical may then covalently bind to either proteins or abstract an electron from unsaturated fatty acids, leading to the formation of fatty acid radicals. These fatty acids may then lead to lipid peroxidation which may ultimately effect the physicochemical integrity of the membrane. This loss of membrane function is presumed to play a key role in cell death.

HISTOPATHOLOGIC CLASSIFICATION

Drug- and toxin-induced hepatocellular necrosis may histologically appear indistinguishable from any form of hepatobiliary disease, including acute or chronic viral hepatitis.[3,4] Hepatocellular necrosis may be either diffuse as occurs with viral hepatitis or appear in discrete acinar zones of the Rapoport model. The appearance of discrete zonal necrosis is highly suggestive of toxin or drug induced injury. Centrizonal necrosis is characteristically produced by carbon tetrachloride, chloroform, acetaminophen, halothane, and other halogenated biphenyls. The susceptibility of the pericentral zone to drug-induced injury has been theorized to be due to the greater concentration of the cytochrome P450 present in this zone. In addition, the lower oxygen concentration in the pericentral zone may potentiate formation of free radicals by the cytochrome P450 system. Ischemic liver disease also produces a similar pattern of injury suggesting a common pathophysiological mechanism. Discrete periportal zonal necrosis rarely occurs and may be produced experimentally by allyl alcohols. Allyl alcohols are metabolized by the nonmicrosomal enzyme alcohol dehydrogenase into the toxic metabolite, acrolein. Inhibition of alcohol dehydrogenase by the specific inhibitor, pyrazole, protects the liver from periportal necrosis. Hepatic infiltration with eosinophils, lymphocytes, and the presence of granuloma formation suggest an immune-mediated process. This pattern of injury is most often found with immune-mediated unpredictable hepatotoxicity.

CLINICAL FEATURES OF DRUG-INDUCED HEPATITIS

The clinical features of drug-induced hepatitis are indistinguishable from typical viral hepatitis. Patients present with fatigue, malaise, fever, and right upper quadrant pain. Jaundice may develop depending on the severity of the liver injury. Drug-induced injury is suggested by a history of recent onset of a therapeutic agent or evidence for an immune-mediated process. Laboratory examination demonstrates transaminase elevation with minimal elevation of the cholestatic marker, alkaline phosphatase. Patients may also present with a mixed picture, with features of both cholestatic and hepatocellular necrosis. The development of fever, rash, eosinophilia, and immunologic markers, such as antimitochondrial antibody (AMA) and antinuclear antibody (ANA) suggest an immune-mediated process. Recognition of toxin- or drug-induced liver disease is an important clinical consideration. Generally, drug-induced disease rapidly improves with discontinuation of the offending agent. Prognosis is usually excellent if the offending drug is stopped before the onset of significant hepatic damage has occurred. Rechallenging of the patient with the suspected drug and development of liver injury remains the most definitive means of confirming a drug-induced liver injury. Careful review of the patient's medical record may reveal inadvertent rechallenging of the patient with subsequent reoccurrence of hepatocellular injury. Patients also need to be closely questioned for the use of other, nonprescription medications that otherwise may be overlooked by the patient or the physician.

With the increasing availability of new and different therapeutic agents, the incidence of drug-induced liver injury continues to increase. Drug-induced liver injury accounts for approximately 5% of hospital admissions for jaundice. In elderly patients, drug-induced liver injury may account for up to 10–20% of these admissions. This chapter reviews some of the primary drugs presenting with an hepatitis pattern. Several excellent reviews summarizing drug-associated hepatic injury have been published and provide an important resource of drug-associated liver injury.[5–20]

Halothane

Halothane is one of the examples of a chemically induced hepatitis. Although the use of halothane has decreased in the United States due to the advent of the newer halogenated agents, enflurane and isoflurane, considerable interest in halothane hepatitis continues to exist. Clinically, halothane hepatitis occurs after multiple exposures, usually during a 1- to 2-month period. Obese females account for 70% of cases. Patients present with clinical symptoms of hepatitis and transaminitis. Fever may be present in 50% of the cases, with eosinophilia (30%) and rash (10%) occurring less frequently.[21,22]

An excellent review article by DeGroot and Noll[23] examines the two major pathways for the metabolism of halothane and discusses the influence of hypoxia on the metabolic route of biotransformation. Approximately 20% of the inhaled halothane is metabolized in the liver by cytochrome P450. In the presence of saturating oxygen tension, halothane is oxidatively metabolized to trifluoroacetyl–halide intermediate. This metabolite may acetylate proteins or react with water to produce trifluoroacetic acid. Trifluoroacetic acid along with the by-products of this conversion, bromide and fluoride, may be detected in the urine and provide a marker for oxidative metabolism. With decreasing oxygen concentrations, the reductive pathway begins to predominate. During reductive metabolism of halothane, one electron is removed followed by release of the bromide ion resulting in the formation of the radical intermediate, 1-chloro-2,2,2-trifluoroethyl $CF_3 \cdot CHCl$. This compound may leave the cytochrome P450 system or undergo removal of a second electron. In rats, the phenobarbital-inducible cytochrome P450 is responsible for catalyzing this reaction. Hypoxia favors the reductive pathway for halothane metabolism and promotes formation of radicals that covalently bind to cytochrome P450 and promote lipid peroxidation. Elegant studies performed by DeGroot and Noll[23] demonstrated that under saturating oxygen tension no lipid peroxidation occurred. With decreasing oxygen tension, reductive metabolism was favored and lipid peroxidation increased. Under anaerobic conditions, reductive metabolism continued, yet little lipid peroxidation occurred since oxygen is required for this reaction. Clinical studies indicate that halothane hepatitis occurs more frequently in obese patients. Also, obese patients have an increase in reductive metabolites of halothane as compared to nonobese patients, suggesting that decreased hepatic oxygen tension is present in these patients. These reductive metabolites may therefore be important for the development of hepatotoxicity.

Recent studies by Kenna et al.[24] have begun to explore the immunologic mechanism of halothane hepatitis. Prior studies have suggested an immune-mediated process because of clinical features and the sensitization of lymphocytes from patients with halothane hepatitis to subcellular fractions of rabbit liver homogenate treated with halothane. These investigators sought the identification of acetylated proteins on membrane structure by the oxidative metabolites of halothane. In order to detect trifluoroacetylated (TFA) adducts in rat liver subcellular fractions, antisera were raised against TFA e-amino groups of lysine residues of rabbit albumin. These investigators identified TFA-adducts in both rat and human liver microsomes after exposure to halothane and went on to demonstrate that this TFA adduct was the specific microsomal cytochrome P450 responsible for halothane metabolism. No TFA adducts were identified in the cytosol. In addition, these antisera recognized a TFA adduct in the plasma membrane of rat hepatocytes treated with halothane with a similar molecular weight as in microsomes. Further work is required to determine whether this adduct is a microsomal contaminant or whether a cytochrome P450–TFA adduct was formed in the plasma membrane. In addition, Kenna et al. identified in the serum of two out of six patients with halothane hepatitis antibodies which recognized adducts of trifluoroacetylated albumin. This work therefore identifies formation of neoantigens in rats exposed to halothane via the oxidative metabolism of halothane with the subsequent TFA adduct formation with cytochrome P450. The authors speculate that patients with halothane hepatitis may develop antibody to TFA adducts on the plasma membrane leading to antibody-mediated hepatocellular damage.

Inapparent exposure to halothane was reported by Varma et al. in patients with a history of halothane hepatitis during anesthesia with nonhalogenated anesthetic agents.[25,26] In their study, these workers suggested that residual halothane present in the vaporizing circuit in anesthetic machinery was responsible for this inapparent exposure to halothane. The capability of halothane to diffuse into rubber and plastic makes it impossible to remove halothane completely from the vaporizing circuit. Varma et al. therefore recommend that anesthetic machinery which has never been exposed to halothane be strictly reserved for patients with a history of halothane hepatitis. The authors also speculate that patients may be unintentionally exposed to halothane and this may present as a mild form of halothane hepatitis postsurgery with fever and abnormal liver tests. This study illustrates the difficulty in excluding halothane from anesthetic equipment.[25]

The histopathologic spectrum of halothane hepatitis was recently reviewed by the Armed Forces Institute of Pathology.[27] Seventy-seven cases of presumed halothane hepatitis defined by their clinical history were reviewed after elimination of other causes for transaminase elevation, such as blood transfusions or episodes of hypotension; 46% of patients were obese and 62% were female. Morphologically, fatal cases tended to exhibit submassive necrosis. Central zonal necrosis was found in 66% of cases with confluent necrosis, the remainder being periportal. It was concluded that the type of surgical procedure was unrelated to the degree of hepatic injury. Repeated exposure to halothane, especially within a 3-month interval, appeared to be a more important factor for the development of liver injury. Interestingly, tissue eosinophilia was associated with spotty necrosis in contrast to zonal necrosis. The discrete zonal pattern is consistent with the generation of a toxic metabolite whereas the eosinophilia suggests an immune-mediated toxicity.

Another line of investigation into the cause of halothane hepatitis used by Farrell and co-workers was to determine if patients with halothane hepatitis possess a genetic susceptibility for cellular injury from toxins.[28] Phenytoin activated to its epoxide reactive metabolite by rat liver microsomes was used as the toxin in the presence of epoxide hydrolase. Susceptibility was defined as an increase in lymphocyte cytotoxicity with decreasing concentrations of the epoxide hydrolase inhibitor 1,1,1-trichloropropene oxide. Patients with halothane hepatitis and 10 of 19 nonaffected family members from four different families demonstrated marked lymphocyte sensitivity to the epoxide metabolite as compared with disease controls. The authors speculate that patients with halothane hepatitis therefore have a genetic predisposition for the development of cellular injury from toxins. Interpretation of these results is highly speculative, since halothane hepatic toxicity is not mediated by epoxide-reactive metabolites. The relationship between susceptibility of lymphocytes to injury and that of hepatocytes is also unclear. Farrell's work is intriguing though and raises important issues about constitutive factors in cellular susceptibility to toxin-induced injury.

Isoniazid

Isoniazid (INH) remains one of the best-recognized causes for drug-induced hepatocellular disease. Since its introduction in 1952, two patterns of INH hepatotoxicity have been identified. The first pattern, occurring within 1–3 months of therapy, consists of an asymptomatic, mild transaminase elevation occurring in 10–20%. Liver biopsy is nondiagnostic. Often, transaminases will return to normal with continuation of INH. The second pattern, occurring in approximately 1% of patients, is the development of significant hepatitis with a fatality rate of approximately 10% in these patients. Risk factors for the development of INH toxicity include increasing age, sex, and race with black females being at increased risk.[16,29]

INH undergoes a complicated route of metabolism. INH is partially converted to acetyl isoniazid, which then is converted to isonicotinic acid and acetylhydrazine. Acetylhydrazine may then be metabolized by cytochrome P450 to form the presumed toxic metabolite. The rate of acetylation determines the rate of elimination of INH. People may be separated into two distinct groups—slow and fast acetylators—which is under genetic control. Much controversy exists regarding the role of acetylator status on the development of INH hepatotoxicity. Mitchell and co-workers initially theorized that rapid acetylators would be at increased risk for hepatotoxicity due to greater formation of acetyl isoniazid. Clinical studies failed to identify rapid acetylators as being at increased risk for hepatotoxicity.[30,31] Investigation into the metabolism of acetyl isoniazid showed that one route of detoxification occurs via secondary acetylation. Thus, although the fast acetylators were capable of producing greater quantities of acetylhydrazine, they were also capable of detoxifying this intermediate by secondary acetylation.

Recent studies have focused on the potentiation of INH toxicity by rifampin. This is an important clinical issue since the combination of these drugs is a major therapeutic modality for tuberculosis. Rifampin by itself is known to be an inducer of cytochrome P450 and to effect the metabolism of a variety of drugs, such as digitoxin, quinidine, corticosteroids, methadone, dapsone, and verapamil. This induction has been reported to increase the formation of hydrazine from INH. Controversy exists regarding the role of acetylator status on the potentiation of INH hepatotoxicity by rifampin.[32] More studies are required to determine whether acetylator status plays a significant role in INH hepatotoxicity.

Sodium Valproate

Sodium valproate hepatitis is a well-recognized clinical entity. Several excellent reviews exist on this subject.[33-36] The pattern for hepatotoxicity of this agent is one of hepatocellular necrosis. Approximately 11% of patients in one study had abnormal transaminases in the range of one to three times their normal value. Other serum tests such as bilirubin and alkaline phosphatase were normal. In more than 90% of the cases, patients were asymptomatic with these liver test abnormalities. At least 42 patients with fatal valproate toxicity have been reported, and the manufacturer has documented a total of 63 fatalities with this agent. Toxicity occurs after several months of use with the majority occurring within 6 months of treatment.

Clinical features of valproate hepatotoxicity indicate a more common occurrence among children, although this may be due to the typical age of onset for epilepsy. Initial clinical appearance is one of loss of efficacy of the drug with onset of epileptic seizures. Often this leads to increased dosage of the medication, which further aggravates the hepatotoxicity. Anorexia, nausea, and vomiting then occur along with hemorrhagic complications. Jaundice is a late occurrence. Typically, there are no features suggestive of an immunologically mediated process, such as eosinophilia, rash, or fever. A Reye's-like syndrome has also been reported in these patients with lethargy, anorexia and vomiting followed by fever, cerebral edema and coma. Hyperammonemia syndrome has also been reported with valproate without liver disease. In addition, valproate administration may induce significant hyperammonemia in patients with an unrecognized ornithine carbamyltransferase deficiency. Other clinical features include the appearance of pancreatitis and a few case reports of associated renal failure with valproate hepatotoxicity. Histologic features of valproate hepatotoxicity include microvesicular fat in approximately 40% of cases found in association with centrilobular necrosis.

The precise mechanism for valproate hepatotoxicity is unknown. Valproate undergoes a complex route of oxidation that involves microsomes, mitochondria, and peroxisomes. The occurrence of valproate hepatotoxicity in patients taking other anticonvulsants, which are known to be microsomal inducers, suggest a P450-catalyzed toxic metabolite. The mechanism of microvesicular fat has been postulated to reflect toxicity to the mitochondrial function via valproate or one of its metabolites. In particular, the 2-n-propyl-4-pentenoic acid metabolite of valproate has been implicated, since it is structurally similar to 4-pentenoic acid, which is capable of producing a Reye's-like syndrome in the rat. Further investigation is required to determine the relationship between microvesicular fat and valproate hepatotoxicity.

Acetaminophen

Acetaminophen hepatotoxicity continues to receive a great deal of attention. The mechanism for acetaminophen toxicity has been extensively examined. The availability of a successful antidote, Mucomyst, is indicative of the extent of our knowledge about acetaminophen hepatotoxicity. Acetaminophen is predominantly biotransformed by either sulfation or glucuronidation when a therapeutic dose of the drug is ingested. Under normal conditions, only a small percentage of the acetaminophen is available for formation of a reactive metabolite by the cytochrome P450 system. Studies suggest that the electrophile N-acetyl-p-benzoquinoneimine can undergo chemical reduction or conjugation with glutathione, which is catalyzed by the cytosolic enzymes, glutathione S-transferases. Hepatotoxicity can occur when the capacity to sulfate or glucuronidate acetaminophen has been overwhelmed, permitting the formation of the reactive metabolite by the cytochrome P450 system. Hepatotoxicity develops when the cellular levels of glutathione have been depleted, allowing for the reactive metabolite to react with thiol groups on essential proteins. Augmentation of the hepatic glutathione pool is therefore the treatment for acetaminophen hepatotoxicity. Glutathione itself is not absorbed by the liver. Therefore, one of its amino acid precursors, cysteine, is provided. Cysteine cannot be administered, since it is rapidly auto-oxidized. The amino acid is therefore provided in the form *N*-acetylcysteine, Mucomyst, which is readily taken up by hepatocytes and converted to cysteine.

Other agents have been used to replenish glutathione levels. A precursor for cysteine, 2-oxothiazolidine-4-carboxylate, which is converted by the enzyme, 5-oxo-L-prolinase, to cysteine has also been successful in increasing hepatic GSH levels.[37] Another approach has been to modify the glutathione chemically so that it may be transported into hepatocytes. The glycl ester of glutathione is taken up by hepatocytes metabolized by esterases to form glutathione and is capable of augmenting the intracellular glutathione concentration.[38] These approaches may eventually be used in clinical practice.

Another approach to acetaminophen hepatotoxicity has been to modulate the activity of the cytochrome P450 system. In particular, the use of H_2-blockers to inhibit cytochrome P450 have been examined in experimental animal models and human subjects.[39] Cimetidine has been shown to decrease acetaminophen hepatotoxicity. In addition, cimetidine is capable of inhibiting glucuronidation of acetaminophen, which would lead to greater metabolism by the cytochrome P450. The therapeutic effect of cimetidine in acetaminophen hepatotoxicity must therefore be a balance between the extent of inhibition of glucuronidation versus inhibition of cytochrome P450. In a careful study by Leonard *et al.*,[40] the dose-dependent effect by ranitidine and cimetidine on acetaminophen toxicity was examined in the rat. At low concentrations of ranitidine, toxicity was potentiated presumably by inhibition of glucuronidation. At high ranitidine concentrations, inhibition of cytochrome P450 prevailed and minimal toxicity was observed. With increasing concentrations of cimetidine, no protection occurred. In this study, cimetidine-treated animals received a greater dose of acetaminophen than did the ranitidine-treated rats. The balance between inhibition of detoxification (glucuronidation) and inhibition of activation (cytochrome P450) will determine the efficacy of H_2-blockers to prevent acetaminophen hepatotoxicity. More work will be required before H_2-blockers can be clinically used for the treatment of acetaminophen hepatotoxicity.

Recent clinical studies have focused on alcoholic patients developing acetaminophen hepatotoxicity while ingesting therapeutic amounts of acetaminophen. In a study of six patients conducted by Seeff *et al.*,[41] with a literature review of 19 additional patients, the average acetaminophen dose was 6.4 g in a range of 2.6–16.5 g/day. In a review from San Francisco General Hospital, Kaysen *et al.*[42] identified five patients who developed both renal and liver disease while ingesting 2.5–10 g acetaminophen per day. The renal disease in these patients was characterized as an acute tubular necrosis pattern clearly distinct from hepatorenal syndrome. In both studies, markedly elevated aminotransferases were noted on admission which clearly differed from the pattern associated with alcoholic hepatitis. Peak levels were recorded on the date of admission and tended to normalize rapidly. AST levels exceeded ALT levels in the majority of cases. A mortality of 20–40% was reported in these two studies. Kaysen and co-workers noted the importance of obtaining a history for acetaminophen ingestion with measurement of serum levels upon admission. These investigators also warned that the colorometric method for measuring acetaminophen may lead to false-positive results in patients with elevated serum creatinine. The combination of renal failure and liver dysfunction in an alcoholic patient must include the determination of acetaminophen serum levels with possible treatment. The mechanism for the potentiation of liver damage in an alcoholic is presumed to be due to induction of the cytochrome P450 system by chronic ethanol ingestion.[43] In addition, a poor nutritional state associated with alcoholism may predispose to a decreased hepatic glutathione concentration thereby limiting the capacity of the liver to detoxify acetaminophen.

Ketoconazole

The antifungal agent, ketoconazole, has been reported to produce hepatocellular injury. A recent report from England summarizes the experience in that country with ketoconozole since its introduction in 1981. The spectrum of clinical disease ranges from asymptomatic serum transaminases elevation to fulminant hepatic failure. In England, 16 cases of probable ketoconazole-related liver disease were identified.[44] Serum transaminases were consistent with hepatocellular damage in 66% of these cases, with the remainder presenting with a mixed hepatocellular and cholestatic pattern. Liver histology in three patients who died and two who survived indicated cholestasis in all five patients. Two of the three patients who expired and one of the two who survived had hepatocellular necrosis. Hepatotoxicity developed within 60 days on average in a range of 5–195 days. Most patients recovered without complication when the medication was terminated. Two of the three fatal cases continued with the medication despite the onset of jaundice. In addition, clinical features did not include fever or rash, suggesting that an immunologically mediated mechanism is not occurring. The estimated occurrence of ketoconazole toxicity is 1 : 15,000. A recent study from Holland suggests an incidence rate of 1 : 1000–3000.[45] Hepatotoxicity occurs after long-term therapy, and therefore a short course (10 days) carries little risk. Current recommendations include measurement of serum liver tests prior to initiation of therapy to exclude underlying hepatitis. Determination of weekly liver tests after 10 days of therapy for two months is recommended followed by bimonthly determinations.

Diphenylhydantoin Hepatotoxicity

The anticonvulsant, diphenylhydantoin, has been associated with multiple systemic effects. Liver toxicity is quite rare, accounting for less than 1% of the reported complications of the drug. In a review article, Mullick and Ishak[47] assessed the histopathologic features of 20 cases of diphenylhydantoin-induced hepatotoxicity. A preponderance of blacks was noted in their series with a 56% incidence of males. Prior studies had identified females as being at increased risk. Most patients present with symptoms after 1–6 weeks of treatment. Clinically, these patients present with a hypersensitivity type of reaction with fever (75%), rash (62.5%), lymphadenopathy and hepatomegaly (60%), eosinophilia (90%), and jaundice (44%). Another pattern of presentation is one that mimics infectious mononucleosis. Exfoliative dermatitis has been reported to occur with hepatomegaly although the reverse is not true.[48] Serum liver tests demonstrated predominantly hepatocellular necrosis with a two- to threefold increase in alkaline phosphatase. Liver histology showed that 13 of 20 patients presented with predominantly hepatocellular necrosis; 4 of the 20 patients presented with a mononucleosislike pattern of injury with increased numbers of lymphocytes in hepatic sinusoids as well as focal hyperplasia and variation in liver cell size. As is typical for most drug-induced lesions, the clinical course was one of resolution after termination of the drug. The pathophysiology of Dilantin hepatotoxicity is one of hypersensitivity, since patients developed fever, rash, adenopathy, and eosinophilia.[48] Rechallenge with the drug reproduced the liver disease. In addition, serum antibodies directed against diphenylhydantoin have been detected and lymphocytic stimulation to diphenylhydantoin in vivo has been noted.

α-Methyldopa

α-Methyldopa is one of the first drugs recognized to produce a clinical syndrome of chronic active hepatitis.[49,50] Since the advent of newer antihypertensive medications, the use of α-methyldopa is decreasing; 2–10% of patients may develop transient, asymptomatic abnormal liver tests that occur within the first 4 weeks of treatment. Another form of more severe hepatitis has been reported more commonly in women. These patients have features of immune-mediated toxicity with autoantibodies (antinuclear and anti-smooth muscle) and positive rechallenge with α-methyldopa. Continuation of the drug in the presence of jaundice may lead to fulminant liver failure. Neuberger *et al.*,[51] sought the presence of antibodies in these patients to drug-altered liver cell membrane antigens using immunofluorescence and antibody-dependent cell-mediated cytotoxicity. The sera of 5 of 9 patients with α-methyldopa hepatitis induced cytotoxicity of hepatocytes from rabbits treated with α-methyldopa and a mixed-function oxidase inducer. In contrast to the lack of cytotoxicity in 32 patients taking methyldopa without evidence for hepatotoxicity, two of the five antibody-positive sera specifically stained the periphery of human hepatocytes from a patient with methyldopa hepatitis. Neuberger and co-workers speculate that antibodies against altered plasma membrane may be mediating the hepatotoxicity. Of note, only one half the patients demonstrated this antibody-mediated cytotoxicity. The investigators[51] response to this lack of antibody is that the antibody may have been bound to the hepatocytes lack of sensitivity of the assay or that methyldopa may mediate its toxicity by an idiosyncratic toxic metabolite.

Pyrimethamine-Sulfadoxine

Pyrimethamine-sulfadoxine (Fansidar) became available in 1982 for the prophylaxis treatment for malaria. In addition, the agent has been used for the prophylactic treatment of *Pneumocystis carinii* pneumonia in patients with acquired immune deficiency syndrome (AIDS) who are unable to tolerate Bactrim. Recently, a case of fatal hepatic necrosis was reported after taking four doses of the medication.[52] Liver biopsy exhibited diffuse extensive necrosis with ductular proliferation. Two prior case reports of granulomatous hepatitis have been reported with Fansidar. Prior reports of severe cutaneous reaction have also appeared associated with a significant mortality (30%). Zitelli *et al.*[52] speculate that the sulfadoxine moiety is the hepatotoxicity agent. The risk for developing hepatocellular disease is approximately 1 : 16,000. Patients require close follow-up while on this medication and should have the medicine discontinued if liver test abnormalities are noted.

CONCLUSION

Case reports of drug-induced hepatitis continue to accumulate with the advent of newer therapeutic agents. Recent advances in our understanding of the pharmacology of hepatotoxicity are beginning to define the precise chemical steps from formation of reactive metabolite to cell death. Future work will continue to determine the metabolites responsible for drug toxicity and the means by which the liver cell detoxifies them.

REFERENCES

1. Farrel GC: Hepatic drug reaction: How predictable are they? *J Gastroenterol Hepatol* **1**:267–271, 1986.
2. Mitchell JR, Smith CV, Hughes H, et al: Overview of alkylation and peroxidation mechanisms in acute lethal hepatocellular injury by chemically reactive metabolites. *Semin Liver Dis* **1**:143–150, 1981.
3. Guidelines for diagnosis of therapeutic drug-induced liver injury in liver biopsy. *Lancet(I)* **4**:854–857, 1974.
4. Rubin E: Iatrogenic hepatic injury. *Hum Pathol* **11**:312–331, 1979.
5. Kolts BE, Langfitt M: Drugs and the liver. *Comp Ther* **10**(12):55–90, 1984.
6. Farrell GC: The hepatic side-effects of drug. *Med J Aust* **145**:600–604, 1986.
7. Sherlock S: Progress report. Hepatic reactions to drugs. *Gut* **20**:634–648, 1979.
8. Black M: Drug induced liver disease. *Postgrad Med J* **59**(suppl 4):116–122, 1983.
9. Ockner RK: Drug-induced liver disease. *West J Med* **131**:36–45, 1979.
10. Maddrey WC, Boitnott JK: Drug-induced chronic liver disease. *Gastroenterology* **72**:1348–1353, 1977.
11. Kaplowitz N, Aw TY, Simon FR, et al: Drug-induced hepatotoxicity. *Ann Intern Med* **104**:826–839, 1986.
12. Kaplowitz N: Drug-induced hepatotoxicity. *Curr Hepatol* **7**:69–102, 1987.
13. Kaplowitz N: Drug-induced hepatotoxicity. *Curr Hepatol* **6**:239–268, 1986.
14. Aw TY, Hanna P, Petrini J, et al: Hepatic drug metabolism and drug-induced liver injury. *Curr Hepatol* **5**:113–196, 1985.
15. Petrini J, Stolz A, Kaplowitz N: Drug metabolism and drug-induced liver injury. *Curr Hepatol* **4**:247–312, 1984.
16. Eberle D, Kaplowitz N: Drug-induced liver disease, in Gitnick GL (ed): *Gastroenterology*. New York, Wiley, 1983, pp. 281–310.
17. Stricker BHCh, Spoelstra P (eds): *Drug-induced Hepatic Injury*, Vol. 1. Amsterdam, Elsevier, 1985.
18. Ludwig J, Axelsen R: Drug effects on the liver: An updated tabular compilation of drugs and drug-related hepatic disease. *Dig Dis Sci* **28**:651–666, 1983.
19. Sharp JR, Ishak KG, Zimmerman HJ: Chronic active hepatitis and severe hepatic necrosis associated with nitrofurantoin. *Ann Intern Med* **92**:14–19, 1980.
20. Black M, Rabin L, Schatz N: Nitrofurantoin-induced chronic active hepatitis. *Ann Intern Med* **92**:62–64, 1980.
21. Stock JGL, Strunin L: Unexplained hepatitis following halothane. *Anesthesiology* **63**:424–439, 1985.
22. Touloukian J, Kaplowitz N: Halothane induced hepatic disease. *Semin Liver Dis* **1**:134–142, 1981.
23. DeGroot H, Noll T: Halothane hepatotoxicity: Relation between metabolic activation, hypoxia, covalent binding, lipid peroxidation and liver cell damage. *Hepatology* **3**:601–606, 1983.
24. Satoh H, Gillette JR, Takemura T, et al: Investigation of the immunological basis of halothane-induced hepatotoxicity. *Adv Exp Med Biol* **197**:657–673, 1986.
25. Varma RV, Whitsell RC, Iskandarani MM: Halothane hepatitis without halothane: Role of inapparent circuit contamination and its prevention. *Hepatology* **5**:1159–1162, 1985.
26. Conn HO, Skornicki J: Halothane hepatitis sans halothane. *Hepatology* **5**:1238–1240, 1985.
27. Benjamin SB, Goodman ZD, Isak KG, et al: The morphologic spectrum of halothane-induced hepatic injury: Analysis of 77 cases. *Hepatology* **5**:1163–1171, 1985.
28. Farrell G, Pendergast D, Murry M: Halothane hepatitis: Detection of a constitutional susceptibility factor. *N Engl J Med* **313**:1310–1314, 1985.

29. Timbrell JA: The role of metabolism in hepatotoxicity of isoniazid and iproniazid. *Drug Metab Rev* **10**(1):125–147, 1979.

30. Gurumurthy P, Krishnamurthy MS, Nazareth O, et al: Lack of relationship between hepatic toxicity and acetylator phenotype in three thousand South Indian patients during treatment with isoniazid for tuberculosis. *Am Rev Respir Dis* **129**:58–61, 1984.

31. Ellard GA: The potential clinical significance of the acetylator phenotype in the treatment of pulmonary tuberculosis. *Tubercle* **65**:211–227, 1985.

32. Gangadharam PRJ: Isoniazid, rifampin and hepatotoxicity. *Am Rev Respir Dis* **133**:963–965, 1986.

33. Powell-Jackson PR, Tredger JM, Williams R: Hepatotoxicity to sodium valproate: A review. *Gut* **25**:673–681, 1984.

34. Gram L, Bentsen KD: Valproate. An update review. *Acta Neurol Scand* **72**:129–139, 1985.

35. Dickinson RG, Bassett ML, Searle T, et al: Valproate hepatotoxicity. A review and report of two instances in adults. *Clin Exp Neurol* **21**:79–91, 1985.

36. Ware S, Millward-Sadler GM: Acute liver disease associated with sodium valproate. *Lancet* **2**:1110–1113, 1980.

37. Williamson JM, Meister A: Stimulation of hepatic glutathione formation by administration of L-2-oxo-thiazolidine-4-carboxylate, a 5-ono-L-prolinase substrate. *Proc Natl Acad Sci USA* **78**:936–939, 1981.

38. Puri RN, Meister A: Transport of glutathione, as gamma-glutamylcysteinylgllycyl ester, into liver and kidney. *Proc Natl Acad Sci USA* **80**:5258–5260, 1983.

39. Mitchell MC, Schenker S, Speeg KU: Selective inhibition of acetaminophen oxidation and toxicity by cimetidine and other histamine H_2-receptor antagonists in vivo and in vitro in the rat and man. *J Clin Invest* **73**:383–391, 1984.

40. Leonard TB, Morgan DG, Dent JG: Ranitidine–acetaminophen interaction: Effects on acetaminophen-induced hepatotoxicity in Fischer 344 rats. *Hepatology* **5**:480–487, 1985.

41. Seeff LB, Cuccherini BA, Zimmerman HJ, et al: Acetaminophen hepatotoxicity in alcoholics. *Ann Intern Med* **104**:399–404, 1986.

42. Kaysen GA, Pond SM, Roper MH, et al: Combined hepatic and renal injury in alcoholics during therapeutic use of acetaminophen. *Arch Intern Med* **145**:2019–2023, 1985.

43. Black M, Rauchy J: Acetaminophen, alcohol and cytochrome P-450. *Ann Intern Med* **104**:427–428, 1986.

44. Lake-Bakaar G, Scheuer PJ, Sherlock S: Hepatic reactions associated with ketoconazole in the United Kingdom. *Br Med J* **294**:419–422, 1987.

45. Sticker B, Blok A, Bronkhort F, et al: Ketoconazole-associated hepatic injury. A clinicopathological study of 55 cases. *J Hepatol* **3**:399–406, 1986.

46. Brown M, Schubert T: Phenytoin hypersensitivity hepatitis and mononucleosis syndrome. *J Clin Gastroenterol* **8**:469–477, 1986.

47. Mullick FG, Ishak KG: Hepatic injury with diphenylhydantoin therapy. *Am J Clin Pathol* **74**:442–452, 1980.

48. Kahn HD, Faguet GB, Agee JF: Drug induced liver injury. In vitro demonstration of hypersensitivity to both phenytoin and phenobarbital. *Arch Intern Med* **144**:1677–1679, 1984.

49. Rodman JS, Deutsch DJ, Gutman SI: Methyldopa hepatitis. A report of six cases and review of the literature. *Am J Med* **60**:941–948, 1976.

50. Wright R: Drug-induced chronic hepatitis. *Springer Semin Immunopathol* **3**:331–338, 1980.

51. Neuberger J, Kenna TG, Aria KN, et al: Antibody mediated hepatocyte injury in methyl dopa induced hepatotoxicity. *Gut* **26**:1233–1239, 1985.

52. Zitelli BJ, Alexander J, Taylor S, et al: Fatal hepatic necrosis due to pyrimethamine-sulfadoxine (Fansidar). *Ann Intern Med* **106**:393–395, 1987.

II

Chronic Hepatitis

Chronic Hepatitis
Classification

GARY GITNICK

BACKGROUND

The first major attempt to differentiate the forms of chronic hepatitis emanated from the relatively recent description of chronic active hepatitis (CAH)[1,2] and chronic persistent hepatitis (CPH). A number of discoveries are now helping to resolve the controversy and confusion that have surrounded efforts to classify the chronic sequelae of acute hepatitis.

Kunkel and co-workers,[1] in 1951, and Waldenstrom,[2] in 1952, first described CAH. They observed young females with hypergammaglobulinemia, plasma cell infiltration of the hepatic parenchyma, and cirrhosis, the causes of which were then unknown. Saint et al.,[3] in 1956, applied the term active chronic hepatitis to this condition in patients of both sexes. Bearn et al.[4] emphasized the prominence of such systemic features as fatigue, fever, arthralgias, acne, and striae. The concept was further expanded in 1956 by Mackay et al.,[5] who initially coined the term lupoid hepatitis when they noted a subset of patients presenting with a positive antinuclear antibody (ANA) or lupus erythematosus (LE) cell test, hyperglobulinemia, fibrosis, and active hepatic necrosis. When Whittingham et al.[6] subsequently developed data suggesting that lupoid hepatitis was not a part of the syndrome of systemic lupus erythematosus (SLE), they suggested the term autoimmune hepatitis. The terms aggressive hepatitis, subacute hepatitis, and active juvenile cirrhosis represent additional nomenclature applied to this spectrum of disease.

More than a decade later, Geall et al.,[7] in 1968, observed the tremendous

GARY GITNICK • Department of Medicine, University of California at Los Angeles School of Medicine, Los Angeles, California 90024.

confusion reigning in all attempts to differentiate the forms of chronic hepatitis with associated active hepatocellular necrosis. These investigators suggested that until a means of differentiation became available, all forms of chronic hepatitis with active cellular necrosis be called chronic active liver disease. This would differentiate patients with lobular or cellular necrosis from those patients who had chronic persistent hepatitis, a chronic liver disease without these sequelae.

Since that time, prospective studies evaluating the long-term sequelae of acute hepatitis, as well as the clinical use of new serologic assays, have made it possible to differentiate more clearly among the forms of CAH and CPH. The time has now come to stop combining the disorders and to identify them as separate entities. This chapter attempts to classify the different forms of chronic hepatitis on the basis of etiology, clinical course, and prognosis.

CHRONIC ACTIVE HEPATITIS

Types Identified and Prognosis

In 1969, Gitnick et al.[8] and Wright et al.[9] described the association of hepatitis B surface antigen (HB$_s$Ag) with CAH. HB$_s$Ag was present in cases that did and that did not progress to cirrhosis. Koretz et al.,[10] in 1976, described the high frequency with which CAH and CPH developed following posttransfusion non-A, non-B hepatitis. These findings, in addition to others related to drugs and immunologic features, have led to the categorization of CAH into four different types, as follows: (1) drug-induced, (2) viral (type B, or non-A, non-B), (3) autoimmune (positive ANA or LE cell tests), and (4) idiopathic.

Drug-Induced CAH

Certain drugs may produce chronic liver disease indistinguishable from CAH. Those that are implicated include α-methyldopa (Aldomet), isoniazid (INH), dantrolene, nitrofurantoin, and laxatives containing oxyphenisatin. Occasionally, the liver biopsy of an alcoholic patient is indistinguishable from that of a patient with CAH. The clinical, biochemical, and histologic features of the drug-induced syndrome are the same as those seen in viral-induced disease. The condition may be symptomatic or asymptomatic, with varying degrees of biochemical activity. If administration of the implicated drug continues, cirrhosis may develop, making it important to discontinue the drug. Corticosteroid therapy is neither helpful nor appropriate for this type of CAH.

Viral CAH

CAH B. Following acute hepatitis B, patients may have total resolution of disease or they may develop the chronic HB_sAg carrier state. These patients may or may not develop CAH or CPH. For those who develop CAH, two clinical courses have been described.

In one course, the patient is usually young, often a drug user, and may be habituated to alcohol. This patient population may develop a chronic low-grade liver disease that either does not progress or that progresses at a very slow rate and is characterized by little clinical symptomatology. The second course may occur at any age and is usually seen in patients with no other underlying liver disease. It may be seen following posttransfusion or sexually transmitted hepatitis B. Among this group of patients, the disease progresses at a more rapid rate with fatigue being a prominent symptom, and serum transaminase levels either significantly or slightly elevated. Patients respond poorly to corticosteroid treatment; in the few who do respond, the disease still progresses to cirrhosis, portal hypertension, and eventual death.

Chronic Active Non-A, Non-B Hepatitis. In 20–60% of patients with non-A, non-B hepatitis CAH or CPH develops.[10,11] Approximately 50% of those who develop chronic hepatitis develop CAH. The illness is frequently characterized by a paucity of clinical symptomatology, although some patients complain of fatigue, and a few develop jaundice.

Controversy exists regarding the long-term prognosis of this type of CAH. The disease follows an indolent or slowly progressive course. It has been observed that, although most patients with the illness are generally asymptomatic and remain stable for long periods, a small but definite group develop cirrhosis and portal hypertension, and eventually die as a result of the illness.[10,11]

Autoimmune CAH

The autoimmune form of CAH is characterized by the presence of hyperglobulinemia and ANA, with or without positive LE cells, and smooth muscle SMA. This type seems to be more common among females than males and may lead to cirrhosis more rapidly than do the other forms of chronic hepatitis. Clinical features may include extreme fatigue, arthritis, arthralgias, rash, and fever.[12]

The autoimmune form of CAH appears to result from unknown causes and is unrelated to prior viral infection or drug ingestion. Thus far, for example, posttransfusion viral hepatitis has not been shown to lead to CAH with immunologic features. Presumably, immune mediation plays a role in its pathogenesis.

Unlike the other forms of CAH, the response of this form of hepatitis to corticosteroid treatment is dramatic and relatively rapid. It may slow down the progression of the disease at least and, at best, bring it into prolonged remission.

Differentiation and Diagnosis

Chronic active hepatitis describes a condition that occurs in either sex, at any age, with persistently high levels of serum transaminase, γ-globulin, or both. SMA and ANA can often be demonstrated.

Chronicity refers to a persistent or fluctuating, but progressive, disease. The presence of cirrhosis establishes chronicity, but, in its absence, the diagnosis depends arbitrarily on clinical assessment of the patient and the duration and degree of activity of documented hepatic disease. Mild abnormalities of laboratory indexes of liver function or hepatic histology may persist for as long as one year, or more, in slowly resolving but self-limited hepatitis. Chronicity is a reasonable assumption, however, when persistent high-grade activity is documented for 6 months or longer. Thus, chronicity is documented by follow-up of more than 24 weeks that shows persistent elevations in liver tests.

Regardless of cause, CAH may be subdivided into symptomatic and asymptomatic forms and into types displaying high-grade activity and with low-grade activity. Arbitrary means of differentiation are used.

Symptoms are subjective and provide an unreliable means of assessing the clinical state of the illness. The most common symptom is fatigue, which is a nonspecific indicator of a variety of conditions.

Activity can be defined more practically and accurately in terms of objective criteria, rather than symptomatology. Thus, the magnitude of elevation of serum transaminase and γ-globulin levels and the degree of hepatocellular necrosis are suitable criteria for determining activity and judging response to therapy.

Activity in chronic liver disease can be defined most readily by establishing arbitrary quantitative biochemical criteria. Biochemical activity provides a mechanism to assess the disease process. Activity can be graded according to serum transaminase values. For example, entrance into the Mayo Clinic treatment trial required a transaminase level greater than 10 times the upper limit of laboratory normal, or greater than 5 times the upper limit of laboratory normal in conjunction with a γ-globulin level greater than twice the upper limit of laboratory normal values.

Some prefer to subdivide the disease into three categories: (1) high-grade activity, as measured by a transaminase level greater than 10 times the upper limit of laboratory normal; (2) intermediate activity, in which the transaminase level is 5–10 times the upper limit of laboratory normal; and (3) biochemical inactivity, in which the enzyme elevation is less than five times the upper limit of laboratory normal. Prospective studies have not been done to determine if this method is reliable. For example, it is not known whether disease exhibiting low-grade activity is less likely to lead to cirrhosis than that of intermediate or high-grade activity.

The biochemical criteria are arbitrary since the level of transaminase may not correlate with the degree of necrosis or severity of disease seen on liver biopsy. Therefore, differentiation is best made by liver biopsy, which shows hepatocellular necrosis, often piecemeal necrosis, and mononuclear cell infiltration, and which may or may not exhibit variable degrees of fibrosis and necrosis.

Hepatocellular necrosis with bridging refers to the disease process expanding from portal tract to portal tract. Some investigators believe that bridging indicates the only progressive lesion in CAH and that liver biopsies that do not show bridging, regardless of other features, indicate less significant liver disease.[13] Prospective studies to determine whether this bridging/nonbridging differentiation is a reliable means of assessing prognosis or need for treatment have not confirmed its validity.

Most of the histologic features of chronic active hepatitis are also in acute hepatitis. A liver biopsy can be interpreted best if obtained a suitable period after the episode of acute hepatitis. When feasible, it is best to wait 6–12 months after the onset of acute hepatitis.

Patients with CAH are frequently found to have chronic hepatitis B antigenemia or to be carriers of non-A, non-B virus. HB_sAg in the sera has been traced from acute hepatitis through the development of CAH. During the course of this illness, the antigen is present, but its titer may rise and fall, and the antigen may or may not be detectable. HB_sAg may be found in 10–50% of patients with CAH. In some instances, circulating antigen–antibody complexes have been demonstrated.

The HB_sAg assay and tests of ANA, SMA, or carcinoembryonic antigen (CEA) may be elevated in this group of patients, but these tests do not replace liver biopsy in terms of usefulness in diagnosing the condition.

A question of great concern is how to determine whether the patient with asymptomatic disease or low-grade biochemical activity has a condition likely to lead to cirrhosis and portal hypertension, and if corticosteroid treatment should be administered. Studies are now under way to answer this question, but a definite answer probably will not be available for several years.

Differential Diagnosis

The differential diagnosis of CAH includes CPH (when the patient has only an elevation of SGOT or SGPT), cirrhosis, alcoholic liver disease, drug-induced liver disease, Wilson's disease, and benign and malignant tumors. In Wilson's disease, liver biopsy may mimic CAH, but the serum ceruloplasmin is reduced.

Diseases associated with nonviral chronic active hepatitis include ulcerative colitis, Hashimoto's thyroiditis, periarteritis, glomerulonephritis, Sjögren's syndrome, vasculitis, pericarditis, and myocarditis. Amenorrhea, hirsutism, stria, cushingoid facies, and acne may be present in young women. A variety of circulating antibodies, including ANA, may be detected.

CHRONIC PERSISTENT HEPATITIS

Types Identified and Prognosis

CAH

Approximately 20% of patients with CAH without treatment spontaneously revert to a clinical, biochemical, and histologic picture of CPH. In addition, of the patients with CAH of high-grade activity brought into remission with treatment, most develop CPH. Approximately one half of these revert to a clinical, biochemical, and histologic picture of CAH within 1 year. Thus, although the lesion of CPH is considered benign, the physician must be aware of the possibility of reversion to a more serious liver problem. Accordingly, such patients merit careful follow-up study.

Idiopathic CPH

Patients without prior documentation of CAH may present with the picture of CPH, with or without knowledge of prior acute hepatitis. Unfortunately, one can never be certain that such patients did not have a previous episode of asymptomatic CAH. Such patients usually have a benign and nonprogressive course, however. The biochemical and histologic abnormalities may resolve spontaneously or may persist for years or for life, but the lesion generally does not progress and does not lead to cirrhosis or signs of portal hypertension.

Etiology

Chronic persistent hepatitis is a histologic and clinical disorder that is seen most frequently following viral hepatitis. Both hepatitis B and non-A, non-B hepatitis are known to progress to this condition. Hepatitis A has not been shown to lead to CPH. The histologic findings can also be associated with a variety of drug-induced liver problems.

A benign prognosis is usually given to this hepatic lesion. However, during the past decade it has been determined that CPH may develop during the natural course of CAH in remission and, accordingly, revert to the more serious lesion of CAH, which carries a more serious prognosis.

Clinical Findings

Chronic persistent hepatitis usually is not associated with symptomatology. Some physicians maintain that fatigue and vague right upper quadrant discomfort may be associated with the condition; however, this has not been the clinical experience of the author. Physical examination indicates no abnormalities attributable to liver disease. The biochemical abnormalities are usually confined to elevation in SGOT and SGPT, with bilirubin, alkaline phosphatase, total protein, albumin, and prothrombin concentrations within the normal range.

Diagnosis

The liver blood tests do not differentiate CPH from CAH. Similarly, a liver scan, ultrasound, and angiography are not of value in establishing the diagnosis; however, they are of value in differentiating this condition.

The essential test for the diagnosis of CPH and for differentiating it from other liver diseases is the liver biopsy, which may be performed by the percutaneous route or by laparoscopy. The latter approach is gaining increasing popularity. It is especially useful in assessing the possible presence of cirrhosis, malignancies, or metastatic lesions by providing a gross view of liver configuration. Since CAH is often a "spotty" lesion (i.e., the lesion may have varying degrees of severity throughout the liver), laparoscopy is especially useful, since it enables the surgeon to secure more than one biopsy from different areas of the organ.

Liver biopsy shows an intact hepatic lobule with normal architecture. There is a prominent mixed inflammatory infiltrate in portal tracts, but generally no significant hepatocellular necrosis is present. Specifically, piecemeal necrosis is not a finding in this condition, as it is in CAH, nor is extensive lobular necrosis. Occasional individual cell necrosis may occur; when this finding becomes prominent or the inflammatory infiltrate is especially heavy, difficulties sometimes occur in differentiating this condition from mild CAH.

Differential Diagnosis

The diagnostic considerations include CAH, drug-induced liver disease, alcoholic liver disease, primary or metastatic malignant processes, mass lesions in the liver (e.g., cysts), and infiltrative disorders, such as Gaucher's disease and lymphomas.

REFERENCES

1. Kunkel HG, Ahrens EH, Jr, Eisenmenger WJ, et al: Extreme hypergammaglobulinemia in young women with liver disease of unknown etiology. *J Clin Invest* **30:**654, 1951 (abst).
2. Waldenstrom J: Leber, Blutproteine und Nahrungseiweiss. *Dtsch Gesellschaft Verdau Stoffwechselkr* **15:**113–119, 1950.
3. Saint EG, King WE, Joske RA, Finckh ES: The course of infectious hepatitis with special reference to prognosis and the chronic stage. *Aust Ann Med* **2:**113–127, 1956.
4. Beam AG, Kunkel HG, Slater RJ: The problem of chronic liver disease in young women. *Am J Med* **21:**3–15, 1956.
5. Mackay IR, Taft LI, Cowling DC: Lupoid hepatitis. *Lancet* **2:**1323–1326, 1956.
6. Whittingham S, Irwin J, Mackay IR, Smalley M: Smooth muscle autoantibody in "autoimmune" hepatitis. *Gastroenterology* **51:**499–505, 1966.
7. Geall MG, Schoenfield LJ, Summerskill WHJ: Classification and treatment of chronic active liver disease. *Gastroenterology* **55:**724–729, 1968.
8. Gitnick GL, Schoenfield LJ, Sutnick AL, et al: Australian antigen in chronic active liver disease with cirrhosis. *Lancet* **2:**285–288, 1969.
9. Wright R, McCollum RW, Klatskin G: Australia antigen in acute and chronic liver disease. *Lancet* **2:**117–121, 1969.
10. Koretz RL, Suffin SC, Gitnick GL: Post-transfusion chronic liver disease. *Gastroenterology* **71:**797–803, 1976.
11. Koretz RL, Stone O, Mousa M, Gitnick GL: Non-A, non-B post-transfusion hepatitis—A decade later. *Gastroenterology* **88:**1251–1254, 1985.
12. Czaja AJ, Davis GL, Ludwig J, et al: Autoimmune features as determinants of prognosis in steroid-treated chronic active hepatitis of uncertain etiology. *Gastroenterology* **85:**713–717, 1983.
13. Boyse KL: Chronic hepatitis—a perspective on classification and determinants of prognosis. *Gastroenterology* **70:**1161–1171, 1976.

History of Chronic Hepatitis

IAN R. MACKAY

Chronic hepatitis, a disease identified around 1950, became of increasing interest to clinicians and pathologists by reason of the introduction of percutaneous liver biopsy for diagnosis, serum transaminase tests for monitoring, serologically defined autoantibodies for pathogenetic insights, and corticosteroid drugs for treatment.[1] Although the cases described initially during the 1950s displayed some particular clinical features, such as predominance among cases of young females and marked hyperglobulinemia, it was widely presumed that the disease was the sequel to a subclinical acute viral hepatitis, and was referred to by some as subacute hepatitis. The term active chronic hepatitis was used to distinguish cases marked by ongoing inflammatory activity from the less frequent inactive chronic cases in which the disease had become quiescent.[2] Active chronic became replaced by chronic active hepatitis (CAH) as the preferred description. Activity in CAH was defined biochemically by elevated serum levels of transaminase enzymes and histologically by inflammatory cellular infiltration within and around portal tracts in the liver with associated hepatocellular damage. The wide range of clinical and pathologic expressions of the disease depend essentially on the degree of inflammatory activity and on the rate of progression to cirrhosis. Initially, the disease was regarded as a single entity of unknown cause.[3] An antecedent hepatitis viral infection was suspected,[2,4] although this could not be readily investigated because of the usually long interval between the presumed infection and the clinical presentation of the disease. By the early 1960s, serologically identifiable autoantibody markers, antinuclear antibody (ANA) and smooth muscle antibody (SMA), raised the possibility that chronic hepatitis depended on autoimmune mechanisms, at least for its perpetuation.[5]

Since the diagnosis of chronic hepatitis depended essentially on biopsy appearances, pathologists had a dominant input during the 1960s, and promul-

---

IAN R. MACKAY • Clinical Research Unit of The Walter and Eliza Hall Institute of Medical Research and The Royal Melbourne University, Victoria 3050, Australia.

gated classifications on the basis of histologic features. Universally accepted is the major subdivision of chronic hepatitis into chronic persistent hepatitis (CPH) and chronic active hepatitis (CAH),[6] histologically established according to whether the limiting plate of the liver lobule is intact (in CPH) or disrupted (in CAH). This subdivision correlates clinically with a benign course (CPH) or progressive course (CAH), and with the absence (CPH) or presence (CAH) of autoimmune serologic markers.

Although hepatitic disease may progress through three stages—acute, chronic active, and cirrhotic[7]—cases of infectious hepatitis usually undergo healing in the acute stage, and some cases of CAH (and all cases of CPH) do not progress to the cirrhotic stage. The three stages might be successively identifiable in the HBV-associated type of CAH but, in autoimmune chronic hepatitis, an acute stage is seldom clinically identifiable.[8] Whether each particular type of acute hepatitis progresses to chronicity by reason of the continuing presence of the initial cause or whether there supervenes new pathogenetic processes common to all types—the notion of a final common pathway—is uncertain.

During the early 1970s heterogeneity was recognized in what histopathologists designated as chronic active hepatitis (CAH).[9] The two major subgroups of the disease comprised the archetypal CAH with autoimmune serologic markers, and the type associated with the then-recognized hepatitis B surface antigen marker (HB_sAg) of infection with hepatitis B virus (HBV). Other etiologies also became identified as causing histologic CAH, including adverse reactions to medicinal drugs (oxyphenisatin, α-methylodopa), copper toxicity (Wilson's disease), ethanol abuse (occasionally), and α_1-antitrypsin deficiency and, later still, other viruses were implicated, including non-A, non-B hepatitis virus(es) and the delta hepatitis virus.

REFERENCES

1. Mackay IR: Chronic active hepatitides. *Front Gastrointest Res* **1:**142–187, 1975.
2. Saint EG, King WE, Joske RA, Finckh ES: The course of infectious hepatitis with special reference to prognosis and the chronic stage. *Aust Ann Med* **2:**113–127, 1953.
3. Beam AG, Kunkel HG, Slater RJ: The problem of chornic liver disease in young women. *Am J Med* **21:**3–15, 1956.
4. Wood IJ, King WE, Parsons PJ, et al: Non-suppurative hepatitis: A study of acute and chronic forms with special reference to biochemical and histological changes. *Med J Aust* **11:**249–261, 1948.
5. Mackay IR: The problem of persisting destructive disease of the liver. *Gastroenterology* **40:**617–626, 1961.
6. De Groote J, Desmet VJ, Gedigk P et al: A classification of chronic hepatitis. *Lancet* **2:**626–628, 1968.
7. Mackay IR: Chronic hepatitis. *Can Med Assoc J* **106:**519–524, 1972.
8. Crapper RM, Bhathal PS, Mackay IR, Frazer IH: "Acute" autoimmune hepatitis. *Digestion* **34:**216–225, 1986.
9. Mackay IR: The prognoses of chronic hepatitis. *Ann Intern Med* **77:**649–651, 1972.

Mechanisms of Chronic Hepatitis

IAN R. MACKAY

INTRODUCTION

There is no clear understanding of the precise "mechanism" for any type of chronic hepatitis, although in given instances a purely virus-mediated or purely immune-mediated type of hepatocellular injury can reasonably be ascribed. This chapter examines derangements (biochemical, histologic, and particularly immunologic) insofar as they bear on mechanisms of liver damage, with particular attention to autoimmune and HBV-associated types of CAH. Ascertainment of HB$_s$Ag and autoantibodies in given cases confirms the individuality of the autoimmune and HBV-associated types of CAH,[1] but this classification is not absolute. For example, Meyer zum Büschenfelde et al.,[2] reporting on 58 cases of CAH, found exclusive reactivity for HB$_s$Ag in 36%, exclusive reactivity for autoantibodies in 34%, reactivity for both HB$_s$Ag and autoantibodies in 7%, and neither reactivity in 23%. Czaja et al.,[3] reporting on 126 cases selected for negativity for HB$_s$Ag, found that 81% had serologic markers of autoimmunity, i.e., lupus erythematosus (LE) cells, antinuclear antibody (ANA) and/or smooth muscle antibody (SMA) and 19% lacked these markers. These two series included a proportion of HB$_s$Ag−ve and autoantibody-negative cases of CAH. It is recognized that some of these cases could include non-A, non-B CAH, and others may be of HBV-associated or autoimmune type but lack the conventional markers; meanwhile, the noncommittal designation of cryptogenic CAH is suggested for this group.

IAN R. MACKAY • Clinical Research Unit of The Walter and Eliza Hall Institute of Medical Research and The Royal Melbourne University, Victoria 3050, Australia.

BIOCHEMICAL DERANGEMENTS

Chronic hepatitis of all types is marked by an increased level of transaminase enzymes in serum, with the degree of increase corresponding to the degree of hepatocellular necrosis; highly raised levels characterize uncontrolled autoimmune CAH. Other biochemical changes, in levels of serum albumin, bilirubin, and alkaline phosphatase or prothrombin index, are not discriminatory for different types of hepatitis and merely reflect impaired liver function consequent either to a phase of exacerbation or to progression to liver insufficiency. Hyperglobulinemia is considered separately under Immunologic Derangements.

HISTOPATHOLOGIC DERANGEMENTS

The appearances that characterize chronic active hepatitis include destruction of the limiting plate of the hepatic lobule and periportal accumulation of lymphoid cells. In the active phases, there is intrahepatic infiltration with lymphoid cells adjacent to damaged or necrotic hepatocytes, and extension of necrosis results in confluent lesions and linking of periportal areas as bridging necrosis.[4] A particular feature of active lesions is the appearance of shrunken eosinophilic hepatocytes, or Councilman bodies, now referred to as apoptotic bodies. Fibrosis develops within the areas of periportal or bridging necrosis, heralding architectural disorganization and cirrhosis. Although histologic appearances per se neither give indications of the particular etiologic type of CAH nor point to causal mechanisms of liver cell destruction, certain features, including prominence of plasma cells in the lymphoid infiltrate and large areas of confluent necrosis point to autoimmune CAH. Other features, including ground-glass hepatocytes, specify HBV-associated CAH, and confirmation is obtainable by the application to liver biopsies of immunohistochemical procedures to demonstrate HBV-encoded structures, core antigen in liver cell nuclei, or surface antigen in cytoplasm. Although immunohistochemical staining shows that HB_sAg is more evidently displayed than HB_cAg at the hepatocyte membrane, it seems likely that HB_cAg provokes the immune attack on HBV-bearing cells.

The lymphoid cell type within the liver infiltrate in CAH has been defined by immunohistochemistry.[5,6] There is an excess, relative to blood, of CD8+ve lymphocytes (cytotoxic-suppressor) over CD4+ve lymphocytes (helper) adjacent to areas of liver cell necrosis, whereas CD4+ lymphocytes predominate in the fibrous tissue scars. However, the excess of CD8+ve lymphocytes is not to a degree that would clearly implicate such cells in cytotoxic damage to hepatocytes.

IMMUNOLOGIC DERANGEMENTS

Humoral Immune Abnormalities

A polyclonal hypergammaglobulinemia occurs in all types of CAH, but particularly in the autoimmune type. The increase is in the immunoglobulin (Ig) G isotype, but studies are lacking on the IgG subclasses responsible for this increase. The possible sites for synthesis of this excess IgG include the liver itself.[7,8]

Autoimmune CAH

The magnitude of the increase in IgG can be extreme, up to 100 g/liter. Contributions to this increase include autoantibodies or polyclonal stimulation of B lymphocytes,[9] or perhaps anti-idiotypic antibody to autoantibody molecules. In the later cirrhotic stage, intestinally derived bacterial antigens bypass the deranged Kupffer cell system in the liver and provoke systemic antibody responses.[9] Also, in autoimmune CAH, there are increased levels of antibodies to viruses, rubella, and measles,[10] with possible connotations for pathogenesis.[11]

The autoantibodies demonstrable in autoimmune CAH are of several types. Antinuclear antibodies (ANA) include antibody to dsDNA, but this is detected infrequently and only transiently in acute phases, anti-ssDNA and antihistone, and antibody to cytoskeletal antigens, conventionally recognized by reactivity with smooth muscle: in autoimmune CAH, the specificity is for actin. These autoantibodies, to nuclei or actin, are the standard diagnostic markers, but neither is readily implicated in pathogenesis, even though actin is abundant in submembranous sites in hepatocytes.[12,13] Subheterogeneity in autoimmune CAH is exhibited, since different types have been defined on the basis of autoantibodies to cell organelles other than the nucleus or cytoskeleton. These organelles include a microsomal antigen that is well represented in liver and renal tubular cells, called liver–kidney microsomal (LKM) antigen,[14] a soluble liver cytoplasmic antigen (SLA) identified by immunoassay but not by immunofluorescence,[15] and the M2 mitochondrial antigen.[16] Thus, cases of autoimmune CAH can be subclassified into classic (ANA+ve, SMA+ve), LKM-associated, SLA-associated, and the CAH-primary biliary cirrhosis overlap type (anti-M2).

Antibodies to a liver-specific autoantigen, or a liver cell membrane structure, have long been sought, with most attention directed to liver-specific protein (LSP) or liver membrane antigen (LMA). LSP is a chromatographically derived macromolecular structure of mol. wt. 4×6 daltons to which antibody can be detected by immunoassay.[17] Much has been written about the significance of anti-LSP in relationship to pathogenesis of autoimmune CAH; LSP itself is no longer held to be liver specific, but it does appear to contain liver-specific antigens, presumably in small amounts[17a] and possibly localized to bile canalicular walls.[17b] The antigenic reactant for LMA is intact liver cells, used in immunofluorescence,[18] radioimmunoassays (RIA),[19] or enzyme-linked immunosorbent assay (ELISA).[20] There is only a degree of specificity for autoimmune CAH in assays for reactivity for antibody to LSP or LMA, since sera from other liver diseases also give reactivity.[19,20] The interpretation of positive results for tests for anti-LSP or anti-LMA in diseases other than autoimmune CAH is problematic; these reactions may merely be a secondary consequence of recurring cycles of liver damage, but they might signify that autoimmunity is a "final common pathway" that contributes to the progression of cirrhosis in most forms of chronic hepatitis. There is some promise of specificity for autoimmune CAH in an immunoassay in which the antigen is a component of LSP, the asialoglycoprotein receptor (asgp-R).[21]

HBV-Associated CAH

Humoral immune abnormalities in HBV-associated CAH are less striking than in autoimmune CAH. Hypergammaglobulinemia is less marked, and autoantibody reactions are usually negative or positive only to low titer. If SMA is present, the cytoskeletal specificity is to vimentin rather than actin.[22] There is serum antibody to the core antigen of HBV (anti-HB_c), which may be of IgM as well as IgG class, but tests for antibody to surface antigen (anti-HB_s) are weak or negative. Circulating antibody to HB_cAg has not been implicated as a cause of hepatocellular damage in HBV-associated CAH.

Cellular Immune Abnormalities: General Remarks

Progress in this aspect of CAH has been slow, since the assays needed are difficult and fickle and, because studies have been done in few centers, much of the published data are uncorroborated. Also, the use of blood lymphocytes in these assays invites the critique that such cells would not reflect the properties of pathogenetically relevant lymphocytes that infiltrate the liver. Other problems include the unsuitability in cytotoxic assays of the conventionally used target cells, including human liver cells, which are fragile in short-term culture, and the need to work within the constraints of major histocompatibility (MHC) restriction, meaning HLA matching in human studies. MHC restriction has the connotation that the same class I MHC molecule must be expressed by the killer T cell and its target, so that human target hepatocytes must be derived by biopsy from the donor of the effector (killer) cells, and maintained in a sufficiently viable state for a cytotoxicity assay to give a meaningful result. Here follows a review of results of assays of cellular immunity in CAH, with a synthesis in the section on mechanisms of hepatocellular injury in CAH.

Helper (CD4+) T Cells

Autoimmune CAH

The activity of CD4+ T cells has been assayed in vitro by the capacity of such cells to release lymphokines on exposure to antigen or by mitogenesis on exposure to liver-derived antigen; results from in vivo tests, based on expression of a cutaneous delayed-type hypersensitivity (DTH) response after intradermal injection of antigen, are not available. Lymphokine-release assays, based on inhibition of migration of indicator cells (macrophages, leukocytes) by lymphokines released when sensitized lymphocytes are exposed to antigen, usually LSP, were reported during the mid-1970s; most publications were in agreement that reactivity (sensitization) of blood T lymphocytes to LSP was demonstrable,[23,24] but these tests lost favor, perhaps because of difficulties in obtaining consistent results in a difficult assay system. A new migration-inhibition assay is described in which T lymphocytes of blood contain both the sensitized population and the indicator population.[25] The test is done in agarose wells and, if sensitized T cells in blood are exposed to antigen, the migration of indicator T lymphocytes from the agarose wells is inhibited. In autoimmune CAH, the lymphokine responsible, T-lymphocyte inhibition factor (T-LIF), is released when T lymphocytes from cases of CAH are exposed to LSP or its constituent, asgp-R. It is to be hoped that these results can be corroborated and that the nature of T-LIF will be clarified, since current technology is allowing biologically active cytokines to be identified and characterized on a molecular basis.

Cell-mediated reactivity to liver antigen preparations including LSP has also been assayed by lymphocyte proliferation.[26] The data are inconsistent, and one well-controlled study reported negative results.[27]

HBV-Associated CAH

Studies on reactivity of lymphocytes from blood with HBV antigens, HB_sAg or HB_cAg, have given variable findings and interpretation of a positive result is difficult since this could reflect either a state of residual protective immunity after past infection, or the presence of clones of T cells with the capacity for reacting with virus-infected hepatocytes. Citations are presented[28,28a] of the reported assays for cell-mediated reactivity of blood lymphocytes in vitro to HB_sAg; most of the recent studies using highly purified antigens do not show sensitization of lymphocytes from blood to HB_sAg, whereas there is sensitization to HB_cAg.[28a]

Cytotoxic (CD8$^+$) T Cells

Autoimmune CAH

The CD8$^+$ subset could be the effectors of the hepatocellular necrosis that occurs in autoimmune CAH, since this subset predominates when liver tissue is studied by immunohistochemistry. However, in a study using autologous hepatocytes as targets, in a 48-hr assay system, in which assessment was by loss of adherence of target cells to the culture dish, cytotoxicity was mediated predominantly by a non-T-cell population.[29] The proposal was that antibody-dependent cytotoxicity (ADCC) (K cells) is operative in vivo[29]; the antibody that attached to hepatocytes to initiate ADCC was assumed to be antibody to LSP or to a constituent of LSP, since LSP was capable of blocking the cytotoxic effect.

HBV-Associated CAH

In the same assay system described above, and using peripheral blood lymphocytes separated into T- and non-T-cell populations, T-cell cytotoxicity was found to be the main effector process.[30] The component of HBV that contributes to the antigen complex presented on the surface of infected hepatocytes is considered to be HB_cAg.[28a]

Suppressor (CD8$^+$) T Cells

The activity of this subpopulation can be determined by assays in which functional effects are measured when putative suppressor T lymphocytes are added to other indicator cell populations. Unfortunately, little is known about the nature of the interaction of antigens with suppressor T cells or about the manner whereby such cells influence immune responses. The assays used measure either non-antigen-specific or antigen-specific suppression. In addition to these functional assays, enumeration can be made of cells in blood with a phenotypic marker of a suppressor population.

Autoimmune CAH

Non-antigen-specific suppressor cell activity in autoimmune disease has been assayed by the capacity of the mitogen concanavalin A (Con A) to recruit from a population of lymphocytes a subset of cells with the capacity to suppress the proliferative response of autologous or allogeneic cells induced by a mitogen. A significantly decreased suppressor cell recruitment from blood lymphocytes was shown in cases of (mostly) HB_sAg−ve CAH,[31] and was corroborated in a subsequent study on cases of autoimmune CAH and SLE.[32] The activity of non-antigen-specific suppressor cells recruited by Con A was also assessed by another readout, the inhibition of IgG secretion by B lymphocytes in vitro; again, decreased non-antigen-specific suppressor function was shown for autoimmune CAH.[33]

Studies on antigen-specific suppression have used LSP or the constituent of LSP, asgp-R. The assay system used was that developed to demonstrate T cells sensitized to LSP or asgp-R, by release of the lymphokine, T-LIF.[25] In an indirect assay, there was inhibition of migration of indicator T cells in cases of autoimmune CAH (and also some cases of PBC) due to release of T-LIF; when T cells from normal subjects were added to the culture system in a ratio of 9 : 1, the inhibited migration of the indicator T cells was normalized. This was taken to indicate that PBL of normal subjects, but not of patients with CAH, contained a T-cell population that could respond to LSP or asgp-R by the specific suppression of the release of T-LIF from LSP-sensitized T cells after exposure to this antigen. The data from this rather complex assay system are yet to be confirmed; should this be accomplished, it would establish that patients with autoimmune CAH have defects in both antigen-nonspecific and antigen-specific suppression as a background on which the disease develops. It is likely that these defects have a genetic basis.

Monoclonal antibodies serve as markers for subsets of T lymphocytes in blood with helper-induced properties (CD4 cells) or cytotoxic and suppressor properties (CD8 cells), and the CD4 : CD8 ratio has been widely used to express imbalance in these populations. However, by reason of the heterogeneity of the CD4 and CD8 populations and the poor correlation between numeric and functional measures of suppression,[34] CD4 and CD8 counts and their ratio have not proved informative in autoimmune disease. More information may come from use of monoclonal antibodies which split CD8 cells into cytotoxic and suppressor subpopulations.[35]

In other diseases, interesting data have been derived from analysis of subpopulations of CD4 lymphocytes. The CD4 subset is divisible into two mutually exclusive populations by monoclonal antibodies (MAb) to markers 4B4 and 2H4[36]; MAb to the 4B4 antigen identifies a helper-inducer subset, and MAb to the 2H4 antigen (and to certain other equivalent antigens) identifies a suppressor-inducer subset that activates CD8 suppressor cells. There is impressive evidence that the suppressor-inducer subset CD4+ 2H4+ is numerically deficient in blood in SLE[37] and active multiple sclerosis[38] and in both blood and synovial fluid in rheumatoid arthritis.[39] There are no reports as yet in autoimmune hepatitis on numbers in the blood of either the suppressor-inducer CD4+ 2H4+ subset or on subpopulations of CD8 cells.

A further approach, using MAb to phenotypic markers for T-cell subsets, would be the examination of liver biopsies by immunohistochemical procedures. Since areas of active piecemeal necrosis show a predominance of CD8+ cells over CD4[+] cells, the use of newer monoclonal markers and immu-nohistochemical staining should enable distinctions between subpopulations of cells with suppressor or cytotoxic phenotypes.

HBV-Associated CAH

There is a report[39a] that non-antigen-specific suppressor regulation is impaired in chronic active and chronic persistent hepatitis associated with HBV infection; the possibility that the changes were secondary was acknowledged.

GENETIC BACKGROUND

Autoimmune hepatitis has a racial–geographic distribution that follows that of the major histocompatibility antigen, HLA B8. The association of CAH with HLA B8 was defined in 1971, and later studies also showed associations with Dw3 and DR3, with published relative risks for these HLA types of 8–15.[40] Explanations for MHC (HLA) and disease associations include molecular mimicry (the MHC molecule closely resembles the structure of a particular pathogen allowing for cross sensitization), MHC-linked immune response genes (coding for a configuration of HLA-DR (Ia) molecules that facilitate presentation of autoantigen to T cells), and MHC-linked immune-suppression genes, the lack of which is a recessively inherited characteristic.[41] Also, it is suggested that the HLA-B8 phenotype is associated with various deficiencies in immune regulatory control of non-antigen-specific type.[42] On the other hand, disease-free first-degree relatives of patients with autoimmune CAH share immune-regulatory defects with patients, both non-antigen-specific[43] and antigen-specific,[44] yet these family studies failed to show that this suppressor defect segregated with genes for HLA or with immunoglobulin allotypes. This seems in keeping with the multiple loci involved in autoimmune diseases in animal models. A genetic locus which may be implicated is that which governs relative proportions of peripheral helper and suppressor T lymphocytes.[45]

COMPARABLE DISEASES

Can data relevant to mechanisms of chronic hepatitis be derived from comparable diseases or other areas of immunopathology? What are the mechanisms of cellular destruction in other organ-specific autoimmune diseases or organ-graft rejection or persisting viral infection? How relevant are these to the autoimmune or HBV-associated types of CAH?

Answers to these questions are not available, and reviewers tend to present diagrams that depict every known type of immune-mediated destruction. Taking autoimmune thyroiditis as an example, the cellular infiltrate shows predominance of T lymphocytes, but there are substantial numbers of B lymphocytes with surface receptors for thyroid antigens,[46] suggesting a role for antibody-mediated damage. In autoimmune type 1 diabetes mellitus, complement-fixing and surface-reactive antibodies to pancreatic islet cells seem to be associated with pancreatic islet cell failure. Certain autoimmune diseases are transmitted transplacentally (e.g., myasthenia gravis) or can be transferred to animals by serum (e.g., pemphigus vulgaris[47]), which implicates humoral antibody as the effector agent.

There are, however, tissue-specific autoimmune diseases that bear a histologic resemblance to autoimmune CAH and in which there are disease-specific marker autoantibodies that cannot be related to cellular damage; examples are primary Sjögren's disease (anti-SS-B/La), primary biliary cirrhosis (anti M-2) and polymyositis (anti-Jo1). Perhaps these diseases are initiated by an extrinsic agent (e.g., Epstein–Barr virus) in the case of primary Sjögren's syndrome,[48] and perpetuated by a cell-mediated immune response to tissue-specific constituents, but the underlying nature of the immune aberrations is unknown.

ANIMAL MODELS

Human autoimmune or virus-induced diseases have models that allow for laboratory investigation of the human equivalent. Within the present context, models that could be considered include induced or spontaneous examples of autoimmune hepatitis or diseases in animals that are carriers of hepatitis DNA (hepadna) viruses.

Models of Autoimmune Hepatitis

Perhaps not the earliest, but the most cited, animal model for experimental CAH was that developed in rabbits by Meyer zum Büschenfelde and colleagues[49] and analyzed in detail in publications in 1974. The protocol included long-term (143 weeks) intraperitoneal immunization of rabbits with human (xenogenic) liver-specific proteins in Freund's complete adjuvant (FCA), the outcome of which was a histologic lesion resembling CAH or liver cirrhosis, depending on antigen dose. Immunized animals developed antibody against allogeneic (rabbit) liver proteins and to a liver membrane antigen on intact hepatocytes, as well as cutaneous DTH against allogenic liver protein. Rabbit liver protein injected in a combined immunization with xenogenic human liver protein had a protective effect.[49] Detailed as the studies have been, the rabbit model described above has not been fully accepted. The immunization protocol differs markedly in duration from that needed for other autoimmune diseases. The animal used (rabbit) is seldom used for establishing autoimmune diseases, and other species (particularly the mouse) appear to be insusceptible to experimental autoimmune hepatitis after immunization with liver protein in FCA, as judged by the scarcity of positive reports over the past 15 years, even though antibody to LSP is readily induced in mice by immunization with LSP.[50] An exception is the report of Mori et al.,[51] who immunized mice with syngenic crude liver protein and detected changes resembling those of human CAH in the C57 BL16 strain particularly; spleen cells from these mice had a high proliferative response to LSP in vitro.

Regulatory mechanisms may operate to control the occurrence of autoimmune reactions to LSP, as judged by the use of cell transfer to immunized mice.[52] These experiments, which showed the presence of naturally occurring suppressor cells that could limit the occurrence of autoimmunity, take on added interest in the light of studies on the experimental induction of autoimmunity in mice by neonatal thymectomy.[53] Without any other treatment, this procedure results in the development of various organ-specific autoimmune diseases, thyroiditis, orchitis, prostatitis, and gastritis and others, each accompanied by organ-specific autoantibodies and characteristic tissue lesions. The explanation given is that effector T cells peripheralize from the thymus earlier than do suppressor T cells, so that the thymectomized animal is unbalanced in terms of helper effects being dominant over suppressor effects; this idea is supported by the capacity of normal adult spleen cells, which contain suppressor cells, to prevent autoimmunity in thymectomized mice.[53] The claim from these experiments that the normal immune system is stocked with a subset of tissue-specific suppressor cells to maintain self-tolerances is convincing. These data recall a report in 1967 on the induction of experimental autoimmune hepatitis in thymectomized mice[54]; equivalent findings were reported in a recent study.[55]

The other type of experimental model that could prove helpful for the understanding of human chronic hepatitis is the natural infection with hepadna viruses of animals, the woodchuck and ground squirrel. Unfortunately these are not readily available models and do not express a precise equivalent of human CAH. The susceptibility of ducks to infection with hepadna virus (DHBV)[56] could provide a more accessible model for investigating issues such as target antigens and cytotoxic effector cells.

MECHANISMS OF HEPATOCELLULAR INJURY IN CAH

The final discussion on mechanisms of hepatocellular damage in CAH can be prefaced by a review of the data and concepts presented above. The two main types of CAH, autoimmune and HBV-associated, differ in so many respects—racial and genetic background, gender, autoimmune serologic markers, HBV markers, and response to treatment—that differences in pathogenesis must be assumed. Furthermore, other mechanisms for chronic persisting liver cell damage must also be considered, independent of autoimmunity or viral infection (e.g., effect of drugs, metabolic disease). The presence of antiliver antibody, anti-LSP and anti-LMA, in different types of CAH[17,19] indicates that autoimmunity could contribute to progression in CAH in general as a "final common pathway."

The pathogenesis of all forms of immunologically mediated tissue injury is complex, whether organ-graft rejection, organ-specific autoimmune damage such as thyroiditis, or pathology associated with persistent viral infection, whether in humans (e.g., subacute sclerosing panencephalitis) or in animal models exemplified by lymphocytic choriomeningitis viral infection of mice or Marek's disease of fowls. Explanations for immunopathologic events in the various types of CAH would certainly be no simpler. The pathogenesis in CAH can be dissected into two major components: immune dysregulation, which provides the background for an immune attack on hepatocytes, and effector mechanisms by which liver cells are destroyed.

Autoimmune CAH

Immune dysregulation detectable as hypofunction of suppressor cell mechanisms is clearly implicated and involves non-antigen-specific and antigen-specific suppression, with genetic determinants for both. The role of deficient non-antigen-specific suppression may be limited, in view of the fact that disease is restricted to the liver in many cases. Various autoimmune or allergic disorders have been attributed to the effects of dominantly inherited MHC (HLA)-linked immune response (Ir) and immune-suppression (Is) genes[41]; deficiency in immune-suppression genes would be a recessive trait in which homozygotes lack Is genes on both chromosomes. However, in the only published study dealing with antigen-specific suppression (to asgp-R), a high-responder state (weak suppression) within families could not be related to HLA alleles.[44] Studies are awaited on counts, from blood or within liver biopsy specimens, of cells of the suppressor-inducer subset CD4$^+$ 2H4$^+$, or the specifically suppressor subset of CD8 cells.

The effector process or processes in autoimmune CAH remains to be clarified since, morphologically, the lymphoid cellular infiltrate consists predominantly (~70%) of T cells. However, from the earliest observations, prominence of plasma cells in the cellular infiltrate has been noted, usually adjacent to damaged hepatocytes, and there is evidence of substantial intrahepatic production of IgG.[7,8] The antigenic specificity of this intrahepatic Ig is unknown, but it could be directed specifically to a disease-relevant liver membrane antigen. However, this was not demonstrable by Western blotting.[57] Complement-dependent antibody lysis is unlikely as a cause of cellular damage in CAH, since complement derangements are inconspicuous. ADCC mediated by K cells has been proposed, based on evidence for intrahepatic IgG synthesis and on studies on cultured hepatocytes exposed to different cell populations from peripheral blood,[29] but immunohistochemical studies indicate that K cells are scanty in the liver infiltrate in CAH.[6] The alternative is that cytoxicity is effected by T lymphocytes. The cytotoxic cell could be of the helper (CD4) or cytotoxic (CD8) class or possibly the lymphokine-activated killer cell familiar in tumor immunology. The CD4 subset, which contains cells that subserve helper-inducer functions and lymphokine release, is not conventionally seen as a killer cell, but the activity of this subset is necessary for the mediation of cytotoxic reactions, as judged by studies on rejection of organ allografts[58] and the occurrence of lesions after transfer of syngeneic cells from animals with experimentally induced autoimmune disease, of brain, testis[59] and other organs. The type of liver cell death, apoptosis, shown histologically as acidophilic bodies and ultrastructurally as cytoplasmic shrinkage and nuclear condensation and fragmentation, reflects immunologic injury, either cellular cytotoxicity or lymphokine-induced cytotoxicity.[60,61]

The more classical type of cytotoxic injury, by the CD8 subset, is exemplified by the killing of virus-infected cellular targets. Although this has not been formally demonstrated in any examples of autoimmune disease, the accumulation of CD8+ lymphocytes at sites of piecemeal necrosis, contiguous with damaged liver cells, is suggestive, and informative data should come from the immunohistochemical use of monoclonal markers that split the cytotoxic and suppressor subsets of CD8 cells. If the CD8 subset were held responsible for hepatocellular death in autoimmune CAH, a target antigen expressed on the liver cell surface, in association with a class I MHC (HLA) molecule, would need to be invoked. This postulated antigen may be a liver-specific autoantigen, but its identification has defied experimental inquiry. It may be a minor constituent of LSP, or the membrane target may be an antigen coded for by a virus that previously infected the liver and became integrated into the liver cell genome; candidates would be HBV or measles virus.[11] Against this is the reported recurrence of autoimmune CAH after orthotopic liver grafting. A 26-year-old woman with autoimmune CAH received an orthotopic liver transplant, after which raised serum IgG levels declined and autoantibodies disappeared but, 18 months later, during tapering of immunosuppressive therapy, there was a recurrence of autoimmune CAH with typical serologic and histologic features.[62] In this instance, at least, recurrent CAH could be attributed to sensitization to an antigen derived from the liver itself rather than to an antigen of extrinsic origin.

HBV-Associated CAH

The existence of HBV carrier states with normal hepatocellular function and morphology indicates that HBV is not of necessity intrinsically cytotoxic, although appearances in acute HBV infection may be those associated with virus-mediated cellular cytotoxicity. Acute hepatitis due to HBV is usually self-limited and associated with cell-mediated and humoral immune responses to antigens of HBV and subsequent lasting immunity to reinfection. With chronic hepatitis due to HBV, the immunological scenario is quite different in that there is no elimination of the virus after the acute attack, and the responses of the immune system range from full tolerance, as in the healthy carrier state, to persisting or recurrent immune attack on noneliminated virus-infected hepatocytes, with progression to cirrhosis.

What determines nonelimination of HBV after acute infection is unknown. It was formerly believed that the incidence of chronicity after acute infection with HBV in adults was ~10%, but this is an overestimate. A follow-up study from Greece on 821 adults with documented acute hepatitis due to HBV showed that 96.8% recovered, 3% died, and only 0.2% had persistent antigenemia[63]; these figures are similar to those of a little-publicized Melbourne report on 336 cases of whom 96.6% recovered, 2.7% died, and 0.7% developed chronic hepatitis.[64]

Persistence of HBV in the liver after acute infection must require special conditions, of which the most would seem to be either immune depression or massive infection, e.g., by blood transfusion, or both. Immune depression would pertain in cases of persisting infection after perinatal infection or of infections in drug abusers, immunodepressed homosexual men, and of subjects infected with the HIV. In states of persisting HBV infection, the pattern of liver disease depends predominantly on the immune status of the host. Liver cell destruction is particularly associated with relief from a state of immune depression, the most familiar example of which would be the rebound exacerbation of hepatitis B after cessation of a course of prednisolone.[65] There are well-documented examples of exacerbation of virus B hepatitis in subjects after relief of immunosuppression from cytotoxic drugs,[66] suggesting that spontaneous episodes of reactivation of chronic hepatitis B in patients not undergoing immunosuppression are due to unexplainable transient subclinical perturbations of the immune system; in this respect, chronic hepatitis B is analogous to other DNA virus infections, particularly herpesvirus infections, which are held in check but not eliminated by the immune system and which become expressed by random immunodepressive events.[66] Such events in the course of chronic infection with HBV become important determinants of the outcome of disease.

The mechanisms of hepatocellular damage are more easily explained in HBV-associated CAH than in autoimmune CAH, although there is uncertainty as to whether HBV may have intrinsically cytolytic activity. Burrell[67] argues for more than one mechanism of hepatocyte injury. In subjects who are HB_eAg+ve and who have cytoplasmic HBV DNA in the liver, hepatocyte injury is associated directly with virus replication and may be caused by it (although the presentation of additional target antigens could provoke an augmented immune attack), whereas in HB_eAg-ve subjects hepatocyte injury occurs in the absence of overt evidence of virus replication. Others hold to the view that damage to HBV-bearing hepatocytes is entirely immune mediated.[68] Of interest, transgenically introduced HB_sAg in mice led in some instances to high concentrations of HB_sAg which were cytotoxic to liver cells.[69]

Progressive HBV-associated CAH tends to be associated with markers of viral replication, i.e., HB_eAg in serum, HB_cAg in liver cells,[69] and HBV DNA in liver cytoplasm and serum, although there are exceptions. Since activity is usually associated with hepatocellular expression of HB_cAg, but not HB_sAg; and since a striking reduction in cytotoxicity in vitro occurred upon preincubation of hepatocytes with anti-Hb_c but not with anti-HB_s, the effector mechanism was taken to be T-cell cytotoxicity directed against HB_cAg on the membrane of hepatocytes,[70] presumably expressed in association with products of class I MHC genes. Further evidence for this was derived by establishing T-cell lines from the hepatic mononuclear infiltrate from 5 patients with HB-CAH; all lines represented mixed populations of $CD4^+$ and $CD8^+$ cells. All responded to HB_cAg and none to HB_sAg preparations, which included the pre-s(2) component.[71]

Of the many accessory factors that may influence intrahepatic events in HBV infection, the capacity for production of cytokines would be one. Important cytokines may be α-interferon (IFN_α) and γ-interferon (IFN_γ), α by reason of its role as a natural virus regulator, and γ by reason of its capacity to influence cellular expression of MHC products. The suggestion could be made that deficient production of IFN_α may facilitate virus replication,[72] and excess production of IFN_γ may augment the immune attack on infected hepatocytes.

REFERENCES

1. Mackay IR: The prognoses of chronic hepatitis. *Ann Intern Med* **77**:649–651, 1972.
2. Meyer zum Büschenfelde K-H, Hütteroth TH: Autoantibodies against liver membrane antigens in chronic active liver disease, in Eddleston AGWF, Weber JCP, Williams R (eds): *Immune Reactions in Liver Disease*. Pitman, Bath, 1979, pp. 12–20.
3. Czaja AJ: Autoimmune chronic active hepatitis, in Czaja AJ, Dickson ER (eds): *Chronic Active Hepatitis, The Mayo Clinic Experience*. Dekker, New York, 1986, pp. 105–126.
4. Mistilis SP: Natural history of active chronic hepatitis. II. Pathology, pathogenesis and clinico-pathological correlations. *Aust Ann Med* **17**:277–288, 1968.
5. Eggink MF, Houthoff HJ, Sippie Huitema CHG, Poppema S: Cellular and humoral immune

reactions in biopsies of patients with untreated idiopathic autoimmune hepatitis, chronic active hepatitis B and primary biliary cirrhosis. *Clin Exp Immunol* **50**:17–24, 1982.

6. Frazer IH, Mackay IR, Bell J, Becker G: Cellular infiltrate in the liver in autoimmune chronic active hepatitis. *Liver* **5**:162–172, 1985.

7. Paronetto F, Rubin E, Popper H: Local formation of γ-globulin in the diseased liver and its relation to hepatic necrosis. *Lab Invest* **11**:150–158, 1962.

8. Kronborg IJ, Knopf PM, Mackay IR: Intrahepatic synthesis of immunoglobulin in liver disease. *Liver* **2**:385–392, 1982.

9. Triger DR, Wright R: Hyperglobulinaemia in liver disease. *Lancet* **1**:1494–1496, 1973.

10. Laitinen O, Vaheri A: Very high measles and rubella virus antibody titres associated with hepatitis, systemic lupus erythematosus and infectious mononucleosis. *Lancet* **1**:194–197, 1974.

11. Robertson DAF, Zhang SL, Guy EC, Wright R: Persistent measles virus genome in autoimmune chronic active hepatitis. *Lancet* **2**:9–11, 1987.

12. Mak WW-N, Sattler CA, Pitot HC: Accumulation of active microfilaments in adult rat hepatocytes cultured on collagen gel/nylon mesh. *Cancer Res* **40**:4552–4564, 1980.

13. Kurki PL, Mittinen A. Linder E, et al: Different types of smooth muscle antibodies in chronic active hepatitis and primary biliary cirrhosis. Their diagnostic and prognostic significance. *Gut* **21**:878–884, 1980.

14. Rizzetto M, Swana G, Doniach D: Microsomal antibodies in chronic hepatitis and other disorders. *Clin Exp Immunol* **15**:331–334, 1973.

15. Manns M, Gerken G, Kyriatsoulis A, et al: Characterization of a new subgroup of autoimmune chronic active hepatitis by autoantibodies against a soluble liver antigen. *Lancet* **1**:292–294, 1987.

16. Berg PA, Wiedmann KH, Sayers TJ, et al: Serological classification of chronic cholestatic liver disease by the use of two different types of anti-mitochondrial antibodies. *Lancet* **2**:1329–1332, 1980.

17. Jensen DM, McFarlane IG, Portmann BS, et al: Detection of autoantibodies directed against a liver-specific membrane lipoprotein in patients with acute and chronic hepatitis. *N Engl J Med* **288**:1–7, 1978.

17a. McFarlane IG: Autoimmunity in liver disease. *Clin Sci* **67**:569–578, 1984.

17b. Helin H, Uibo R, Paronen I, Krohn K: Immunohistochemical localization of human liver specific protein using rabbit antisera and the avidin-biotin complex technique. *Clin Exp Immunol* **59**:371–376, 1985.

18. Hopf U, Meyer zum Büschenfelde K-H, Arnold W: Detection of a liver membrane autoantibody in HbsAg-negative chronic active hepatitis. *N Engl J Med* **294**:574–582, 1976.

19. Frazer IH, Kronborg IJ, Mackay IR: Autoantibodies to liver membrane antigens in chronic active hepatitis. II. Specificity of high titres for autoimmune chronic active hepatitis. *Clin Exp Immunol* **54**:213–218, 1983.

20. Ohtani Y, Kakumu S, Fuje A, Murase K: Autoantibodies against liver cell membrane antigens detected by enzyme-linked immunosorbent assay in acute and chronic liver disease. *Clin Immunol Immunopathol* **43**:9–22, 1987.

21. McFarlane BM, McSorley CG, McFarlane IG, Williams R: Serum autoantibodies reacting with the hepatic asialoglycoprotein receptor (hepatic lectin) in acute and chronic liver disorders. *J Hepatol* **3**:196–205, 1986.

22. Pedersen JS, Toh BH, Mackay IR, et al: Segregation of autoantibody to cytoskeletal filaments, actin and intermediate filaments, with two types of chronic active hepatitis. *Clin Exp Immunol* **48**:527–532, 1982.

23. Meyer zum Büschenfelde K-H, Knolle J, Berger J: Celluläre Immunoreactionen gegenüber

homologem leberspezifischen Antigenen (HLP) bei chronischen Leberentzündungen. *Klin Wochenschr* **52**:246–257, 1974.

24. Miller J, Smith MGM, Mitchell CG, et al: Cell-mediated immunity to a human liver-specific antigen in patients with active chronic hepatitis and primary biliary cirrhosis. *Lancet* **2**:296–297, 1972.

25. Vento S, O'Brien CJ, McFarlane BM, et al: Lymphocyte sensitization to hepatocyte antigens in autoimmune chronic active hepatitis and primary biliary cirrhosis. Evidence for different underlying mechanisms and different antigenic targets. *Gastroenterology* **91**:210–217, 1986.

26. Nouri-Aria KT, Anastassakos C, Eddleston ALWF, Williams R: Immunological responses in liver disease, in Arias IM, Frenkel M, Wilson SHP (eds): *The Liver Annual*, Vol. 5. Elsevier, Amsterdam, 1986, pp. 192–209.

27. Feighery C, McDonald GSA, Greally JF, Weir DG: Histological and immunological investigation of liver specific protein (LSP) immunized rabbits compared with patients with liver disease. *Clin Exp Immunol* **45**:143–151, 1981.

28. Ferrari C, Penna A, Fiaccadori F: Cellular immune response to hepatitis B virus. *J Hepatol* (in press).

28a. de Moerloose PA, Frazer IH, Sewell WA, et al: Cell-mediated immunity to hepatitis B virus antigens in mice: correlation of *in vivo* and *in vitro* assays. *Clin Exp Immunol* **64**:285–295, 1986.

29. Miele-Vergani G, Vergani D, Jenkins PJ, et al: Lymphocyte cytotoxicity to autologous hepatocytes in HBsAg-negative chronic active hepatitis. *Clin Exp Immunol* **38**:16–21, 1979.

30. Mondelli M, Vergani GM, Alberti A, et al: Specificity of T lymphocyte cytotoxicity to autologous hepatocytes in chronic hepatitis B infection: evidence that T cells are directed against the HBV core antigen expressed on hepatocytes. *J Immunol* **129**:2773–2778, 1982.

31. Hodgson HSF, Wands JR, Isselbacher KJ: Alteration in suppressor cell activity in chronic active hepatitis. *Proc Natl Acad Sci USA* **75**:1549–1553, 1978.

32. Coovadia HM, Mackay IR, d'Apice AJF: Suppressor cells assayed by three different methods in patients with chronic active hepatitis and systemic lupus erythematosus. *Clin Immunol Immunopathol* **18**:268–275, 1981.

33. Nouri-Aria KT, Alexander GJM, Portmann B, et al: *In vitro* study of IgG production and concanavalin A induced suppressor cell function in acute and chronic hepatitis B virus infection. *Clin Exp Immunol* **64**:50–58, 1986.

34. Alexander GJM, Nouri-Aria KT, Eddleston ALWF, Williams R: Contrasting relations between suppressor-cell function and suppressor-cell number in chronic liver disease. *Lancet* **1**:1291–1293, 1983.

35. Kansas GS, Engleman EG: Phenotypic identification of suppressor-effector, suppressor-amplifier and suppressor-induced T cells of B cell differentiation in man. *Eur J Immunol* **17**:453–457, 1987.

36. Morimoto C, Letvin NL, Distaso JA, et al: The isolation and characterisation of the human suppressor inducer T cell subset. *J Immunol* **134**:1508–1515, 1985.

37. Morimoto C, Steinberg AD, Letvin NL, et al: A defect in immunoregulatory T cell subsets in systemic lupus erythematosus patients demonstrated with anti-2H4 antibody. *J Clin Invest* **79**:762–768, 1987.

38. Rose LM, Ginsberg AH, Rothstein TL, et al: Selective loss of a subset of T helper cells in active multiple sclerosis. *Proc Natl Acad Sci USA* **82**:7389–7395, 1985.

39. Emery P, Gentry KC, Mackay IR, et al: Suppressor-inducer subset of T lymphocytes is deficient in rheumatoid arthritis. *Arth Rheumatism* **30**:849–856, 1987.

39a. Nouri-Aria KT, Alexander GJM, Portmann D, et al: *In vitro* study of IgG production and concanavalin A induced suppressor cell function in acute and chronic hepatitis B virus infection. *Clin Exp Immunol* **64**:50–58, 1986.

40. Mackay IR: Genetic aspects of immunologically mediated liver disease. *Sem Liver Dis* **4:**13–25, 1984.

41. Sasazuki T, Nishimura Y, Muto M, Ohta N: HLA-linked genes controlling immune response and disease susceptibility. *Immunol Rev* **70:**52–75, 1983.

42. Ambinder JM, Chiorazzi N, Gibofsky A, et al: Special characteristics of cellular immune function in normal individuals of HLA-DR3 type. *Clin Immunol Immunopathol* **23:**269–374, 1982.

43. Krawitt EL, Kilby AE, Albertini RJ, et al: An immunogenetic study of suppressor cell activity in autoimmune chronic active hepatitis. *Clin Immunol Immunopathol* **46:**249–257, 1988.

44. O'Brien CJ, Vento S, Donaldson PT, et al: Cell-mediated immunity and suppressor cell defects to liver-derived antigens in families of patients with autoimmune chronic active hepatitis. *Lancet* **1:**350–353, 1986.

45. Crapper RM, Mathews JD, Clifford C, et al: A genetically determined setting of the CD4/CD8 (T helper/T suppressor) ratio in men: evidence from monozygous and dizygous twins. 1988, (submitted)

46. Tötterman TH: Distribution of T-, B-, and thyroglobulin-binding lymphocytes infiltrating the gland in Graves' disease, Hashimoto's thyroiditis, and de Quervains thyroiditis. *Clin Exp Immunol* **10:**270–277, 1978.

47. Diaz LA, Roscoe JT, Eaglstein NF, et al: Human pemphigus antibodies are pathogenic to squamous epithelium. *Ann NY Acad Sci* **475:**181–190, 1986.

48. Whittingham S, McNeilage LJ, Mackay IR: Epstein-Barr virus as an etiological agent in primary Sjögrens syndrome. *Medical Hypotheses* **22:**373–386, 1987.

49. Meyer zum Büschenfelde K-H, Hopf U: Studies on the pathogenesis of experimental chronic hepatitis in rabbits. I. Induction of the disease and protective effect of allogenic liver specific proteins. *Brit J Exp Path* **55:**498–508, 1974.

50. Bartholomaeus WN, Reed WD, Joske RA, Shilkin KB: Autoantibody response to liver-specific lipoprotein in mice. *Immunology* **43:**219–226, 1981.

51. Mori Y, Mori T, Yoshida H, et al: Study of cellular immunity in experimental autoimmune hepatitis in mice. *Clin Exp Immunol* **57:**85–92, 1984.

52. Bartholomaeus WA, Reed WD, Joske RA: Autoantibody to liver-specific lipoprotein in the mouse: regulation by naturally occurring autoantigen-specific suppressor cells. *Immunology* **58:**307–316, 1984.

53. Taguchi O, Nishizuka Y: Self-tolerance and localized autoimmunity. Mouse models of autoimmune disease that suggest tissue-specific suppressor T cells are involved in self-tolerance. *J Exp Med* **165:**146–156, 1987.

54. Scheiffarth F, Warnatz H, Schmidt HJ: Immunological studies on the development of experimental hepatitis in thymectomized mice. *Int Arch Allergy* **32:**308–317, 1967.

55. Watanabe T, Masucla K, Ikemoto Y, et al: J Gastroenterol Hepatol (in press), 1988.

56. Omata M, Yokosuka O, Imazeki F, et al: Transmission of duck hepatitis B virus from Chinese carrier ducks to Japanese ducklings: a study of viral DNA in serum and tissue. *Hepatology* **4:**603–607, 1984.

57. Frazer IH, Jordan TW, Collins EC, et al: Antibody to liver membrane antigens in chronic active hepatitis. IV. Exclusion of specific reactivity to polypeptides and glycolipids by immunoblotting. *Hepatology* **7:**4–10, 1987.

58. Charpentier BM, Bach MA, Lang P, et al: Phenotypic composition and in vitro functional capacities of unmodified fresh cells infiltrating acutely rejected human kidney allografts. *Transplantation* **44:**38–43, 1987.

59. Mahi-Brown C, Yule TD, Tung KSK: Adoptive transfer of murine autoimmune orchitis to naive recipients with immune lymphocytes. *Cell Immunol* **106:**408–419, 1987.

60. Bhathal PS, Powell LW, Mackay IR: Apoptosis in autoimmune chronic active hepatitis (CAH) (abstract). *Hepatology* **2:**154, 1982.

61. Searle J, Harmon BV, Bishop CJ, Kerr IFR: The significance of cell death by apoptosis in hepatobiliary disease. *J Gastroenterol Hepatol* **2:**77–96, 1987.
62. Neuberger J, Portmann B, Calne R, Williams R: Recurrence of autoimmune chronic active hepatitis following orthotopic liver grafting. *Transplantation* **37:**363–365, 1984.
63. Tassopoulos NC, Papaevangelou GJ, Sjogren MH, et al: Natural history of acute hepatitis B surface antigen-positive hepatitis in Greek adults. *Gastroenterology* **92:**1844–1850, 1987.
64. Lucas CR, Gust ID: Acute hepatitis B—four-and-a-half years' experience at Fairfield Hospital, Melbourne, in Logan GE (ed): *Hepatitis B, Proceedings of the First Australasian Hepatitis Symposium, 1974.* Abbott Laboratories, Sydney, 1975.
65. Hanson RG, Peters MG, Hoofnagle JH: Effects of immunosuppressive therapy with prednisolone on B and T lymphocyte function in patients with Type B hepatitis. *Hepatology* 173–179, 1986.
66. Davis GL, Hoofnagle JH: Reactivation of chronic hepatitis B virus infection. *Gastroenterology* **92:**2028–2031, 1987.
67. Burrell CJ: Cell virus relationships in persistent hepatitis B infection in man: implications from *in situ* hybridization studies, in Chisari FV (ed). *Advances in Hepatitis Research.* Masson, New York, 1984, pp. 62–68.
68. Hoofnagle JH, Shafritz DA, Popper H: Chronic type B hepatitis and the "healthy" HBsAg carrier state. *Hepatology* **7:**758–763, 1987.
69. Chisari FV, Filipi P, Buras J, et al: Structural and pathological effects of synthesis of hepatitis B large envelope polypeptide in transgenic mice. *Proc Nat Acad Sci USA* **84:**6909–6913, 1987.
70. Vento S, Eddleston ALWF: Immunological aspects of chronic active hepatitis. *Clin Exp Immunol* **68:**225–232, 1987.
71. Ferrari C, Penna A, Giuberti T, et al: Intrahepatic, nucleocapsid antigen-specific T cells in chronic active hepatitis B. *J Immunol* **139:**2050–2058, 1987.
72. Jelbert AR, Burrell EJ, Gowans EJ, et al: Cellular localization of α-interferon in hepatitis B virus-infected liver tissue. *Hepatology* **6:**957–961, 1986.

Chronic Hepatitis
Histopathology

SWAN N. THUNG, MICHAEL A. GERBER, and HANS POPPER

INTRODUCTION

Chronic hepatitis is defined as a group of primary diseases of the liver characterized by hepatocellular damage, inflammation, and fibrosis continuing without improvement for at least 6 months.[1-3] The disease may be attributable to viral infections, particularly by hepatitis viruses B, B and D, parenteral NANB, drug reactions, autoimmune processes, alcoholism, genetic diseases, chronic hepatic allograft rejection, or unknown causes. Hepatitis A and enteric hepatitis NANB do not cause chronic hepatitis.

The term chronic hepatitis is relatively recent. At the time that the histologic diagnosis was almost entirely based on autopsy specimens, the process had usually progressed to cirrhosis. Therefore, such designations as active or decompensated cirrhosis were applied to instances with conspicuous inflammatory reaction and severe clinical manifestations referable to liver disease. German hepatologists, under the leadership of H. Kalk, one of the pioneers of laparoscopy, used the term chronic hepatitis earlier than it was used by Anglo-American clinicians. In the middle of this century, several factors shifted the emphasis in nomenclature from cirrhosis to chronic hepatitis. One was the widespread use of blind liver needle biopsy which visualized earlier stages of the disease in which

SWAN N. THUNG and HANS POPPER • The Lillian and Henry M. Stratton–Hans Popper Department of Pathology, Mount Sinai School of Medicine of the City University of New York, New York 10029.   MICHAEL A. GERBER • Department of Pathology, Tulane University School of Medicine, New Orleans, Louisiana 70112.

cirrhosis was not yet or just barely visible. The second factor was the growing application of hepatic tests, particularly of the aminotransferases, which led to routine diagnosis or at least suspicion of milder degrees of liver injury and permitted one to follow its evolution prospectively. This was particularly important, since the clinical manifestations of milder degrees of chronic hepatitis are rather nonspecific and mainly fatigability. A third factor was the development of immunosuppressive therapy, predominantly corticosteroids. This therapy stimulated the attempt to identify conditions in which it was indicated. The resulting, originally therapeutic, classification is today, almost ironically, still the most widely used, although the use of immunosuppressive therapy is now greatly restricted.

The classification of chronic hepatitis is commonly based on morphologic criteria. Clinical information is often needed for the diagnosis, particularly the time of onset of the disease, but an accurate diagnosis is usually not possible on clinical and biochemical grounds alone. Thus, liver biopsy is essential for the diagnosis, but clinical information and results of biochemical tests must be taken into account before a final diagnosis is reached.

Two main forms of chronic hepatitis have been widely accepted: (1) chronic active hepatitis (CAH), also known as chronic aggressive hepatitis and chronic periportal hepatitis, and (2) chronic persistent hepatitis (CPH), also known as chronic portal hepatitis. The major difference between these two forms is the location of the inflammatory infiltrate. In CPH it is confined to the portal tracts, whereas in CAH it extends into the periportal parenchyma, usually accompanied by hepatocellular destruction and by fibrosis. This distinction plays a major role in diagnosis and management of patients with chronic hepatitis. There are also important differences between the prognoses for CAH and CPH, particularly with respect to the development of cirrhosis, which may follow CAH but not necessarily CPH.

CHRONIC ACTIVE HEPATITIS

Chronic active hepatitis is not a single entity, but rather a morphologic reaction pattern that may be seen in liver diseases from a variety of causes. Therefore, the etiologic factor should be specified whenever possible.

The morphologic hallmark of CAH is piecemeal necrosis (Fig. 1). This is defined as the destruction of liver cells at an interface between parenchyma and connective tissue together with a predominantly lymphocytic and plasma cell infiltrate. The characteristic lesion is seen at the edge of portal tracts and septa where various types of lymphocytes and macrophages, as well as segmented leukocytes infiltrate the limiting hepatocellular plate. The hepatocytes undergo gradual destruction by this process of piecemeal necrosis, as indicated by hydro-

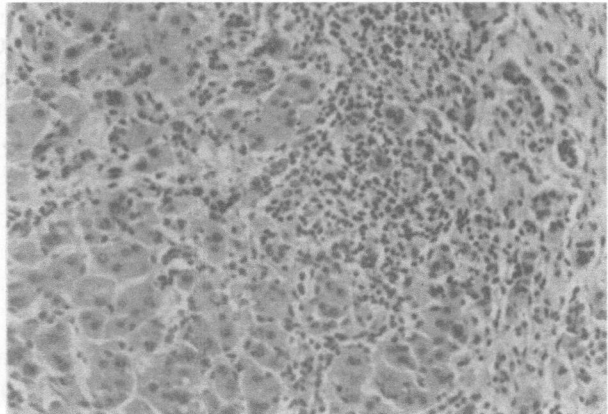

FIGURE 1. Extension of the inflammatory exudate into the periportal zone, accompanied by necrosis of periportal hepatocytes in chronic active hepatitis. (H&E.)

pic swelling, focal necrosis, formation of acidophilic bodies, and apoptosis. Lymphocytes in close contact with hepatocytes (peripolesis), and within them (emperipolesis—lymphocytes penetrating and destroying hepatocytes) may be seen. Simple spillover of inflammatory cells into the periportal parenchyma without hepatocellular necrosis may be seen in acute hepatitis, but also focally in CPH, and has no prognostic significance. Destruction of a sleeve of periportal hepatocytes may be recognized, if surviving liver cells are trapped behind the advancing edge of piecemeal necrosis or if connective tissue stains distinguish the original portal tract from the collapsed periportal parenchyma. With appropriate stains, the thick birefringent fibers of preexisting type I collagen may be distinguished from recently formed pliable collagen, mainly of type III, which is lighter in color. The hepatocytes in the vicinity of portal tracts and fibrous septa often are arranged in glandlike or pseudorosette formations. Piecemeal necrosis is also accompanied by formation of new collagen fibers and ingrowth of blood vessels and bile ductules.

The portal tracts appear to be enlarged, owing to the periportal piecemeal necrosis and to connective tissue septa. They are infiltrated by lymphocytes, plasma cells, macrophages, and segmented leukocytes; the latter often accompany proliferating bile ductules.

The lobular architecture is initially preserved. Small foci of spotty necrosis, ballooned cells, and eosinophilic bodies are usually present within the lobules (lobular necrosis). Larger intralobular foci of hepatocellular degeneration and necrosis surrounded by more or less normal parenchyma may correspond to acute flare-ups of chronic hepatitis or superinfection by a second virus. These circumscribed necroinflammatory lesions may favor rapid progression of CAH to cirrhosis.[4,5] Morphologic findings show a wide spectrum in CAH, ranging from mild lesions resembling CPH to active cirrhosis. The extent of piecemeal necrosis and lobular and portal inflammation varies considerably. Indeed, cirrhosis is often already present when the diagnosis of CAH is made. Thus, it is not surprising that the prognosis in CAH is variable.

CHRONIC PERSISTENT HEPATITIS

Chronic persistent hepatitis is a primary hepatic disease, usually viral in origin, characterized by chronic inflammatory infiltration, mostly portal, with preserved lobular architecture and little or no portal fibrosis, although the tracts are expanded (Fig. 2). The portal infiltration by lymphocytes and plasma cells may be associated with a variety of extrahepatic or intrahepatic diseases. Therefore, the histologic picture is not pathognomonic for CPH and the diagnosis can be established only within the context of clinical manifestations after exclusion of other causes.[6]

Connective tissue stains disclose little or no portal fibrosis, with occasional short septa radiating into the parenchyma and sometimes linking portal tracts. Proliferation of bile ductules is usually absent.

The hepatic parenchyma is histologically normal or shows a few foci of hepatocellular necrosis and inflammatory infiltration. The lobular architecture is

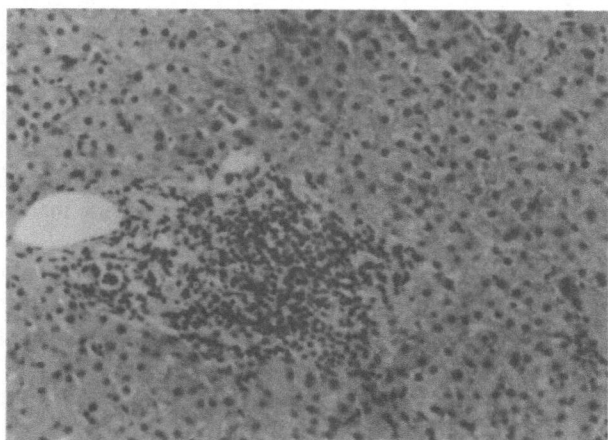

FIGURE 2. Mononuclear cell infiltrate in an enlarged portal tract in chronic persistent hepatitis. (H&E.)

preserved or the hepatic plates are uneven, producing a cobblestone appearance. Cholestasis is usually absent. The sinusoidal lining cells, including Kupffer cells, are activated to varying degrees. Ground-glass hepatocytes may be found in hepatitis B surface antigen (HB_sAg)-positive patients. When features of acute hepatitis are superimposed on CPH, it becomes impossible to distinguish CPH from chronic lobular hepatitis (CLH) histologically, and it should be designated as such.

The significance of the diagnosis CPH lies in its distinction from CAH, and not in the lesion itself. CPH is mostly stationary. In many instances, it resolves after many months or years spontaneously, far more frequently than CAH.[7] Lymphoid follicles with germinal centers or damaged interlobular bile ducts in CPH are thought to be associated with progression to more serious liver disease, such as CAH or cirrhosis.[8] CPH that develops in the course of treatment of CAH has a tendency to relapse if treatment is discontinued.

CHRONIC LOBULAR HEPATITIS

In 1971, the term chronic lobular hepatitis (CLH) was proposed for parenchymal necroinflammation resembling acute hepatitis but persisting for more than 6 months.[3] This new category has been adopted by the International Group as one form of chronic hepatitis. Piecemeal necrosis and bridging necrosis are not part of CLH. The severity of the hepatocellular damage may vary from mild spotty necrosis and inflammation to severe hepatocellular injury reflected in swelling, eosinophilic bodies, diffuse inflammatory infiltration and cholestasis. This form of chronic hepatitis is distinguished from acute hepatitis only by the duration of disease. Follow-up studies indicate that CLH may last for several years with remissions and relapses, but without evidence of progression to cirrhosis. The prognosis is generally good and specific therapy is not required.

CHRONIC SEPTAL HEPATITIS

Chronic septal hepatitis is a form of chronic hepatitis characterized by noninflammatory septa, sometimes representing the residual lesion of CAH, or more commonly CPH.[9]

IMMUNOPATHOLOGY

Immunohistochemically, a variety of expression patterns of hepatitis B virus (HBV) antigens has been observed in different forms in chronic B infection.[10]

Variable focal expression of HB_sAg and of hepatitis B core antigen (HB_cAg) is usually seen in CAH type B, whereas large numbers of HB_sAg-positive hepatocytes are observed in inactive cirrhosis, in CPH, and in "healthy" carriers with little or no liver damage. Abundant HB_cAg with little HB_sAg is often found in immunosuppressed patients with mild liver disease, such as those on hemodialysis or with acquired immune deficiency syndrome (AIDS). Thus, there appears to be a rough correlation between the expression pattern of HBV antigens in liver tissue and the type of hepatitis. Overall, there is an inverse relationship between the amount of HBV antigens, particularly HB_sAg, in hepatocytes and the severity of liver damage suggesting that HBV is not directly cytopathic.

As a result of combined serologic and immunohistochemical studies for HBV markers and molecular hybridization for HBV DNA in serum and liver, it has been proposed that the natural history of chronic HBV infection is characterized by two sequential virologic phases: an early replicative or permissive phase (various nonintegrated forms of replicative HBV DNA in serum and liver, infectious virions in serum, HB_cAg and HB_sAg in liver) and a later nonreplicative or nonpermissive phase (integrated HBV DNA in liver, no infectious virions in serum, HB_sAg but no HB_cAg in liver). In general, active HBV replication appears to be associated with necroinflammation in the liver. These findings are consistent with the hypothesis that HBV-induced hepatocellular injury is mediated by the host immune response to virus-encoded or -induced target antigens expressed on the hepatocyte surface during viral replication. There is increasing evidence that HLA-restricted cytotoxic T lymphocytes directed against a molecular complex of viral and histocompatibility antigens on the hepatocyte surface represent the effector cells. Predominance of T8-positive lymphocytes reacting with HLA class I antigens in areas of intraparenchymal and piecemeal necrosis support this hypothesis.[11,12]

VARIANTS OF CHRONIC ACTIVE HEPATITIS

CAH with Abnormal Bile Duct Epithelium

Abnormal bile duct epithelium in CAH has been noted by several observers, most commonly in hepatitis NANB. The affected bile ducts are of medium size (with lumen ~100 nm) and show multilayered rounded epithelium with pale cytoplasm and pyknotic nuclei, indistinct basement membrane, and infiltration by chronic inflammatory cells. The changes are segmental in the bile ducts and focal in the liver and are therefore found only if step sections are made. They are associated with heavy mononuclear cell infiltration in the vicinity, with occasional formation of lymphoid follicles. Cholestasis may be present. CAH with abnormal biliary epithelium has a worse prognosis than CAH without this lesion, progressing more quickly and more frequently to cirrhosis.[13]

CAH with Confluent Necrosis

Boyer and Klatskin,[14] in 1970, described confluent necrosis forming bridges between the various vascular canals of the liver in acute viral hepatitis. This lesion, also classified as subacute hepatic necrosis, was assumed to lead to fatal hepatic failure or to development of cirrhosis in a significant number of patients. Recently, the prognostic significance of bridging necrosis has been questioned.

In CAH with bridging necrosis, the lobules are dissected by broad or narrow bands of necrosis bridging between central veins and, more importantly, between central veins and portal tracts. Necrosis linking portal tracts with each other probably represents extensive piecemeal necrosis. Collapse of the necrotic bridges produces passive septa. Necroinflammation is usually present in all parts of the parenchyma. The bridging necrosis may progress to involve entire lobules and lead to multilobular necrosis and collapse. In the presence of piecemeal necrosis, bridging necrosis appears to predispose to more rapid development of cirrhosis.[15,16] This may be related to the formation of portal–systemic vascular shunts inducing ischemia of parts of the lobules with uneven distribution of regeneration and to extension of the relevant immune reaction from the portal areas deep into the lobules.

TRANSITION TO CIRRHOSIS

In contrast to CPH, CAH often progresses to cirrhosis. With continuation of the disease, regeneration occurs first periportally and subsequently without relation to acinar structure and eventually obscuring the latter, and is recognized as foci of hepatocellular plates more than one cell thick. The regenerated nodules are surrounded by fibrous septa, and transition to cirrhosis, usually macronodular, develops. A liver biopsy specimen obtained at this stage of the disease demonstrates cirrhosis with features of CAH (Fig. 3). The activity of the cirrhosis may be estimated from the amount of hepatocellular necrosis and inflammation. There is no sharp border between CAH and cirrhosis. CAH may occur alone or in combination with cirrhosis, which may eventually become inactive (cirrhosis without CAH or inactive cirrhosis). Depending on the predominant lesion, the terms CAH with cirrhosis or cirrhosis with CAH or activity (active cirrhosis) are used.

The histologic criteria for the diagnosis of cirrhosis are important because the liver biopsy provides the best objective proof for the presence of cirrhosis. The diagnosis is established if (1) parenchymal nodules surrounded by fibrous septa, or (2) septa linking portal tracts and central veins are observed. Frequently, however, these features are absent from needle biopsy specimens because the needle may be diverted from the dense fibrous septa or obtain tissue

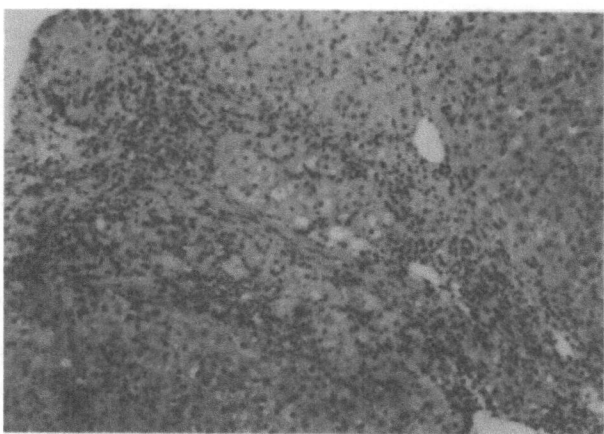

FIGURE 3. Nodules of hepatocytes surrounded by fibrous septa with mononuclear cell infiltrate. Piecemeal necrosis is also seen in this liver with chronic active hepatitis and cirrhosis. (H&E.)

from a large nodule only. Therefore, the following criteria suggestive of cirrhosis are used: (1) fragmentation of the liver tissue into small rounded pieces; (2) fibrous septa covering more than one half the circumference of a parenchymal fragment; (3) variations in the degree of regeneratory activity (differential regeneration) reflected in thickening of cell plates or compression of one area by another; (4) concentric arrangement of liver cell plates with disturbance of lobular architecture; (5) variations in different parenchymal areas, e.g., degree of atypism or amount of fat, iron, cholestasis, lipofuscin, inflammation; and (6) disproportion between sparse portal tracts and excess of hepatic veins. Some of these features are best seen on reticulin or connective tissue stains.

After the diagnosis of cirrhosis has been made, the activity of the process should be specified by the degree of hepatocellular damage and in inflammatory infiltration of the lobular or nodular parenchyma or at interface with the connective tissue. The etiology of cirrhosis cannot always be determined from the histologic appearance; however, etiologic hints, particularly when the specific manifestations of the precursor hepatitis persist or have reappeared, may be observed. Special stains for HB_sAg, iron, copper and DPAS-positive globules or immunoperoxidase stains may be helpful. Conspicuous hepatocellular atypism is suggestive but not diagnostic for transition to hepatocellular carcinoma. Classification of cirrhosis into macronodular, micronodular, and mixed types is not particularly helpful clinically.

ROLE OF THE LIVER BIOPSY IN DIFFERENTIAL DIAGNOSIS

Morphologic examination in cases of chronic hepatitis is important because it may (1) establish the diagnosis of hepatitis in general; (2) provide clues for the etiologic agent; (3) offer information about the pathogenesis; (4) assist in prognosis; and, most important for the patient, (5) monitor therapy.[2]

Histologically, CAH must be distinguished from several other primary hepatic diseases. Differentiation from acute hepatitis may be difficult, particularly from the form that may resemble CLH, with possible transition to CAH or bridging necrosis. Information as to the duration of the disease is the deciding factor. The distinction between mild CAH and CPH is often very difficult. Some portal tracts may show changes characteristic of CPH, while others are typical of CAH and frequently piecemeal necrosis involves only part of the circumference of the tract. Again clinical, biochemical, and immunologic data have all to be considered for a definitive diagnosis aiding in prognosis and therapy.

Piecemeal necrosis alone does not diagnose CAH. This lesion may be observed in liver diseases of many different causes, such as primary biliary cirrhosis, prolonged biliary tract disease (both extra- and intrahepatic), Wilson's disease, α_1-antitrypsin deficiency, alcohol- or drug-induced liver disease, and autoimmune hepatitis.

In prolonged large bile duct obstruction, cholestasis is prominent in the periportal zone and is associated with feathery degeneration and necrosis of hepatocytes, rather than with true mainly lymphocytic piecemeal necrosis. Segmented leukocytes predominate over mononuclear cells in the portal tracts, and there is usually considerable proliferation of bile ductules, particularly along the margins of the portal tracts.

Primary biliary cirrhosis and CAH share many histologic features. They can usually be distinguished by a combination of all manifestations. The histologic differentiation becomes more difficult when the diagnostic lesion of nonsuppurative destructive cholangitis is missing, and primary biliary cirrhosis progresses to more advanced stages. The distinction of CAH from primary biliary cirrhosis becomes particularly difficult when CAH is associated with bile duct damage or cholestasis, but may be made by determination of trypsin-sensitive mitochondrial antibodies.

Sclerosing cholangitis has many morphologic features in common with CAH. Distortion, atrophy, and vanishing of bile ducts with concentric periductal fibrosis and formation of bile duct scars, as well as irregular proliferation of bile ductules and cholestasis, including the deposition of copper and copper–protein complexes in periportal hepatocytes, are characteristic of sclerosing cholangitis.

Malignant lymphoma in the liver may resemble CPH. The neoplastic lymphocytes of well-differentiated lymphocytic lymphoma cannot be distinguished histologically from inflammatory lymphocytes in routine paraffin sections. However, in malignant lymphoma, some of the smaller portal tracts are often spared, and only part of the larger portal tracts is infiltrated. By contrast, all portal tracts are usually affected in chronic hepatitis, the smaller portal tracts to a greater extent than the larger ones.

Nonspecific reactive hepatitis represents an inflammatory response in the liver as a reaction to a variety of extrahepatic diseases. It can be distinguished from CPH only sometimes, on the basis of clinical information.

In chronic orthotopic liver transplant rejection,[17] the portal tracts may show fibrosis with loss of bile ducts. The hepatic arteries contain cells with foamy cytoplasm and have thickened walls.

Finally, autoimmune hepatitis is a significant histologic problem from the point of view of diagnosis.[18,19] The pathogenesis of primary autoimmune hepatitis is not fully established; a defect in one of the repertoires of specific suppressor T cells appears to be a reasonable assumption,[20] and specific autoantibodies in the serum are gradually becoming diagnostic.[21] Moreover, an autoimmune reaction to hepatic antigens complicates all chronic liver diseases, including viral hepatitides. This secondary autoimmune hepatitis is also reflected particularly in piecemeal necrosis, creating the most frequent diagnostic quandary for pathologists, i.e., hepatitis NANB; chronic drug-induced hepatitis, particularly on a hypersensitivity basis; and autoimmune hepatitis. Plasma cells need not be in excess in primary autoimmune hepatitis and may be found in similar amounts in the two other diseases. Eosinophils are not particularly common in autoimmune hepatitis and may be found to equal degrees in any form of hepatitis. An abundance of portal eosinophils characterizes Hodgkin's disease and some parasitic infestations.

REFERENCES

1. DeGroote J, Gedigk P, Popper H, et al: A classification of chronic hepatitis. *Lancet* 2:626–628, 1968.
2. Gerber MA, Thung SN: Viral hepatitis: Pathology, in Berk JE (ed): *Bockus Gastroenterology*. Vol. 5. WB Saunders, Philadelphia, 1985, pp. 2825–2855.
3. Popper H, Schaffner F: The vocabulary of chronic hepatitis. *N Engl J Med* 284:1154–1156, 1971.
4. Popper H: Changing concepts of the evolution of chronic hepatitis and the role of piecemeal necrosis. *Hepatology* 3:758–762, 1983.
5. Scheuer PJ: Changing views on chronic hepatitis. *Histopathology* 10:1–4, 1986.
6. Peters RL: Viral hepatitis: A pathologic spectrum. *Am J Med Sci* 270:17–31, 1975.
7. Becker MD, Scheuer PJ, Baptista A, Sherlock S: Prognosis of chronic persistent hepatitis. *Lancet* 1:53–56, 1970.
8. Chadwick RG, Galizzi J, Heathcote J, et al: Chronic persistent hepatitis: Hepatitis B virus markers and histological follow-up. *Gut* 20:372–377, 1979.
9. Gerber MA, Vernace S: Chronic septal hepatitis. *Virchows Arch Pathol Anat* 363:303–309, 1983.

10. Gerber MA, Thung SN: The diagnostic value of immunohistochemical demonstration of hepatitis viral antigens in the liver. *Hum Pathol* **18**:771–774, 1987.
11. Alexander G, Williams R: Characterization of the mononuclear cell infiltrate in piecemeal necrosis. *Lab Invest* **50**:247–249, 1984.
12. Paronetto F: Cell-mediated immunity in liver disease. *Hum Pathol* **17**:168–178, 1986.
13. Christoffersen P, Poulsen H, Scheuer PJ: Abnormal bile duct epithelium in CAH and cirrhosis. *Hum Pathol* **3**:227–235, 1972.
14. Boyer JL, Klatskin G: Pattern of necrosis in acute viral hepatitis. Prognostic value of bridging (subacute hepatic) necrosis. *N Engl J Med* **283**:1063–1071, 1970.
15. Cooksley WG, Bradbear RA, Robinson W, et al: The prognosis of chronic active hepatitis without cirrhosis in relation to bridging necrosis. *Hepatology* **6**:345–348, 1986.
16. Sakaguchi S: Clinical and histopathological studies on hepatitis with bridging necrosis. *Acta Hepatol Jpn* **27**:1043–1055, 1986.
17. Ludwig J, Wiesner RH, Batts K, et al: The acute vanishing bile duct syndrome (acute irreversible rejection) after orthotopic liver transplantation. *Hepatology* **7**:476–483, 1987.
18. Waldenström J: Leber Blutproteine und Nahrunsein-weisz (Sonderband XV Tagung, Bad Kissingen). *Dtsch Verdau Stoffwechselkr* **1950**:8–15, 1950.
19. Mistilis SP, Blackburn CRB: Active chronic hepatitis. *Am J Med* **48**:484–495, 1970.
20. Thomas HC, Brown D, Labrooy J, et al: T-cell subsets in autoimmune and HBV-induced chronic liver disease: A review of the abnormalities and the effects of treatment. *Liver* **2**:266–269, 1982.
21. Doniach D, Rott M, Walker JG, et al: Tissue antibodies in primary biliary cirrhosis, active chronic (lupoid) hepatitis, cryptogenic cirrhosis and other liver disease and their clinical implications. *Clin Exp Immunol* **1**:237–262, 1966.

Chronic Persistent Hepatitis and Chronic Lobular Hepatitis

JORGE RAKELA and JURGEN LUDWIG

INTRODUCTION

Chronic persistent hepatitis (CPH) and chronic lobular hepatitis belong to the clinicopathologic spectrum of chronic hepatitis. Both have a benign connotation in the sense that they do not progress, by definition, to serious forms of chronic liver diseases, e.g., chronic active hepatitis and cirrhosis.

CHRONIC PERSISTENT HEPATITIS

Definition

In 1968, De Groote et al.[1] described a characteristic liver biopsy finding from a patient with chronic persistent hepatitis (CPH) as consisting of chronic inflammatory infiltration, mostly portal, with preserved lobular architecture and little or no fibrosis; absent or slight piecemeal necrosis and features of acute hepatitis may be superimposed. The initial impression was that this lesion did not have the potential to evolve to either chronic active hepatitis (CAH) or cirrhosis, or both. Therefore, the prognosis of CPH was considered generally good. As Bianchi et al.[2] later pointed out, the importance of this diagnosis lies in its distinction from CAH rather than in the lesion itself.

Morphologically, CPH also can be indistinguishable from slowly resolving acute viral hepatitis and nonspecific reactive hepatitis.[3] When features of acute

JORGE RAKELA and JURGEN LUDWIG • Departments of Medicine and Pathology, Mayo Clinic and Foundation, Rochester, Minnesota 55905.

hepatitis are superimposed on the portal lesion of CPH, the distinction from chronic lobular hepatitis (CLH) may become moot. Clinically, CPH is characterized by persistence past 6 months after onset of serum aminotransferases elevation without hyperbilirubinemia and minimal symptomatology.

Clinicopathologic Features

This condition is probably related in the majority of the cases to the clinical course of viral hepatitis; it can be hypothesized that it is closely linked to the ability of hepatitis viruses to cause a persistent infection. Hepatitis A virus (HAV) may relapse in 8–10% of patients; the association of this clinical course with IgM-HAV positivity has been demonstrated.[4] Another prolonged course associated with acute type A hepatitis is characterized by persistent intrahepatic cholestasis with pruritus, fever, diarrhea, weight loss, and serum bilirubin levels >10 mg/dl.[5] However, CPH type A is currently not recognized.

Kao and co-workers[6] described four patients with prolonged elevated serum alanine aminotransferases (>120 days) and positive IgM-anti-HAV; the longest recorded duration of elevated ALT before a normal result was observed was 364 days. This patient was reported to be asymptomatic for several months prior to ALT normalization and IgM-anti-HAV disappearance. Although Kao et al. did not describe histologic findings among these patients, it is likely they would have had findings consistent with CPH.

The commonest histopathologic finding among patients with prolonged hepatitis A has been marked centrilobular cholestasis[5]; three of the five patients who underwent liver biopsy also showed prominent portal inflammation. Therefore, these patients presented a cholestatic form of CPH until their disease resolved.

Chronic hepatitis B virus infection, i.e., hepatitis B surface antigen (HB_sAg) persistence greater than 6 months, occurs in 5–10% of adult patients who present with acute type B hepatitis.[7] The proportion of CPH among these patients will depend on such factors as the existence of superinfection with hepatitis delta virus, as Rizzetto recently observed,[8] and co-infection with human immunodeficiency virus (HIV).[9] Chronic delta infection in a patient with chronic hepatitis B infection usually determines a progressive clinical and pathologic course; by contrast, chronic HBV infection without delta infection in patients who are anti-HIV positive seems to have a more indolent clinical course with less severe histopathologic findings. Therefore, the pathologic expression in this patient population is modulated by the status of host immunity and by co-infection with other viral agents.

The prognosis of CPH is regarded as good because it does not seem to progress to CAH or cirrhosis. However, Aldershvile et al.[10] studied 53 patients with CPH HB_sAg positive. Fourteen patients with HB_sAg and HB_eAg positivity were followed for 12–120 months (mean, 38 months), 11 of whom were persistently HB_eAg positive and five of whom developed CAH or cirrhosis. It was concluded that the persistence of HB_eAg in patients with CPH is associated with a frequent transition to CAH or cirrhosis. This group does not mention the incidence of delta infection and its possible association with progressive disease.

Transfusion-associated non-A, non-B viral hepatitis is associated with more than 50% of patients with persistent (more than 6 months) serum alanine aminotransferase elevation. Most of them develop CAH, but 25–30% present with clinical and pathologic features of CPH.[11]

Rarely, patients infected with delta virus may also present with CPH. Most cases rapidly evolve into more serious forms of liver disease.[12]

Differential Diagnosis

The differentiation between CAH and CPH is quite difficult to establish in some patients and is therapeutically important to establish. The diagnosis of either condition depends mainly on the interpretation of the degree of periportal inflammation. Intraobserver variation in the grading of piecemeal necrosis, however, may be greater than 40%. Therefore, additional methods are being tested to make the distinction.

Redeker[7] presented preliminary data suggesting that portal pressure determinations may discriminate between these two conditions. In his experience, the net wedged hepatic vein pressure was normal in 22 of 23 patients with CPH, and it was only 6 mm Hg in one instance. Contrastingly, this pressure was elevated in 24 of 25 patients with CAH. Determinations of fasting and postprandial serum cholylglycine and sulfolithocholylglycine bile acid concentrations and [^{14}C]aminopyrine metabolism have also shown promise in the separation of these two disorders.[13] Prospective studies should be conducted to define their role in the clinical management of patients with chronic hepatitis.

Chronic persistent hepatitis has also been described as a stage in the natural history of CAH and as an end point in steroid-treated CAH.[14] Although patients in both groups may have the same degree of portal hepatitis in liver biopsy samples, the prognosis is different from those patients with CPH without evidence of previous episodes of CAH.

Chronic persistent hepatitis that results from steroid treatment of severe CAH often exacerbates after treatment has been stopped and may even progress asymptomatically to cirrhosis.[14] Because of this difference in prognosis and the need for continuous observation of patients who have had CAH, we classify the portal hepatitis in such instances as CAH in remission.

CHRONIC LOBULAR HEPATITIS

Definition

Popper and Schaffner,[15] in an editorial published in 1971, proposed the name chronic lobular hepatitis (CLH) to describe spotty hepatocellular necrosis with associated inflammation indistinguishable from cases of uncomplicated acute viral hepatitis. These workers also stated that the clinical and laboratory features may be mild with elevated serum aminotransferases and fatigue or indistinguishable clinically from classic acute viral hepatitis. They considered this picture to be acute hepatitis lasting longer than 3 months. They mentioned the possibility of the chronicity being due to persistent viral infection or unrecognized etiologic agents and suggested that it may last for years and suddenly disappear. The clinical importance of this newly discovered syndrome was that it did not require specific therapy (corticosteroids), unless it was associated with periportal hepatitis, in which case it probably should not be classified as CLH.

Later, Bianchi et al.[2] echoed the general feeling that the then prevailing classification of chronic hepatitis between two neat categories (CPH and CAH) did not encompass all the clinical situations and included CLH to provide more flexibility in our nomenclature.

Clinicopathologic Features

Two publications[16,17] have since attempted to better define the clinical characteristics of CLH.

Wilkinson and co-workers[16] described the clinical course and biochemical, immunologic, and liver histologic changes in five patients with CLH. All were males ranging in age from 17 to 44 years. Their initial presentation was similar to that of acute viral hepatitis. Four of the five patients were successfully treated with prednisone in an attempt to induce remission of the disease. Two required prednisone to maintain control of the disease but, despite prolonged treatment, the results of their liver tests did not return to normal, although they stayed at a level that was better than pretreatment. In the other two patients, prednisone had been necessary to induce lasting remission.

Pathologic studies performed during relapse demonstrated findings indistinguishable from those of acute viral hepatitis. None of the patients showed histologic evidence of progression to cirrhosis even after 8½ years of follow-up. Interestingly, all patient had non-organ-specific autoantibodies in serum and four had hyperglobulinemia. All were HB_sAg negative. Wilkinson et al. postulated that the initial presentation, findings on liver biopsy, and clinical course were consistent with a persistent viral infection. By contrast, the presence of autoantibodies and hypergammaglobulinemia and the excellent biochemical and clinical response to prednisone were consistent with CAH, autoimmune type. The histologic findings were indistinguishable from acute viral hepatitis in repeated liver biopsies, and the lack of progression to cirrhosis despite relapses of disease activity also weighed against being a variant of CAH.

Liaw et al.,[17] from Taiwan, later reported a series of 80 patients with CLH. They also found a predominance of males (81.3%). They were able to demonstrate an etiopathogenic relationship to HBV in 67.5% of patients, 58% of whom presented as acute viral hepatitis. It was concluded that the clinical and laboratory features were indistinguishable from acute viral hepatitis during the acute phase or convalescence. No evidence of progression to cirrhosis was observed at least in a 4½-year period of follow-up. Liaw et al. concluded that despite disease persistence (clinical, laboratory, and liver biopsy findings), there was no progression to more serious forms of liver diseases (CAH or cirrhosis). No treatment with corticosteroids was required in any of the patients. These 80 cases corresponded to 30.9% of patients with biopsy-proven chronic hepatitis in a period of 4 years of observation. This communication is one of the few that provides an idea of the prevalence of this condition. The most characteristic clinical course of CLH was mono- or multiphasic elevation of serum aminotransferases without clinical symptoms.

Ludwig et al.[18] studied 47 patients whose initial biopsy had been previously classified as unresolved viral hepatitis, CLH, or CAH with viral features. It was concluded that lobular hepatitis of unresolved viral hepatitis was indistinguishable from CLH. Ludwig et al. also observed that CLH has a good prognosis with or without steroids unless this condition was complicated by bridging necrosis or multilobular necrosis. In this latter instance, resolution is least likely in a steroid-treated patient with unresolved viral hepatitis.

Differential Diagnosis

The differential diagnosis of CLH from CAH is therapeutically important and probably difficult to establish prospectively, particularly when a patient presents with elevated serum aminotransferases for more than 3 months, hypergammaglobulinemia, and is symptomatic. Wilkinson et al.[16] treated four of their five patients with steroids; by contrast, Liaw et al.[17] did not treat any patient with corticosteroids without apparent failure. However, in a preliminary communication, Ludwig et al.[18] reported fatalities in the long-term follow-up of this condition and concluded that the good prognosis of CLH characterized by lack of disease progression was mainly determined by the selection of cases with inflammation confined to the lobules with spotty necrosis and without bridging necrosis or confluent necrosis.

On the other side of the spectrum, the distinction of CLH from CPH should be simpler because in the latter, the pathologic changes are circumscribed to the portal area and the lobular changes are nonexistent. It is very likely that the paucity of clinical reports describing CLH is due to the inclusion of this subset of patients under other categories such as unresolved viral hepatitis or persistent viral hepatitis or even as CPH.

FINAL COMMENTS

When a clinician faces a patient with chronic hepatitis, it must be decided whether to treat, using corticosteroids or antiviral therapy. The clinician will also be requested to provide a prognosis regarding progression of the disease. Does the establishment of the diagnosis of CLH help? Probably not. If the patient is HB_sAg negative and has presented elevated serum aminotransferases for more than 3 months and is symptomatic, a trial with corticosteroids is unavoidable, which was what Wilkinson et al.[16] opted to do in four of their five patients. If the patient is HB_sAg positive or if HB_sAg negative with a clear background of exposure to non-A, non-B hepatitis, such as blood transfusion, the patient may be placed on a form of antiviral therapy,[19,20] in an attempt to eradicate or diminish significantly the degree of viral replication with the hope of influencing the pathologic features and ultimately improving clinical symptoms.

The histopathologic spectrum of chronic viral hepatitis that encompasses unresolved viral hepatitis, CPH, some cases of fulminant hepatitis with a subacute course, CLH, and CAH without or with cirrhosis may be looked on as a clinical continuum, and various factors may determine the transition from one pathologic condition to another. The prevailing concept has been that chronic persistent viral hepatitis was a condition that did not evolve into CAH and cirrhosis. Discovery of the delta hepatitis virus has shown that some cases evolving as CPH for years, once infected with the delta agent, may progress rapidly into CAH, developing into hepatic failure.[12] The histopathologic status probably reflects the interaction between viral replication and the host immune response to the chronic viral infection and modulation of this interaction is likely to be reflected in variable degrees of necrosis and inflammatory changes in the hepatic acinus.

The classification of chronic hepatitis, established in 1968,[1] and revisited in 1977,[2] when the term CLH was officially accepted, will adopt its final form once we complete our growing knowledge of chronic HBV infection and its consequences in the host and when non-A, non-B hepatitis will no longer be a diagnosis of exclusion.

REFERENCES

1. DeGroote J, Desmet VJ, Gedigk P, et al: A classification of chronic hepatitis. *Lancet* 2:626–628, 1968.
2. Bianchi L, DeGroote J, Desmet VJ, et al: Acute and chronic hepatitis revisited. *Lancet* 2:914–919, 1977.
3. Peters RL: Viral hepatitis: A pathologic spectrum. *Am J Med Sci* 270:17–31, 1975.
4. Sjogren MH, Tanno H, Fay O, et al: Hepatitis A virus in stool during clinical relapse. *Ann Intern Med* 106:221–226, 1987.
5. Gordon SC, Reddy KR, Schiff L, Schiff ER: Prolonged intrahepatic cholestasis secondary to acute hepatitis A. *Ann Intern Med* 101:635–637, 1987.
6. Kao HW, Ashcavai M, Redeker AG: The persistence of hepatitis A IgM antibody after acute clinical hepatitis A. *Hepatology* 4:933–936, 1984.
7. Redeker AG: Advances in clinical aspects of acute and chronic liver disease of viral origin, in Vyas GN, Cohen SN, Schmid R (eds): *Viral Hepatitis*. The Franklin Institute Press, Philadelphia, 1978, pp. 425–429.
8. Rizzetto M: The delta agent. *Hepatology* 3:729–737, 1983.
9. Krogsgaard K, Lindhardt BO, Nielsen JO, et al: The influence of HTLV-III infection on the natural history of hepatitis B virus infection in male homosexual HB_sAg carriers. *Hepatology* 7:37–41, 1987.
10. Aldershvile J, Dietrichson O, Skinhoj P, et al, and the Copenhagen Hepatitis Acute Programme: Chronic persistent hepatitis: serological classification and meaning of the hepatitis B e system. *Hepatology* 2:243–246, 1982.
11. Rakela J, Taswell HF, Ludwig J: Chronic non-A, non-B hepatitis, in Czaja AJ, Dickson ER (eds): *Chronic Active Hepatitis. The Mayo Clinic Experience*. Dekker, New York, 1986, pp. 153–170.
12. DeCock KM, Govindarajan S, Chin KP, Redeker AG: Delta hepatitis in the Los Angeles area: A report of 126 cases. *Ann Intern Med* 105:108–114, 1986.
13. Rakela J, Czaja AJ: Clinical, biochemical, and histologic features of HB_sAg-negative chronic active hepatitis, in Czaja AJ, Dickson ER (eds): *Chronic Active Hepatitis. The Mayo Clinic Experience*. Dekker, New York, 1986, pp. 69–82.
14. Czaja AJ, Ludwig J, Baggenstoss AH, Wolf A: Corticosteroid-treated chronic active hepatitis in remission. *N Engl J Med* 304:5–9, 1981.
15. Popper H, Schaffner F: The vocabulary of chronic hepatitis. *N Engl J Med* 284:1154–1156, 1971.
16. Wilkinson SP, Portmann B, Cochrane AMG, et al: Clinical course of chronic lobular hepatitis. *QJ Med* 188:421–429, 1978.
17. Liaw YF, Chu CM, Chen TJ, et al: Chronic lobular hepatitis: A clinicopathological and prognostic study. *Hepatology* 2:258–262, 1982.
18. Ludwig J, Czaja AJ, Wolff AM: Prognosis of lobular hepatitis in patients with unresolved viral or chronic hepatitis. *Gastroenterology* 79:1034, 1980 (abst).
19. Dooley JS, Davis GL, Peters M, et al: Pilot study of recombinant human alpha-interferon for chronic type B hepatitis. *Gastroenterology* 90:150–157, 1986.
20. Hoofnagle JH, Mullen KD, Jones DB, et al: Treatment of chronic non-A, non-B hepatitis with recombinant human alpha interferon: A preliminary report. *N Engl J Med* 315:1575–1578, 1986.

III

Chronic Active Hepatitis

Clinical Features of Chronic Active Hepatitis

ALBERT J. CZAJA

INTRODUCTION

The clinical features of chronic active hepatitis (CAH) are familiar to most physicians. Similar symptoms, physical findings, and laboratory abnormalities are found in virtually all forms of acute and chronic liver disease. The diagnosis of CAH is possible only if these nonspecific features are clustered into characteristic patterns. The mettle of the clinician is measured by the ability to recognize these patterns.

Chronic active hepatitis can be asymptomatic with only mild biochemical changes, or it can be incapacitating with rapidly evolving manifestations of liver failure. The nature and number of clinical findings depend on the etiology of the disease, duration of illness, and, most importantly, the severity of inflammatory activity. Variations in the degree of inflammatory activity reflect differences in the immunologic tolerance of the host for viral or self-antigens on the hepatocyte surface. These differences, in turn, influence the clinical expression of the disease and the clinician's ability to suspect and secure the diagnosis. The very presence of symptoms and physical findings implies a moderate to severe inflammatory process.

DEMOGRAPHIC FEATURES

Autoimmune CAH is typically an insidious disease of young females.[1] Women constitute at least 70% of all cases, and as many as 50% of patients are

ALBERT J. CZAJA • Division of Gastroenterology, Mayo Clinic and Mayo Medical School, Rochester, Minnesota 55905.

under 30 years old (Table I). Onset is usually between the third and fifth decades, but patients may range in age from 9 months to 81 years. Fifteen percent of patients have a history of contact with acute hepatitis, and up to 40% experience an abrupt onset of illness. Familial occurrences are infrequent, but the disease may be found in siblings, parents, and grandparents of propositi. In one series, 3 of 55 families (5%) had more than one member with overt chronic liver disease.[2] By contrast, serologic abnormalities are common among relatives. Serum immunoglobulin abnormalities (47%), circulating autoantibodies (42%), hypergammaglobulinemia (34%), and elevated serum alkaline phosphatase levels (14%) are frequently found.[2]

Chronic active hepatitis due to hepatitis B virus (HBV) infection, or CAH B, is mainly a disease of men (89%) and patients with severe inflammatory activity are usually older than autoimmune counterparts (median age, 52 versus 35 years).[3] CAH B, however, can develop at any age and age distinctions may simply reflect differences in patterns of referral. Most adult patients (71%) describe an abrupt onset of illness compatible with acute hepatitis.[4] Intrafamilial spread of the virus is possible by perinatal transmission, sexual activity, and

TABLE 1. Distinguishing Features between Autoimmune CAH, CAH B, and Non-A, Non-B CAH[a]

Distinguishing features	Autoimmune CAH	CAH B	Non-A, non-B CAH
Sex	Female	Male	Male
Onset	Insidious	Abrupt	Abrupt
Age (years)	≤30	≥35	≥35
Symptoms	Arthralgias	Numbness	None
Physical findings	Jaundice, thyromegaly, synovitis	Purpura, hypesthesia	Anicteric
Biochemical findings	Hypergammaglobulinemia	Sudden AST elevation	None specific
Immunoserologic markers	Common	Infrequent	Rare (if any)
HLA tests	B8, Dw3	Bw15, 17, 35	None
Histologic features	None	Ground-glass cells, sanded nuclei	Intrasinusoidal cells, steatosis, giant cells, clear cells, bile duct cell proliferation, "naked" acidophilic bodies

[a]CAH, chronic active hepatitis; AST, serum aspartate aminotransferase level.

household contact and familial occurrences of CAH B have been described, typically among the males of the family.[5]

Chronic active hepatitis attributable to non-A, non-B virus infection (non-A, non-B CAH) usually develops after blood transfusion (29%) or illicit self-injection (27%), but in 44% of cases there may be no obvious source of disease.[6] Seventy-five percent of the transfusion-related cases and 66% of those without an obvious source are over 35 years of age. Conversely, only 10% of the addiction-related cases are over 35 years of age. As in CAH B, most patients with non-A, non-B CAH are male (78%).[6] Since the disease may be transmitted by perinatal or sexual contact, intrafamilial spread is possible. Familial occurrences of non-A, non-B CAH, however, are rare in the United States.

SYMPTOMS

The symptoms of CAH have little etiologic specificity; they reflect mainly the severity of hepatocellular inflammation. Easy fatigability is the major complaint of 85% of patients with severe CAH.[1] The symptom does not correlate closely with specific biochemical abnormalities, and it cannot be quantitated or monitored objectively. Its inexplicable persistence, variable severity, and subjectivity are sources of frustration for patient and physician, and each must guard against skepticism about the integrity of the other. Children seem more tolerant of the symptom than are adults. Importantly, easy fatigability does improve during corticosteroid therapy in patients with autoimmune CAH, and this symptom alone is sufficient justification for a treatment trial. Unfortunately, few patients admit to a full recovery of their stamina and any improvement may be unsustained after termination of therapy.

As many as 77% of patients describe features of jaundice, such as scleral icterus or change in the color of urine and stool.[1] Pruritus occurs in 36% of patients, but prominent features of cholestasis are uncommon. Prolonged jaundice and intense pruritus have been reported in 12–28% of patients with CAH, but other biochemical and histologic features in these patients have suggested the possibility of the primary biliary cirrhosis syndrome.[7,8]

Mild upper abdominal discomfort occurs in 48% of patients.[1] The pain is usually localized to the hepatic region, and it is either transient and sharp or, more commonly, protracted and dull. The cause of the pain is unknown, although it is easy to speculate that hepatic enlargement, distention of the liver capsule, liver cell necrosis and regeneration, and increased patient awareness of the right upper quadrant of the abdomen contribute to the sensation. Importantly, other diagnostic considerations, such as biliary tract disease, primary hepatocellular carcinoma, peptic ulcer disease, and pancreatitis, must be excluded before the pain is ascribed to CAH. The discomfort may persist throughout the clinical illness and may recur even when the disease is inactive by biochemical and histologic criteria.

Other common complaints are anorexia (30%), polymyalgia (30%), diarrhea (28%), and delayed menarche or amenorrhea (89%).[1] Hematochezia suggests ulcerative colitis that may occur concomitantly with CAH but that is more typical of the syndrome of primary sclerosing cholangitis.[9] Features of sicca syndrome can be discovered in 22% of patients with autoimmune CAH and an obscure fever (rarely as high as 40°C) recurs in 18%. Cosmetic changes, including facial rounding, hirsutism, and acne, the classic features of autoimmune CAH, occur in 19% of such patients, typically in young women. Weight loss is unusual in all forms of CAH despite the frequent complaint of anorexia. In fact, patients may actually gain weight.[1]

Rare symptoms at presentation that have an etiologic connotation are distal extremity numbness and abnormal gait. The findings can usually be ascribed to a polyarteritis syndrome associated with HBV infection.[10] Features of mononeuritis multiplex may also occur, however, in conjunction with non-B disease. Findings of serum sickness (synovitis and urticaria) are unusual in CAH B, although they are features of acute hepatitis B. Their presence suggests the diagnosis of autoimmune CAH (Table I). Patients with non-A, non-B CAH rarely if ever have serum sickness-like symptoms despite the presence of circulating immune complexes.[11]

PHYSICAL FINDINGS

Physical findings reflect the duration and severity of the disorder. Patients with severe autoimmune CAH and cirrhosis invariably have physical manifestations of their disease, whereas 26% of patients without cirrhosis have normal physical examinations.[12] Hepatomegaly is the most common finding (78%) and jaundice is detected frequently (69%). Patients with cirrhosis have splenomegaly more commonly than do those without cirrhosis (56% versus 32%, $p<0.05$), but splenomegaly occurs so commonly in patients with severe hepatocellular inflammation (42%) that the finding lacks specificity for cirrhosis.[12]

Spider nevi occur in 58% of patients with severe autoimmune CAH; they can be identified with similar frequency in patients with and without cirrhosis (67% versus 52%).[12] In CAH B, the presence of spider nevi has been recognized as an independent factor associated with a poor prognosis.[13]

Ascites is detectable at presentation in 17% of patients with severe autoimmune CAH; this finding is highly specific for cirrhosis (92%).[12] Like spider nevi, ascites has been associated with a poor prognosis in patients with CAH B.[13]

Features of hepatic encephalopathy are unusual at presentation, occurring in only 14% of patients.[12] In 92% of instances, however, the findings connote cirrhosis. Endogenous hepatic encephalopathy augurs a poor prognosis with greater certainty than do any of the other physical findings.

Hyperpigmentation (≤1%) and xanthelasma (2%) are such unusual findings in CAH that their presence militates against the diagnosis.[1] Slit-lamp examination of the eyes may rarely disclose Kayser–Fleischer rings in severe cholestatic forms of the disease, but rings are never discernible by gross visual inspection.[1]

Thyromegaly (7%), synovitis (2%), pleuritis, and pericarditis are uncommon features of autoimmune CAH but, when present, strongly support the diagnosis[14] (Table I). Acne, facial rounding, dorsal hump formation, and hirsutism may be early symptoms or physical findings of CAH. Esophageal varices are uncommon at presentation (8%),[15] and jaundice seems to be less frequent in the viral forms of CAH, especially in non-A, non-B disease.[16]

ASSOCIATED AUTOIMMUNE DISORDERS

Circulating immune complexes have been demonstrated in viral and nonviral CAH and autoimmune manifestations have been described in each type. Disorders of a possible immunologic nature occur most commonly in autoimmune CAH (≤48%) and least commonly in non-A, non-B disease.

In autoimmune CAH, almost any organ system can be involved. Hashimoto's thyroiditis is diagnosed in 7% of cases; ulcerative colitis in 4%, rheumatoid arthritis in 2%; and systemic lupus erythematosus (SLE), iritis, pernicious anemia, idiopathic thrombocytopenic purpura, or Sjögren's syndrome in 4%.[14] Thyromegaly does not always connote Hashimoto's thyroiditis, and Graves' disease may be present in some patients. Additional associations have included myasthenia gravis, urticaria, pyoderma gangrenosum, neutropenia, hyperplastic gingivitis, peripheral neuropathy, hemolytic anemia, eosinophilia, membranoproliferative glomerulonephritis with distal and proximal renal tubular acidosis, fulminant secretory diarrhea, fibrosing alveolitis, pleuritis, pericarditis, and cryoglobulinemia.[1] The pathogenetic relationship between these various clinical findings and autoimmune CAH is uncertain. In some instances, the occurrence of the immunologic disorder is so infrequent that its association with autoimmune CAH may be coincidental. In other instances, the liver disease may be a secondary finding in a systemic disorder involving multiple organs, such as SLE. Lastly, the liver disease may be misdiagnosed as CAH and wrongly associated with an immunologic feature that is more appropriately included in the syndrome of primary biliary cirrhosis or primary sclerosing cholangitis. In this regard, ulcerative colitis may have a closer association with primary sclerosing cholangitis than with autoimmune CAH.[9]

Viral CAH is infrequently complicated by manifestations of immune-complex disease. Pancreatitis, membranous nephritis, pericarditis, and mononeuritis multiplex are parts of a polyarteritis syndrome associated with hepatitis B surface antigenemia.[10] Arthralgia, purpura, nephritis, and chronic liver disease constitute the syndrome of essential mixed cryoglobulinemia, which has also been linked to HBV infection.[17] Similar associations have not been described in non-A, non-B CAH, which is typically devoid of immunologic trappings. Purpura, urticaria, arthralgia, and aplastic anemia are unusual features of acute non-A, non-B infection. They have not as yet been recognized as manifestations of chronic disease.[11,18]

BIOCHEMICAL FEATURES

Serum aminotransferase levels are the major biochemical indices of inflammatory activity. Although these tests are not predictive of the pattern of histologic abnormality, they do correlate with disease severity and prognosis. In most cases, the level of serum aspartate aminotransferase does not exceed 500 IU/liter.[19] Markedly elevated aminotransferase levels ($\geq$1000 IU/liter), however, may occur in 16% of patients with hepatitis B surface antigen (HB_sAg)-negative CAH,[19] and the abnormality may suggest acute hepatocellular necrosis of viral, toxic, ischemic, or drug-induced origin. Differentiation of CAH with extreme aminotransferase elevation from acute viral hepatitis depends on the presence of chronic symptoms, recognition of physical findings compatible with chronic disease (i.e., ascites, spider nevi, esophageal varices), and demonstration of hypoalbuminemia or hypergammaglobulinemia.[19] Patients with extremely active CAH and high aminotransferase concentrations have lower serum albumin levels (2.3 ± 0.3 g/dl versus 3.1 ± 0.2 g/dl, $p<0.02$) and higher γ-globulin concentrations (4.1 ± 0.3 g/dl versus 1.4 ± 0.1 g/dl, $p<0.001$) than do patients with fulminant viral hepatitis.[20]

Patients with CAH B and non-A, non-B CAH generally have lower levels of serum aminotransferase activity than do patients with autoimmune disease.[4,16] An abrupt elevation of serum aspartate aminotransferase activity in patients with CAH B suggests a superimposed infection with delta[21] or non-A, non-B agents.[11] Aminotransferase levels may also increase in patients undergoing a spontaneous seroconversion from HB_eAg to anti-HB_e and in anti-HB_e-positive patients who suddenly reactivate their disease and undergo a backconversion from anti-HB_e to HB_eAg.[23] Patients with CAH B who present with high aminotransferase levels (i.e., greater than tenfold normal) may well have a superimposed or reactivated viral infection or an immunologic intolerance of viral antigens that will ultimately terminate their HBV infection (Table I). Such considerations in these patients may explain variations in their disease behavior as well as differences in their responses to treatment. Patients with non-A, non-B CAH are also at risk of superimposed viral infections, but these occurrences are poorly documented. Nevertheless, decompensation in a patient with non-A, non-B CAH always justifies an assessment of this possibility.

Cholestatic findings may be present in all forms of CAH, but they are less prominent than the biochemical features of hepatocellular inflammation. Hyperbilirubinemia can be documented in 83% of patients with severe autoimmune CAH, but the serum bilirubin level exceeds 3.0 mg/dl in only 46%.[1] In non-A, non-B CAH, hyperbilirubinemia occurs in only 4% and it does not exceed 1.8 mg/dl.[16] Elevation of the serum alkaline phosphatase level occurs in 81% of patients with severe hepatocellular inflammation, but it is greater than two times normal in only 33% and more than fourfold normal in only 10%.[1]

The serum γ-globulin concentration reflects the severity and duration of hepatocellular inflammation. Hypergammaglobulinemia is a hallmark of autoimmune CAH (Table I) and it is present in more than 80% of patients with severe disease.[12] Serum levels >3 g/dl occur in 48% of patients, and they are more common in those with cirrhosis (67% versus 35%, $p<0.01$).[12] A polyclonal increase in the concentrations of the serum immunoglobulins is typical of autoimmune CAH, and the immunoglobulin G (IgG) fraction is the predominant abnormality.[1] Hypergammaglobulinemia is less frequent and less pronounced in the viral forms of CAH, probably because of less severe inflammatory activity. In one series of 25 patients with non-A, non-B CAH, only 16% had elevated globulin levels.[16]

Hypoprothrombinemia, hypoalbuminemia, and thrombocytopenia are features of advanced liver disease. Prolongation of the prothrombin time beyond 3 sec of control (30%), reduction of the albumin level to <3 g/dl (49%), and decrease in the platelet count below 100,000/mm³ (10%) are common features of severe autoimmune CAH; most of these patients (56%) have cirrhosis.[12] Thrombocytopenia has the lowest sensitivity for cirrhosis (23%) but the highest specificity for the diagnosis (90%). In patients with viral CAH, these findings are less frequent. Hypoprothrombinemia and hypoalbuminemia have been described in only 8% and 16%, respectively, of patients with non-A, non-B CAH.[16]

Anemia (hemoglobin level <12 g/dl) occurs in 32% of patients with severe autoimmune CAH.[12] Patients with cirrhosis are more commonly anemic than those without cirrhosis (49% versus 21%, $p<0.01$), and the finding probably reflects hypersplenism in most cases. A Coombs positive hemolytic anemia, however, can be documented in 1% of cases.[24]

In patients with nonviral CAH, urinary copper excretion may exceed normal levels in nearly 50% of instances. The abnormality, however, is infrequently at a level suggesting Wilson's disease (>100 μg/day). Hepatic copper content may also be increased, but it rarely exceeds 100 μg/g dry tissue weight.[25] The rhodamine stain for tissue copper is routinely negative in patients with CAH lacking antimitochondrial antibody (AMA). In 19% of patients with histologic features of CAH and AMA seropositivity, however, there will be a positive stain. These patients typically respond to corticosteroid therapy.[26]

IMMUNOSEROLOGIC FEATURES

Serologic markers of a possible autoimmune nature are characteristic but not pathognomonic of autoimmune CAH (Table I). Antinuclear antibody (ANA) may be detected in acute viral hepatitis (43%), alcoholic hepatitis (50%), primary biliary cirrhosis (23%), primary sclerosing cholangitis (11%), and CAH B (6%).[3,27] Anti-smooth muscle antibody (anti-SMA) is similarly characteristic but nondiagnostic of autoimmune CAH, occurring commonly in acute viral hepatitis (80%), alcoholic hepatitis (50%), and primary biliary cirrhosis (66%).[27] Despite the nonspecificity of the findings, the demonstration of immunoserologic abnormalities solidifies the diagnosis of autoimmune CAH.

Most patients with severe autoimmune CAH (81%) will have the LE cell phenomenon (27%), ANA (28%), or SMA (40%), and many (30%) will have two or more markers.[1] AMA can be demonstrated in 20% of patients, but the titer is usually less than 1 : 40. Only 15% of AMA-positive patients have titers exceeding 1 : 160. These patients are distinguished from those with primary biliary cirrhosis syndrome by the presence of histologic features characteristic of CAH.[26]

Antibodies to double-stranded (native) DNA are present in more than 40% of patients with autoimmune CAH.[1] Similar frequencies have been reported in acute and chronic hepatitis B, and the finding has been attributed to the release of DNA from damaged hepatocytes. When the development of an immunofluorescence assay with *Crithidia luciliae* as substrate failed to detect biologically relevant antibody to double-stranded DNA in autoimmune hepatitis, it was reported that this test would separate the syndromes of SLE and autoimmune CAH.[28] Additional experiences with this assay and others of similar specificity and superior sensitivity, however, have demonstrated the presence of IgG antibody to double-stranded DNA in patients with drug-induced CAH (37%), autoimmune CAH (64%), HB$_s$Ag-positive CAH (43%), and idiopathic (ANA-negative) CAH (46%).[29] Importantly, immunoserologic abnormalities have not been closely linked to immunologically mediated pathogenetic mechanisms of disease, and they should continue to be regarded as nonspecific manifestations of inflammatory activity.

Multiple paraproteins displaying antibody activity have been described in severe autoimmune CAH, and their etiologic and clinical significance remains uncertain. Antibodies to bacterial *(Escherichia coli, Bacteroides,* and *Salmonella)* and viral (measles, rubella, and cytomegalovirus) agents may be present.[1] The inability of the damaged liver to sequester exogenous antigens normally and prevent antibody production may explain the heterogeneous antibody response. Alternatively, a genetically predetermined nonspecific increase in immunologic responsiveness or an abnormal immunologic defense against infection may account for the phenomena. Rarely, extremely high levels of immunoglobulin may produce coagulation abnormalities, renal insufficiency, and mental disturbances consistent with a hyperviscosity syndrome.

In 20% of patients with severe CAH, there are neither immunoserologic markers nor epidemiologic factors for viral infection.[14] Although these patients may well have sporadic non-A, non-B disease, they are best classified under the rubric of idiopathic CAH. Recent studies with sera obtained from patients with non-A, non-B CAH have indicated the absence of significant autoimmune serologic reactions in this patient population.[30] All samples lacked smooth muscle antibody, and only low-titer reactions were demonstrated for ANA and cytofilament antibody (11% and 22% of specimens, respectively). Perhaps the absence of immunoserologic markers will have greater diagnostic specificity than their presence in some forms of CAH. Firm conclusions about the diagnostic value of immunoserologic tests must await the development of a reliable assay for non-A, non-B infection and the performance of critical studies in well-defined etiologic subgroups matched for disease severity.

GENETIC PREDISPOSITIONS

The histocompatibility antigen HLA-B8 can be identified in more than 60% of patients with autoimmune CAH,[1] and there is evidence that such patients may respond more frequently to corticosteroids than counterparts without this antigen (100% versus 47%).[31] Other studies have demonstrated a higher than normal occurrence of HLA-Dw3 in severe autoimmune CAH (68% versus 24%, $p <$ 0.001), linking the presence of this antigen to an unsatisfactory response to corticosteroids.[32] The increased prevalence of HLA-B8 in immunologic disorders, such as celiac disease, childhood asthma, Addison's disease, Graves' disease, myasthenia gravis, Coombs test positivity, and dermatitis herpetiformis, as well as its association with defects in suppressor lymphocyte function suggest that an enhanced immunologic reactivity to self-antigens may be genetically determined and important in the development of autoimmune CAH. In addition, the HLA associations indicate that the ability to respond to corticosteroids may be influenced by genetic factors.

Susceptibility to viral CAH may also have a genetic control (Table I). Both CAH B and non-A, non-B CAH have a male predisposition and hepatitis B surface antigenemia has been associated with Bw15, Bw17, and Bw35.[33] Adequate studies have not as yet been performed in non-A, non-B CAH, but there is evidence that this disease may be distinguishable from autoimmune CAH by its low prevalence of HLA A1 (5% versus 56%, $p<0.01$) and HLA B8 (10% versus 44%, $p<0.05$).[31]

CLINICAL IMPLICATIONS OF HISTOLOGIC FINDINGS

In untreated patients with nonviral CAH, the histologic pattern at presentation has prognostic importance. Patients with bridging or multilobular necrosis have an 82% incidence of cirrhosis within 5 years and a mortality of 45%, while those with similar clinical and biochemical abnormalities but periportal necrosis have less than a 17% incidence of cirrhosis during the same interval and a normal survival probability.[34] In patients with clinical and biochemical evidence of severe autoimmune CAH, the histologic patterns of active cirrhosis, periportal hepatitis, bridging necrosis, and multilobular necrosis occur with similar freqency (25%) and are distinguishable only by tissue examination.[34] Bridging necrosis with portal–portal linkage seems to be a more benign lesion than central–portal linkage in that progression to cirrhosis occurs less commonly in the former condition (10% versus 29%).[35]

DIAGNOSTIC PITFALLS

Since the findings of CAH are nonspecific and the diagnosis requires a careful cluster analysis, diagnostic difficulties can be encountered. The differential diagnosis of CAH includes Wilson's disease, primary biliary cirrhosis, alcoholic liver disease, primary sclerosing cholangitis, α_1-antitrypsin deficiency, and hemochromatosis. A careful clinical history, expert interpretation of the liver biopsy tissue, routine serum studies (e.g., ceruloplasmin, ferritin, and α_1-antitrypsin concentrations), diagnostic procedures (e.g., endoscopic cholangiography), and special tissue tests (e.g., iron and copper analyses) will usually establish the diagnosis. The major diagnostic pitfalls are in distinguishing CAH from slowly resolving acute viral hepatitis, impaired regeneration syndrome, chronic lobular hepatitis, and primary biliary cirrhosis syndrome.

Slowly resolving acute viral hepatitis is distinguished from CAH mainly by the duration of illness and histologic examination. Disease of more than 6 months duration is chronic by international criteria, and this finding alone should separate the entities. Estimates of disease duration, however, can be variable, and the option of observing for 6 months may defer institution of a potentially lifesaving therapy. The presence of spider nevi, ascites, hypoalbuminemia, hypergammaglobulinemia, thrombocytopenia, or esophageal varices supports the diagnosis of CAH.[12] Unfortunately, the morphologic examination may also be confusing, since both CAH and slowly resolving acute viral hepatitis can have periportal hepatitis and lobular changes, such as acidophilic cell necrosis, Kupffer cell hyperplasia, and hepatic cord disarray. In these instances, the diagnosis hinges on the extent of portal versus lobular change and the uniformity of lobular involvement. In CAH, inflammatory activity and regenerative changes vary from lobule to lobule, in contradistinction to acute viral hepatitis.

Impaired regeneration syndrome is a variant of slowly resolving viral hepatitis.[36] The disease usually occurs in older patients (mean age, 62 years). The diagnosis is made by liver tissue examination. Although the portal tracts are often widened by destruction of the limiting plate, extension of the inflammatory exudate beyond this limit is unusual. The lobular architecture is preserved, the hepatic cords are usually straight and somewhat shrunken, and cholestasis may be severe late in the course. Periportal bile plugs, bile infarcts, and bile lakes may suggest extrahepatic biliary obstruction.[36]

Chronic lobular hepatitis poses the same diagnostic problems as slowly resolving acute viral hepatitis.[37] In this disease, the morphologic features are identical to those of slowly resolving viral hepatitis, but the duration of illness is at least 6 months. Chronic lobular hepatitis is distinguished from CAH chiefly by the extent of lobular change.

Primary biliary cirrhosis is rarely confused with autoimmune CAH but, if the confusion prevents institution of corticosteroid therapy, the significance of the error is great. Routine laboratory tests can facilitate the distinction. Patients with CAH infrequently have AMA titers greater than 1 : 160 (17%), alkaline phosphatase elevations greater than fourfold normal (18%), immunoglobulin M concentrations greater than 6 mg/ml (13%), or cholesterol levels above 300 mg/dl (23%).[26] The keystone of the diagnosis is the histologic evaluation. Granulomatous cholangitis (florid duct lesion) is specific for primary biliary cirrhosis,[35] while the absence of tissue copper, especially in the cirrhotic stage of disease, supports the diagnosis of CAH.[26] AMA-positive CAH can be consistently differentiated from primary biliary cirrhosis by histologic assessment and tissue copper staining in 91% of instances.[26]

REFERENCES

1. Czaja AJ: Natural history, clinical features, and treatment of autoimmune hepatitis. *Semin Liver Dis* **4:**1–12, 1984.
2. Galbraith RM, Smith M, Mackenzie RM, et al: High prevalence of seroimmunologic abnormalities in relatives of patients with active chronic hepatitis or primary biliary cirrhosis. *N Engl J Med* **290:**63–69, 1974.
3. Schalm SW, Summerskill WHJ, Gitnick GL, Elveback LR: Contrasting features and responses to treatment of severe chronic active liver disease with and without hepatitis Bs antigen. *Gut* **17:**781–786, 1976.
4. Bulkley BH, Heizer WD, Goldfinger SE, et al: Distinctions in chronic active hepatitis based on circulating hepatitis-associated antigen. *Lancet* **2:**1323–1326, 1970.

280

CHAPTER 20

5. Eliakim M, Ligumski M, Sandler SG, Zlotnick A: Familial clustering and immune response in family contacts of patients with HB$_s$Ag-positive liver cirrhosis. *Am J Dig Dis* **23**:407–412, 1978.
6. Rakela J, Redeker AG: Chronic liver disease after acute non-A, non-B viral hepatitis. *Gastroenterology* **77**:1200–1202, 1979.
7. Cooksley WG, Powell LW, Kerr JF, Bhathal PS: Cholestasis in active chronic hepatitis. *Am J Dig Dis* **17**:495–504, 1972.
8. Shouval D, Levij IS, Eliakim M: Chronic active hepatitis with cholestatic features. *Am J Gastroenterol* **72**:542–550, 1979.
9. Wiesner RH, LaRusso NF: Clinicopathologic features of the syndrome of primary sclerosing cholangitis. *Gastroenterology* **79**:200–206, 1980.
10. Kohler PF: Clinical immune complex disease. Manifestations in systemic lupus erythematosus and hepatitis B virus infection. *Medicine (Baltimore)* **52**:419–429, 1973.
11. Czaja AJ, Davis GL: Hepatitis non-A, non-B. Manifestations and implications of acute and chronic disease. *Mayo Clin Proc* **57**:639–652, 1982.
12. Czaja AJ, Wolf AM, Baggenstoss AH: Clinical assessment of cirrhosis in severe chronic active liver disease. Specificity and sensitivity of physical and laboratory findings. *Mayo Clin Proc* **55**:360–364, 1980.
13. Weissberg JI, Andres LL, Smith CI, et al: Survival in chronic hepatitis B. An analysis of 379 patients. *Ann Intern Med* **101**:613–616, 1984.
14. Czaja AJ, Davis GL, Ludwig J, et al: Autoimmune features as determinants of prognosis in steroid-treated chronic active hepatitis of uncertain etiology. *Gastroenterology* **85**:713–717, 1983.
15. Czaja AJ, Wolf AM, Summerskill WHJ: Development and early prognosis of esophageal varices in severe chronic active liver disease (CALD) treated with prednisone. *Gastroenterology* **77**:629–633, 1979.
16. Hoofnagle JH, Alter HJ: Chronic non-A, non-B hepatitis. *Prog Clin Biol Res* **82**:63–69, 1985.
17. Levo Y, Gorevic PD, Kassab HJ, et al: Association between hepatitis B virus and essential mixed cryoglobulinemia. *N Engl J Med* **296**:1501–1504, 1977.
18. Fagan EA, Williams R: Non-A, non-B hepatitis. *Semin Liver Dis* **4**:314–335, 1984.
19. Davis GL, Czaja AJ, Baggenstoss AH, Taswell HF: Prognostic and therapeutic implications of extreme serum aminotransferase elevation in chronic active hepatitis. *Mayo Clin Proc* **57**:303–309, 1982.
20. Czaja AJ, Rakela J, Ludwig J: Rapidly fatal idiopathic chronic active hepatitis (RF-CAH). A valid clinical entity? *Hepatology* **5**:1051, 1985.
21. Shiels MT, Czaja AJ, Taswell HF, et al: Frequency and significance of delta antibody in acute, and chronic hepatitis B. A United States experience. *Gastroenterology* **89**:1230–1234, 1985.
22. Liaw Y-F, Chu C-M, Su I-J, et al: Clinical and histological events preceding hepatitis B e antigen seroconversion in chronic type B hepatitis. *Gastroenterology* **84**:216–219, 1983.
23. Davis GL, Hoofnagle JH, Waggoner JG: Spontaneous reactivation of chronic hepatitis B virus infection. *Gastroenterology* **86**:230–235, 1984.
24. Hall S, Czaja AJ, Kaufman DK, et al: How lupoid is lupoid hepatitis? *J Rheumatol* **13**:95–98, 1986.
25. LaRusso NF, Summerskill WHJ, McCall JT: Abnormalities of chemical tests for copper metabolism in chronic active liver disease. Differentiation from Wilson's disease. *Gastroenterology* **70**:653–655, 1976.
26. Kenny RP, Czaja AJ, Ludwig J, Dickson ER: Frequency and significance of antimitochondrial antibodies in severe chronic active hepatitis. *Dig Dis Sci* **31**:705–711, 1986.
27. Ludwig RN, Deodhar SD, Brown CH: Autoimmune tests in chronic active disease of the liver. *Cleve Clin Q* **38**:105–112, 1971.

28. Gurian LE, Rogoff TM, Ware AJ, et al: The immunologic diagnosis of chronic active "autoimmune" hepatitis. Distinction from systemic lupus erythematosus. *Hepatology* **5**:397–402, 1985.
29. Wood JR, Czaja AJ, Beaver SJ, et al: Frequency and significance of antibody to double-stranded DNA in chronic active hepatitis. *Hepatology* **6**:976–980, 1986.
30. Mackay IR, Frazer IH, Toh B-H, et al: Absence of autoimmune serologic reactions in chronic non-A, non-B viral hepatitis. *Clin Exp Immunol* **61**:39–43, 1985.
31. Kilby AE, Albertini RJ, Krawitt EL: HLA typing and autoantibodies in hepatitis B surface antigen-negative chronic active hepatitis. *Tissue Antigens* **28**:214–217, 1986.
32. Opelz G, Vogten AJM, Summerskill WHJ, et al: HLA determinants in chronic active liver disease. Possible relations of HLA Dw3 to prognosis. *Tissue Antigens* **9**:36–40, 1977.
33. Hillis WD, Hillis A, Bias WB, Walker WG: Associations of hepatitis B surface antigenemia with HLA locus B specificities. *N Engl J Med* **296**:1310–1314, 1977.
34. Schalm SW, Korman MG, Summerskill WHJ, et al: Severe chronic active liver disease. Prognostic significance of initial morphologic patterns. *Am J Dig Dis* **22**:973–980, 1977.
35. Cooksley WGE, Bradbear RA, Robinson W, et al: The prognosis of chronic active hepatitis without cirrhosis in relation to bridging necrosis. *Hepatology* **6**:345–348, 1986.
36. Peters RL, Omata M, Aschavai M, Liew CT: Protracted viral hepatitis with impaired regeneration, in Vyas GN, Cohen SN, Schmid R (eds): *Viral Hepatitis.* Franklin Institute Press, Philadelphia, 1978, pp. 79–84.
37. Liaw Y-F, Chu C-M, Chen T-J, et al: Chronic lobular hepatitis. A clinicopathological and prognostic study. *Hepatology* **2**:258–262, 1982.
38. Ludwig J, Czaja AJ, Dickson ER, et al: Manifestations of nonsuppurative cholangitis in chronic hepatobiliary diseases. Morphologic spectrum, clinical correlations and terminology. *Liver* **4**:105–116, 1984.

Associated Conditions in Chronic Hepatitis

CHRISTOPHER D. LIND and GARY L. DAVIS

INTRODUCTION

Chronic hepatitis is a syndrome characterized by clinical, biochemical, and/or histologic evidence of unresolving hepatic inflammation.[1] Our understanding of this syndrome has come a long way since the initial description by Waldenstrom more than 35 years ago.[2] Astute clinical observations detected the heterogeneity in the group of patients assigned the diagnosis of chronic hepatitis. Development of sophisticated laboratory tests, such as serological assays for hepatitis antigens, and radiographic studies, such as endoscopic retrograde cholangiopancreatography, confirmed the clinical suspicion that chronic hepatitis was in fact a generic syndrome composed of several distinct hepatic diseases[1] (Table I).

The realization that chronic hepatitis is an etiologically diverse syndrome is of more than academic importance. The accurate determination of the cause of chronic hepatitis in such patients allows the physician to determine prognosis more accurately and prescribe the most appropriate treatment. While specific treatment may be effective in some of these disorders (e.g., idiopathic hepatitis, hemochromatosis, and Wilson's disease), for others, such as chronic viral hepatitis, no effective treatment presently exists. Furthermore, a treatment that is clearly effective in one form of chronic hepatitis may be without benefit or may be detrimental in another etiologic form of the syndrome. For example, corticosteroids, which may be lifesaving in severe idiopathic (autoimmune) chronic hepatitis,[3] may result in prolongation and progression of chronic type B hepati-

CHRISTOPHER D. LIND and GARY L. DAVIS • Division of Gastroenterology, Hepatology, and Nutrition, University of Florida College of Medicine, Gainesville, Florida 32610.

TABLE I. Causes of Chronic
Hepatitis

Idiopathic
    Autoimmune chronic hepatitis
Viral
    Chronic type B hepatitis
    Chronic non-A, non-B hepatitis
Inflammatory
    Primary biliary cirrhosis
    Primary sclerosing cholangitis
Metabolic
    Genetic hemochromatosis
    Wilson's disease
    α_1-Antitrypsin deficiency
Iatrogenic
    Chronic drug-induced hepatitis

---

tis.[4] Thus, it is essential to identify the etiology of chronic hepatitis before considering treatment of the disease.

Because liver histology alone does not usually differentiate the major causes of chronic hepatitis, an etiologic diagnosis often depends on the laboratory and clinical features of the disease. The association of certain unusual clinical conditions or laboratory test abnormalities can provide important assistance in confirming the etiologic subtype of chronic hepatitis and thus determining prognosis and appropriate therapeutic options. Furthermore, the presence of associated clinical and laboratory findings may lead to a better understanding of the pathogenesis of the various forms of chronic hepatitis.

This chapter reviews the clinical conditions and distinctive laboratory abnormalities associated with chronic hepatitis, emphasizing the implications that these conditions may have on the diagnosis and treatment of these disorders.

IDIOPATHIC (AUTOIMMUNE) CHRONIC HEPATITIS

Idiopathic chronic hepatitis refers to chronic hepatitis not associated with viral infection, drugs, toxins, or metabolic disorders. It was previously referred to as autoimmune or lupoid hepatitis because, like systemic lupus erythematosus (SLE), it occurred predominantly in female patients and was occasionally associated with acne, malar rash, and a variety of so-called autoimmune conditions, such as thyroiditis and Sjögren's syndrome.[5,6] It is important to identify this form of chronic hepatitis, since its severe form can be controlled with corticosteroid treatment yet tends to be progressive and associated with a poor prognosis if left untreated.[7]

Although the diagnosis of idiopathic chronic hepatitis is made by excluding other possible causes of hepatitis, the occurrence of associated clinical conditions or laboratory abnormalities may permit a more confident diagnosis. A wide range of associated conditions have been reported to occur in patients with idiopathic chronic hepatitis.[8-12] As initially reported, amenorrhea, acne, hirsuitism, and gynecomastia are common features.[2,5,6,8-12] Table II lists the most commonly associated conditions in this form of hepatitis. Between 17 and 63% of patients have been reported to have extrahepatic signs and symptoms thought to be related to the presence of chronic hepatitis. Early reports found that approximately 40% of patients had such associated conditions.[8,9] Nonspecific arthritis and rash were most frequent (11–27% and 19–27%, respectively). Thyroiditis, ulcerative colitis, and pleuropericarditis were seen less commonly. The King's College Hospital report found a high percentage of patients with associated Sjögren's syndrome, renal tubular defects, and/or pulmonary diffusion defects.[10] This differs from other reports. Less frequently observed associations are listed in Table III. The significance of most of these associated conditions remains unclear, but all have in common a presumed autoimmune pathogenic mechanism.

Unfortunately, many of the above clinical data are derived from early studies and, although patients are presumed to have idiopathic (autoimmune) hepatitis, the available technology precluded the ability to eliminate patients with other forms of hepatitis. For example, the presence of chronic ulcerative colitis in 3–11% (Table II) suggests the possibility of primary sclerosing cholangitis.[21] Certainly, ulcerative colitis occurs in some patients with idiopathic hepatitis,[20] but

TABLE II. Conditions Associated with Chronic Hepatitis

Condition	Royal Free[a] (N = 81) (%)	Prince Alfred[b] (N = 82) (%)	King's College[c] (N = 108) (%)	Yale University[d] (N = 67) (%)	Mayo Clinic[e] (N = 126) (%)
Arthritis	11	18	27	6	2
Rash	27	20	19	—	—
Thyroid disease	4	4	8	—	7
Ulcerative colitis	6	11	6	3	4
Sjögren's syndrome	—	—	35	—	1
Renal tubular defects	—	—	25	—	—
Pericarditis/pleurisy	—	11	—	6	—
Pulmonary diffusion defects	—	—	17	—	—
Neuropathy/myopathy	—	—	15	—	—
Total (%)	40	41	63	20	17

[a]Read et al.[8] [b]Mistilis et al.[9] [c]Golding et al.[10] [d]Klatskin[11] [e]Czaja et al.[12]

TABLE III. Other Conditions Reported
in Chronic Hepatitis

Condition	References
Autoimmune hemolytic anemia	10, 13, 17
Diabetes mellitus	8, 9
Glomerulonephritis	8, 9, 15, 17
Iritis, uveitis	11, 12, 18
Myasthenia gravis	11, 20
Systemic lupus erythematosus	12
Pernicious anemia	12
Idiopathic thrombocytopenia purpura	12, 17
Fibrosing alveolitis	13
Cryoglobulinemia	14, 15
Hairy cell leukemia	16
Erythema nodosum	9
Pyoderma gangrenosum	19
Cutaneous vasculitis	9
Urticaria	10, 20
Lichen planus	10
Scleroderma	8

our own experience would suggest that it is unusual, perhaps at the lower end of the above range. The high prevalence of Sjögren's syndrome, renal tubular defects, and pulmonary diffusion defects in another series[10] suggests primary biliary cirrhosis. Later studies attempted to eliminate other forms of chronic liver disease that might simulate idiopathic chronic hepatitis. Thus, patients with primary sclerosing cholangitis or primary biliary cirrhosis were eliminated by appropriate laboratory and radiographic studies. Furthermore, the development of serologic assays for hepatitis B surface antigen (HB_sAg) permitted the exclusion of patients with chronic type B hepatitis. Although the possibility exists that some of the remaining patients have other forms of liver disease, such as chronic non-A, non-B hepatitis, these later studies certainly describe a more homogeneous group of patients than did earlier reports. Not surprisingly, these studies[12] also find a smaller, yet still significant, proportion of patients with associated autoimmune disease (20% versus >40% in earlier reports) (Table II). A large number of isolated reports relating idiopathic chronic hepatitis to a wide variety of less common immunologically mediated diseases are listed in Table III.

The presence of associated autoimmune disorders does not appear to affect prognosis or response to treatment in patients with idiopathic chronic hepatitis.[20] The only exception in this regard is the presence of ulcerative colitis.[20] These patients entered remission less frequently (25% versus 66%) and failed treatment more commonly (62% versus 19%). However, because of the frequent association of primary sclerosing cholangitis and ulcerative colitis,[21] it would be interesting to reevaluate these patients to ensure the accuracy of the initial diagnosis.

Serologic abnormalities suggestive of an immunologically mediated condition, autoimmunity if you will, are common in idiopathic chronic hepatitis. The most common of these are hypergammaglobulinemia, the presence of the LE cell phenomenon, and the presence of organ-nonspecific antibodies to nuclear components, i.e., antinuclear antibody (ANA) or smooth muscle antibody (SMA). The prevalence of these features in patients with idiopathic chronic hepatitis is summarized in Table IV. In the Mayo Clinic study, at least one of these features was present in 81% of patients.[12] Several other autoantibodies, including rheumatoid factor (RF), antimitochondrial antibody (AMA), and the antibodies against parietal cells, renal tubular cells, and thyroid have been described.[22,23] Furthermore, liver membrane antigen (LMA) and antibodies against other apparently organ-specific liver-derived antigens, i.e., anti-liver-specific protein (LSP), have also been noted.[24] Although LMA and antibodies to LSP were thought to be specific for idiopathic (autoimmune) hepatitis, they have now been reported to occur in patients with a wide variety of acute and chronic liver diseases, including acute hepatitis A and B, chronic type B hepatitis, halothane hepatitis, alcoholic liver disease, primary biliary cirrhosis, α_1-antitrypsin deficiency, and cystic fibrosis.[24]

It is tempting to consider autoantibodies as specific disease markers that might also provide clues to the immunopathogenesis of this condition. This is unlikely, however, as these antibodies are, for the most part, not organ-specific and occur in patients with chronic liver diseases of many varied etiologies. In addition, the fact that autoantibodies often disappear as the disease improves

TABLE IV. Frequency of Autoantibodies
in Idiopathic Autoimmune
Chronic Hepatitis

Condition	Percentage
Antinuclear antibody (ANA)	30–60
Antibody in double-stranded DNA	40–60
Smooth muscle antibody (SMA)	50–70
Lupus preparation (LE cell)	10–20
Antimitochondrial antibody (AMA)	0–30
Antibody to liver-specific protein	90
Liver membrane antigen (LMA)	40–60
Rheumatoid factor	20–70
Immune complexes	0–35
False-positive VDRL	5–10

(spontaneously or because of treatment) suggests that they may be an epi-phenomenon secondary to severe hepatic necrosis with release of self-antigens into the systemic circulation. Alternatively, they may be a manifestation of a disease-induced alteration in immunoregulation. Nevertheless, the high prevalence of autoantibodies in the idiopathic form of chronic hepatitis is noteworthy. Finally, histocompatibility antigen testing has identified HLA-A1 and B8 in more than 60% of patients with idiopathic chronic hepatitis.[25] The prevalence of DRw3 is also increased.[26] The frequent association of HLA-B8 and DRw3 with other immunologically mediated disorders such as celiac disease, myasthenia gravis, and Graves' disease suggests that this antigen marker may identify patients with a genetically determined reactivity to self-antigens.[27]

IDIOPATHIC HEPATITIS VERSUS CHRONIC CHOLESTATIC DISEASE

Some patients with chronic hepatitis have clinical, serologic or histologic features of both idiopathic hepatitis and chronic cholestatic diseases, such as primary biliary cirrhosis or primary sclerosing cholangitis.[28] The correct diagnosis may be elusive, since the classical histologic features are usually not present on liver biopsy. These patients have been categorized as having an overlap syndrome, although their true diagnosis usually becomes apparent with time. Associated serologic studies and clinical conditions may assist in making the appropriate diagnosis in these difficult cases.

Early studies in idiopathic hepatitis and primary biliary cirrhosis found the presence of AMA in 28% and 98% of cases, respectively.[29] More recent reports have confirmed the presence of AMA in 20% of patients with idiopathic hepatitis, but the titer of the antibody is generally low ($<1 : 40$) in contrast to that in patients with primary biliary cirrhosis.[30] Furthermore, the presence of low-titer AMA in patients with histologic features of chronic idiopathic hepatitis does not influence the response to corticosteroid treatment. Further serologic characterization of patients with chronic liver diseases comes from clinical studies in patients with idiopathic chronic hepatitis, primary biliary cirrhosis, and primary sclerosing cholangitis, conducted at the Mayo Clinic.[28] Primary sclerosing cholangitis is infrequently associated with autoantibodies, AMA being present in 4% and SMA in 9%. Primary biliary cirrhosis is most frequently associated with autoantibodies: AMA in 96%, SMA in 66%, rheumatoid factor in 70%, and ANA in 23%. Of note, however, is that the SMA in patients with primary biliary cirrhosis is usually of the IgM class, while in idiopathic hepatitis it is IgG. Autoantibodies in these and other diseases are outlined in Table V.

In addition to serologic changes, the associated autoimmune conditions

TABLE V. Frequency of Autoantibodies in Various Forms
Chronic Hepatitis and Other Disease States[a]

Condition	ANA (%)	AMA (%)	SMA (%)
Chronic hepatitis			
Chronic type B hepatitis	0–10	0–10	10–30
Chronic non-A, non-B hepatitis	0–30	10–30	20–30
Primary biliary cirrhosis	25–50	90–100	0–65
Primary sclerosing cholangitis	5–10	0–5	5–10
Metabolic liver diseases	0–1	0–1	0–10
Other diseases			
Alcoholic liver disease	0–15	0–1	5–15
Extrahepatic biliary obstruction	0–1	0–1	0–1
Systemic lupus erythematosus (SLE)	80	5–10	0
Normal	0–1	0–1	0–1

[a]ANA, antinuclear antibody; AMA, antimitochondrial antibody; SMA, smooth muscle antibody.

found in primary biliary cirrhosis, primary sclerosing cholangitis, and idiopathic chronic hepatitis have been documented by the Mayo Clinic group.[28] Inflammatory bowel disease was found in 89% of patients with primary sclerosing cholangitis when carefully sought by radiologic and endoscopic methods.[31] By contrast, inflammatory bowel disease is unusual in the other conditions (6%). Similarly, keratoconjunctivitis sicca was seen in 69% of patients with primary biliary cirrhosis, yet in only 1% of patients with idiopathic hepatitis. Thyroid disorders and polyarthritis were seen in all three diseases but were more common (19%) in primary biliary cirrhosis. In patients with chronic liver disease and suspected idiopathic hepatitis, the presence of associated inflammatory bowel disease, especially ulcerative colitis, or keratoconjunctivitis sicca therefore suggests the alternative diagnoses of primary sclerosing cholangitis or primary biliary cirrhosis, respectively. Ultimately, careful evaluation of the histologic features will best help separate these different disease states.

CHRONIC TYPE B HEPATITIS

Early series of chronic hepatitis patients (prior to 1970) were unable to distinguish viral causes, particularly hepatitis B, from idiopathic (autoimmune) chronic hepatitis. Since 1970, however, HB_sAg testing has permitted identification of this major subset of patients. This clarification of patient identity is most important, since HB_sAg positivity not only influences treatment options and prognosis, but also, with respect to the present discussion, is related to a distinctly different set of associated conditions. It is generally accepted that the majority of conditions associated with chronic type B hepatitis are due to immune-complex deposition.

Soon after the description of the Australia antigen by Blumberg[32] and its subsequent association with serum hepatitis, the presence of circulating antigen–antibody immune complexes was reported. These complexes were assigned importance in causing the prodromal symptoms of the acute disease (e.g., myalgia, arthralgia, rash) and many of the associated conditions of the chronic form of the illness.[33,34] Characterization of the circulating immune complexes in HB_sAg-positive patients with arthritis demonstrated within cryoproteins the presence of HB_sAg, IgM, IgG, IgA, and several components of complement that were capable of activating the classic or alternate complement pathways.[35] Similar studies have subsequently defined most of the extrahepatic manifestations of chronic type B hepatitis to be immune-complex related. Localized HB_sAg-containing immune complexes and evidence of complement activation have been found in involved organs in HB_sAg-positive patients with extrahepatic manifestations.[36,37]

The major associated conditions identified with chronic type B hepatitis are shown in Table VI and include arthritis, polyarteritis nodosa, membranous or membranoproliferative glomerulonephritis, cryoglobulinemia, peripheral neuropathy, and cutaneous vasculitis. The prevalence of these associated conditions is low, certainly less than 10%.[11,41] The Mayo Clinic found associated immune-complex-related conditions in 2 of 18 patients with chronic type B hepatitis.[41] Polyarteritis nodosa was present in one and glomerulonephritis in the other. The presence of autoantibodies such as ANA, AMA, SMA, and LE cells is unusual (<5%) in patients with chronic type B hepatitis (Table V).

TABLE VI. Extrahepatic Manifestations
of Chronic Type B Hepatitis

Condition	Reference
Polyarthritis	35
Polyarteritis nodosum	36
Chronic glomerulonephritis	37
Papular acrodermatitis: Gianotti–Crosti	38
Mixed cryoglobulinemia	39, 40
Peripheral neuropathy	39

CHRONIC NON-A, NON-B HEPATITIS

Chronic non-A, non-B hepatitis, like idiopathic chronic hepatitis, is a diagnosis of exclusion. The presence of epidemiologic risk factors for acquisition of the disease, such as blood transfusion, intravenous drug use, or needlestick exposure, is helpful in supporting the diagnosis.[42] The distinction from idiopathic chronic hepatitis is therapeutically important, since corticosteroid treatment appears to have little beneficial effect in chronic non-A, non-B hepatitis and may accelerate progression of the disease.[43]

The clinical features of chronic non-A, non-B hepatitis are generally minimal, with most patients having asymptomatic hypertransaminasemia. Autoantibodies such as ANA and SMA are not typically present in patients with chronic non-A, non-B hepatitis but are occasionally seen.[44,45] No specific autoimmune or immune-complex conditions have been associated with this disease. Although circulating immune complexes are commonly found in patients with chronic non-A, non-B hepatitis,[46] symptoms and signs attributable to deposition in tissues are generally lacking. Perrillo et al.[47] described the presence of a serum sickness-like syndrome in one patient with circulating immune complexes. Extrahepatic features such as arthritis and rash are rare. Rash, urticaria, or purpura occur in fewer than 3% of cases and are usually present only in the acute phase of the illness.[48] Aplastic anemia, while a rare complication of viral hepatitis, is usually attributable to non-A, non-B hepatitis and should support that diagnosis.[49]

METABOLIC CAUSES OF CHRONIC HEPATITIS

Idiopathic genetic hemochromatosis is a rare but important cause of chronic hepatitis. Its recognition is essential, since early treatment prevents the clinical manifestations of the disease and results in normal survival.[50] Despite the fact that most patients with hemochromatosis are cirrhotic when they develop clinical manifestations of the disease, the hepatic manifestations of the disease are often subtle.[51] It is therefore essential to be alert to the extrahepatic features of the condition. Bronze or grayish pigmentation of the skin is apparent in 75% of patients and diabetes in 60%,[51,52] hence the descriptive term bronze diabetes. Anterior pituitary infiltration by iron leads to loss of trophic hormone release in two thirds and to hypogonadism and loss of body hair in one half of patients.[51,52] Arthropathy involving the metacarpophalangeal and larger joints is present in one half of the patients.[53] In addition, acute calcium pyrophosphate deposition (pseudogout) and chondrocalcinosis are features of hemochromatosis. Approximately 40% of patients will develop cardiac involvement characterized by either heart failure or arrhythmias.[54] Although cardiac dysfunction typically improves with appropriate treatment (phlebotomy), hypogonadism and arthritis do not respond.[50] Autoimmune diseases and autoantibodies are not features of idiopathic hemochromatosis.

Wilson's disease is another rare cause of chronic hepatitis. Like hemochromatosis, it is extremely important to recognize, since early treatment improves survival. Also like hemochromatosis, the extrahepatic features of the disease are related to tissue overload by the involved metal; copper in the case of Wilson's disease. The most prominent nonhepatic features of Wilson's disease are the neuropsychiatric manifestations, including tremor, grimacing, fine motor and speech impairment, dystonia, and personality change.[55] Hemolytic anemia may lead to confusion with drug-induced or idiopathic (autoimmune) hepatitis, although hemolysis in Wilson's disease is due to direct effects of high red cell copper and is Coombs negative.[56] Renal tubular defects causing aminoaciduria, glycosuria, phosphaturia, and uricosuria may mistakenly suggest idiopathic hepatitis or primary biliary cirrhosis.[57] Finally, the premature osteoarthritis of Wilson's disease may suggest hemochromatosis.[58] Physical signs attributable to tissue copper overload include Kaiser–Fleischer rings of the cornea, sunflower cataracts, and azure blue lunulas of the fingernails. As with hemochromatosis, autoimmune diseases or antibodies are not commonly associated. The diagnosis is confirmed by the presence of low serum ceruloplasmin and elevated hepatic copper.[59] Finally, α_1-antitrypsin deficiency is a rare cause of chronic hepatitis. Chronic obstructive lung disease is commonly present in these patients.[60]

DRUG-INDUCED CHRONIC HEPATITIS

Several drugs are known to cause chronic liver injury and may account for a considerable proportion of cases of chronic hepatitis.[61,62] Indeed, in one series, 14 of 21 cases (67%) of chronic nonviral hepatitis were attributed to drugs.[63] Although the laxative oxyphenisatin is the classical offender, it is no longer available in this country. Most cases today are caused by α-methyldopa, nitrofurantoin, isoniazid, sulfonamides, and dantrolene.[61,62] The clinical, histologic, and biochemical features of chronic drug-induced hepatitis mimic chronic idiopathic (autoimmune) hepatitis,[62,64] although a detailed history will usually prevent confusion. Autoantibodies, in particular ANA, SMA, and the LE cell, are common.[65] Antibodies to thyroid and glomerular membranes are reported in macrodantin-induced hepatitis.[66] Red cell antibodies are occasionally reported in macrodantin and α-methyldopa hepatitis, but they are unrelated to the hepatic injury and may occur independently.[67] Associated clinical conditions and signs include rash (most common in sulfonamide injury), autoimmune hemolytic anemia (α-methyldopa), serum sickness (sulfonamides), and pulmonary disease resembling Loeffler's syndrome or pulmonary fibrosis (macrodantin).[61,62,65]

SUMMARY

Chronic hepatitis is an etiologically diverse syndrome manifested by unresolving hepatic inflammation. Hepatic histology is frequently not helpful in identifying the cause of chronic hepatitis. Therefore, the diagnosis is usually derived from serologic testing for disease markers such as hepatitis virus antigens and antibodies. Appropriate clinical management and treatment depend on precise identification of the cause of chronic hepatitis in the individual patient. Recognition of associated conditions or extrahepatic manifestations of the primary disease may facilitate diagnosis and direct treatment in some cases. These associated conditions may also provide useful clues to the pathogenesis of the disease.

REFERENCES

1. Davis GL: Chronic active hepatitis, in Fauci AS, Lichtenstein LM (eds): *Current Therapy in Allergy, Immunology, and Rheumatology.* Decker, New York, 1985, pp. 126–129.
2. Waldenstrom J: Leber, blutproteine und nahrungseiweiss. *Dtsch Gesell Verdau Stoffwechselkr* 2:113–119, 1950.
3. Wright EC, Seeff LB, Berk PD, et al: Treatment of chronic active hepatitis: An analysis of 3 controlled trials. *Gastroenterology* 73:1422–1430, 1977.
4. Lam KC, Lai CL, Ng RP, et al: Deleterious effect of prednisolone in HBsAg-positive chronic active hepatitis. *N Engl J Med* 304:380–386, 1981.
5. Joske RA, King WE: The "LE cell" phenomenon in active chronic viral hepatitis. *Lancet* 2:477–479, 1955.
6. Mackay IR, Taft LI, Cowling DC: Lupoid hepatitis. *Lancet* 2:1323–1326, 1956.
7. Davis GL, Czaja AJ: Immediate and long-term results of corticosteroid therapy for severe idiopathic chronic active hepatitis, in Czaja AJ, Dickson ER (eds): *Chronic Hepatitis: The Mayo Clinic Experience.* Dekker, New York, 1986, pp. 269–283.
8. Read AE, Sherlock S, Harrison CV: Active "juvenile" cirrhosis considered as part of a systemic disease and the effect of corticosteroid therapy. *Gut* 4:378–393, 1963.
9. Mistilis SP, Skyring AP, Blackburn CRB: Natural history of active chronic hepatitis. I. Clinical features, course, diagnostic criteria, morbidity, mortality and survival. *Aust Ann Med* 17:214–223, 1968.
10. Golding PL, Smith M, Williams R: Multisystem involvement in chronic liver disease: Studies on the incidence and pathogenesis. *Am J Med* 55:772–782, 1973.
11. Klatskin G: Persistent HB antigenemia: Associated clinical manifestations and hepatic lesions. *Am J Med Sci* 270:33–40, 1975.
12. Czaja AJ, Davis GL, Ludwig J, et al: Autoimmune features as determinants of prognosis in

steiod-treated chronic active hepatitis of uncertain etiology. *Gastroenterology* **85**:713–717, 1983.

13. Williams AJ, Marsh J, Stableforth DE: Cryptogenic fibrosing alveolitis, chronic active hepatitis and autoimmune haemolytic anemia in the same patient. *Br J Dis Chest* **79**:200–203, 1985.

14. Jori GP, Buonanno G: Chronic hepatitis and cirrhosis of the liver in cryoglobulinaemia. *Gut* **13**:610–613, 1972.

15. Feizi T, Gitlin N: Immune-complex disease of the kidney associated with chronic hepatitis and cryoglogulinemia. *Lancet* **2**:873–876, 1969.

16. Begley CG, Mackay IR, Bhathal PS: Another immune-mediated disease associated with hairy cell leukemia: Chronic active hepatitis. *Acta Haematol* **73**:104–105, 1985.

17. Cuesta B, Fernandez J, Pardo J, et al: Evan's syndrome, chronic active hepatitis and focal glomerulonephritis in IgA deficiency. *Acta Haematol* **75**:1–5, 1986.

18. Bloom JN, Rabinowicz IM, Shulman ST: Uveitis complicating autoimmune chronic active hepatitis. *Am J Dis Child* **137**:1175–1176, 1983.

19. Green LK, Hebert AA, Jorizzo JL, et al: Pyoderma gangrenosum and chronic persistent hepatitis. *J Am Acad Dermatol* **13**:892–897, 1985.

20. Czaja AJ, Wolf AM: Immunopathic diseases (ID) associated with severe chronic active liver disease (CALD): Determinants of treatment response. *Gastroenterology* **78**:1152, 1980 (abst).

21. Wiesner RH, LaRusso NF: Clinicopathologic features of the syndrome of primary sclerosing cholangitis. *Gastroenterology* **79**:200–206, 1980.

22. Gurian LE, Rogoff TM, Ware AJ, et al: The immunologic diagnosis of chronic active "autoimmune" hepatitis: Distinction from systemic lupus erythematosis. *Hepatology* **5**:397–402, 1985.

23. Hodges JR, Millward-Sadler GH, Wright R: Chronic active hepatitis: The spectrum of disease. *Lancet* **1**:550–552, 1982.

24. Meyer zum Buschenfelde KH, Manns M: Mechanisms of autoimmune liver disease. *Semin Liver Dis* **4**:26–35, 1984.

25. Page AR, Sharp HL, Greenberg LJ, Yunis EJ: Genetic analysis of patients with chronic active hepatitis. *J Clin Invest* **56**:530–535, 1975.

26. Mackay IR, Tait BD: HLA associations with autoimmune-type chronic active hepatitis: Identification of B8-DRw3 haplotype by family studies. *Gastroenterology* **79**:95–98, 1980.

27. Roitt I, Brostoff J, Male D: Autoimmunity and autoimmune disease, in Roitt I, Brostoff J, Male D (eds): *Immunology*. 1st ed. CV Mosby, St. Louis, 1985, pp. 1–12.

28. Linder KD, Wiesner RH, LaRusso NF, Dickson ER: Chronic active hepatitis: Overlap with primary biliary cirrhosis and primary sclerosing cholagitis, in Czaja AJ, Dickson ER (eds): *Chronic Active Hepatitis: The Mayo Clinic Experience*. Dekker, New York, 1986, pp. 171–187.

29. Doniach D, Roitt IM, Walker JG, Sherlock S: Tissue antibodies in primary biliary cirrhosis, active chronic (lupoid) hepatitis, cryptogenic cirrhosis and other liver diseases and their clinical implications. *Clin Exp Immunol* **1**:237–262, 1966.

30. Kenny RP, Czaja AJ, Ludwig J, Dickson ER: Frequency and significance of antimitochondrial antibodies in severe chronic active hepatitis. *Dig Dis Sci* **31**:705–711, 1986.

31. LaRusso NF, Wiesner RH, Ludwig J, et al: Randomized trial of penicillamine in primary sclerosing cholangitis. *Hepatology* **6**:1205, 1986, (abst).

32. Blumberg BS: Polymorphism of serum proteins and the development of iso-precipitins in transfused patients. *Bull NY Acad Med* **40**:377–386, 1964.

33. Sabesin SM, Levinson MJ: Acute and chronic hepatitis: Multisystem involvement related to immunologic disease. *Adv Intern Med* **22**:421–454, 1977.

34. Almeida JD, Waterson AP: Immune complexes in hepatitis. *Lancet* **2**:983–986, 1969.

35. Wands JR, Alpert E, Isselbacher KJ: Arthritis associated with chronic active hepatitis: Complement activation and characterization of circulating immune complexes. *Gastroenterology* **69**:1286–1291, 1975.

36. Gocke DJ, Morgan C, Lockshin M, et al: Association between polyarteritis and Australia antigen. *Lancet* **2:**1149–1153, 1970.
37. Combes B, Stastny P, Shorey J, et al: Glomerulonephritis with deposition of Australia antigen–antibody complexes in glomerular basement membrane. *Lancet* **2:**234–237, 1971.
38. Gianotti F: Papular acrodermatitis of childhood—an Australia antigen disease. *Arch Dis Child* **48:**794–799, 1973.
39. Farivar M, Wands JR, Benson GD, et al: Cryoprotein complexes and peripheral neuropathy in a patient with chronic active hepatitis. *Gastroenterology* **71:**490–493, 1976.
40. Levo Y, Gorevic PD, Kassab HJ, et al: Association between hepatitis B virus and essential mixed cryoglobulinemia. *N Engl J Med* **296:**1501–1504, 1977.
41. Schalm SW, Summerskill WHJ, Gitnick GL, Elveback LR: Contrasting features and responses to treatment of severe chronic active liver disease with and without hepatitis Bs antigen. *Gut* **17:**781–786, 1976.
42. Dienstag JL. Non-A, non-B hepatitis. I. Recognition, epidemiology, and clinical features. *Gastroenterology* **85:**439–462, 1983.
43. Koretz RL, Stone O, Mousa M, Gitnick GL: Non-A, non-B post-transfusion hepatitis—A decade later. *Gastroenterology* **88:**1251–1254, 1985.
44. Mackay IR, Frazier IH, Toh BH, et al: Absence of autoimmune serological reactions in chronic non-A, non-B viral hepatitis. *Clin Exp Immunol* **61:**39–43, 1985.
45. Berman M, Alter HJ, Ishak KG, et al: The chronic sequelae of non-A, non-B hepatitis. *Ann Intern Med* **91:**1–6, 1979.
46. Dienstag JL, Bhan AK, Alter HJ, et al: Circulating immune complexes in non-A, non-B hepatitis: Possible masking of viral antigen. *Lancet* **1:**1265–1267, 1979.
47. Perrillo RP, Pohl DA, Roodman ST, Tsai CC: Acute non-A, non-B hepatitis with serum sickness-like syndrome and aplastic anemia. *JAMA* **245:**494–496, 1981.
48. Koff RS, Pannuti CS, Periera MLG, et al: Hepatitis A and non-A, non-B viral hepatitis in Sao Paulo, Brazil: Epidemiological, clinical, and laboratory comparisons in hospitalized patients. *Hepatology* **2:**445–448, 1982.
49. Zeldis JB, Dienstag JL, Gale RP: Aplastic anemia and non-A, non-B hepatitis. *Am J Med* **74:**64–68, 1983.
50. Niederau C, Fischer R, Sonnenberg A, et al: Survival and causes of death in cirrhotic and in noncirrhotic patients with primary hemochromatosis. *N Engl J Med* **313:**1256–1262, 1985.
51. Milder MS, Cook JD, Stray S, Finch CA: Idiopathic hemochromatosis, an interim report. *Medicine (Baltimore)* **59:**34–49, 1980.
52. Stocks AE, Martin FIR: Pituitary function in haemochromatosis. *Am J Med* **45:**839–845, 1968.
53. Dymock IW, Hamilton EBD, Laws JW, Williams R: Arthropathy of haemochromatosis: Clinical and radiological analysis of 63 patients with iron overload. *Ann Rheum Dis* **29:**469–476, 1970.
54. Lewis HP: Cardiac involvement in haemochromatosis. *Am J Med Sci* **227:**544–558, 1954.
55. Cartwright GE: Diagnosis of treatable Wilson's disease. *N Engl J Med* **298:**1347–1350, 1978.
56. McIntyre N, Clink HM, Levi AG, et al: Hemolytic anemia in Wilson's disease. *N Engl J Med* **276:**439–444, 1967.
57. Bearn AG, Tu TF, Gutman AB: Renal function in Wilson's disease. *J Clin Invest* **36:**1107–1114, 1957.
58. Golding DN, Walshe JM: Arthropathy of Wilson's disease. Study of clinical and radiologic features in 32 patients. *Ann Rheum Dis* **36:**99–111, 1977.
59. Gollan JL: Copper metabolism, Wilson's disease and hepatic copper toxicosis, in Zakim D, Boyer TD (eds): *Hepatology: A Textbook of Liver Disease.* WB Saunders, Philadelphia, 1982, pp. 1138–1158.

60. Eriksson S, Hagerstrand I: Cirrhosis and malignant hepatoma in α-1 antitrypsin deficiency. *Acta Med Scand* **195:**451–458, 1974.
61. Seeff LB: Drug-induced chronic liver disease with emphasis on chronic active hepatitis. *Semin Liver Dis* **1:**104–115, 1981.
62. Maddrey WC, Boitnott JK: Drug-induced chronic liver disease. *Gastroenterology* **72:**1348–1353, 1977.
63. Goldstein GB, Lam KC, Mistilis SP: Drug-induced active chronic hepatitis. *Am J Dig Dis* **18:**177–184, 1973.
64. Reynolds TB, Peters RL, Yamada S: Chronic active and lupoid hepatitis caused by a laxative, oxyphenisatin. *N Engl J Med* **285:**813–820, 1971.
65. Zimmerman HJ: Drug-induced liver disease, in Zimmerman HJ (ed): *Hepatotoxicity.* Appleton-Century-Crofts, New York, 1978, pp. 349–369.
66. Bach O, Lundgren R, Wiman LG: Nitrofurantoin-induced pulmonary fibrosis and lupus syndrome. *Lancet* **1:**930, 1974.
67. Glontz GE, Saslaw S: Methyldopa fever. *Arch Intern Med* **122:**445–447, 1968.

Chronic Active Hepatitis
Diagnostic Approach

ROGER D. SOLOWAY

INTRODUCTION

Most frequently, the physician is faced with the necessity to examine a patient with the possibility of chronic active hepatitis (CAH) because the referring physician has detected abnormalities of the aminotransferases. These elevations are usually detected during periodic screening in seemingly healthy persons or during a medical evaluation for unrelated problems. Since aminotransferases and alkaline phosphatase have become an important part of such screening packages, this represents the most frequent type of patient referral to the gastroenterologist or hepatologist for evaluation of the possibility of liver disease.

CLINICAL CONSIDERATIONS

For the patient with an elevation of aminotransferase who has not undergone liver biopsy (for additional, detailed information concerning the management of patients without biopsy, see section on management without biopsy in Chapter 23), it is advisable, after a thorough history and physical examination, to postpone liver biopsy until the patient has had at least 6 months of documented aminotransferase elevation. This is important, since the physician should try to minimize the incidence of conditions, such as slowly resolving hepatitis, which might obscure or confuse interpretation. If the patient is taking any medications, the first step is to change or delete them if at all possible, since almost all drugs

ROGER D. SOLOWAY • Department of Medicine, University of Texas Medical Branch, Galveston, Texas 77550-2778.

have been incriminated in liver disease. The list of medications that have not been suspected of hepatotoxicity is much shorter than those for which an association has been proposed.

The next step, if the patient weighs more than 20% above ideal weight, is institution of a vigorous weight reduction program and a series of graded exercises. If the patient consumes even a modest amount of alcohol, this must be discontinued for two months. These steps will ensure that the maximum amount of fat will be mobilized from the liver. This is important because fat can obscure the pattern of lobular hepatitis or patchy necrosis within the lobule and may make difficult the diagnosis of piecemeal necrosis or even bridging necrosis.

If only two or three elevations of transaminase have been obtained over a period of 1–2 months, the additional 4-month waiting period can be devoted to minimization of hepatic fat content and to resolution of slowly resolving hepatitis. If the transaminases return to normal during this waiting period, caution should be observed because the course of Non-A, Non-B acute hepatitis is undulating and because the condition frequently progresses to CAH. Such patients must be rechecked four to six times during the first year of follow-up after biochemical normality has been achieved to ensure that chronic non-A, non-B hepatitis does not continue undetected.

LIVER BLOOD TESTS

Aminotransferase

A number of investigators have discussed the frequency with which aspartate aminotransferase (AST, SGOT) is higher than alanine aminotransferase (ALT, SGPT) in alcoholic hepatitis compared with other forms of chronic hepatitis in which the reverse relationship is frequently present. Although this relationship between the aminotransferases is usually correct, I have encountered a sufficient number of patients for whom this relationship is misleading, so I do not try to make a decision on this basis.

γ-Glutamyltransferase

Similarly, although the level of γ-glutamyltransferase has been demonstrated to be a sensitive indicator of alcohol induction in populations with a high frequency of increased alcohol intake, in the general population, so many other stimuli induce this enzyme that an elevation cannot be assumed to be diagnostic.

Globulin

Although the level of serum globulins, especially γ-globulin, has been closely associated with autoimmune CAH, the low incidence of elevation in patients with other forms of CAH, especially Non-A, Non-B viral disease, indicates that antibody production is not a prominent feature of this condition.

Albumin

In the absence of excessive protein loss or malnutrition, a reduction in the level of albumin serves as an indicator of chronic disease and of a condition more severe than chronic persistent hepatitis (CPH). However, decreased serum albumin is not a sensitive indicator of liver disease. Patients can have established cirrhosis with normal levels of albumin.

Alkaline Phosphatase

Only a few patients with CAH have a greater than threefold elevation of alkaline phosphatase. However, this elevation does identify about 15% of patients in whom an overlap of CAH and primary biliary cirrhosis may be difficult or impossible to separate by biochemical criteria.

Bilirubin

Total bilirubin has not been a sensitive indicator of early CAH. The direct-reacting level of bilirubin (formerly thought to represent only conjugated bilirubin) is more sensitive but not specific enough to be diagnostically reliable. The newer tests for bilirubin that measure unconjugated, monoconjugated, diconjugated, and albumin-bound bilirubin have recently been introduced[1] and have not been tested for their sensitivity in the detection of CAH or minimal cirrhosis. A source of confusion is in the isolated elevation of unconjugated bilirubin, most commonly measured as total bilirubin, which occurs in about 5% of the population. It indicates primarily the presence of Gilbert's syndrome,[2] several closely related congenital defects in hepatic bilirubin handling, which should be correctly identified because of the completely benign prognosis associated with this condition. This diagnosis is more difficult to establish when CPH is also present but should be considered. Such patients have normal handling of bile salts and indocyanine green, a dye that is not conjugated by the liver before secretion into bile.

A series of studies have noted that fasting and postprandial levels of serum bile acids are among the most sensitive tests in detecting minimal cirrhosis.[3]

These tests seem to be more sensitive than standard liver tests including the aminotransferases.

INITIAL EVALUATION

In addition to the liver blood studies, a number of blood studies should be obtained at the initial evaluation to help categorize the condition, assess its severity, and determine whether there are treatable causes of CAH once this pattern has been recognized histologically. It is now clear that this pattern is the picture of hepatic necrosis for a number of separate conditions, since the liver responds to injury in only a limited number of ways.

DIFFERENTIAL DIAGNOSIS

Viral Hepatitis

Hepatitis A and B should be ruled out by appropriate antigen and antibody testing. Hepatitis A has not been demonstrated to progress to CAH but is now recognized to persist sometimes for longer periods than the usual 4- to 8-week course of acute hepatitis A and may produce a variety of chronic clinical syndromes. Hepatitis B is eliminated in all but a few cases if serum tests are negative. A final diagnostic tool remains reaction of the unstained liver biopsy section with fluorescent-tagged monoclonal antibodies to the surface and core antigens of the B virus. It is possible that patients with chronic viral hepatitis B may have a variable degree of viral genome incorporated into the host hepatocyte nucleus. Since this may frequently occur and persist following acute infection, identification of such incorporation does not establish an etiology for the chronic active hepatitis found on the present biopsy. Obtaining serum hepatitis B virus (HBV) DNA levels will help in most, but not all, cases. Patients with isolated hepatitis B core antibody (HB_cAb) may have a false-positive reaction; thus, the presence of the antibody alone cannot be assumed as diagnostic of past hepatitis B. Similarly, until recently, it was assumed that the presence of the antibody to hepatitis B surface antigen (HB_sAg) meant that the host had developed immunity to the virus and that the progressive CAH was due to another cause; recent reports indicate that a small number of these patients have progressive CAH due to hepatitis B and that, when titered, low levels of antibody to the surface antigen may be nonspecific. High titers of the antibody are still thought to be diagnostic of the development of immunity, and one should attempt to use laboratories that report titers when these questions arise.

Non-A, Non-B Hepatitis

Non-A, Non-B CAH remains the major obstacle to efficient diagnosis. We arbitrarily assign patients to this category when there is a history of blood transfusion in historical proximity to a clinically apparent episode of acute hepatitis.[4] If these criteria are not satisfied, we make arbitrary assumptions, if there has been a history of transfusion of blood products or if the patient has abused intravenous substances at any time in the past. If all other markers are negative, many assign this diagnosis to cases of nonspecific CAH. This is unfortunate, since it cannot be ascertained which proportion of these patients have lost the markers of autoimmune CAH or have had undetected drug or toxin exposure. We continue to await specific tests for the viruses that cause Non-A, Non-B CAH. Until then, it is best to label patients without a very suggestive history as having nonspecific CAH.

Wilson's Disease

In any patient with a low ceruloplasmin, irrespective of age, Wilson's disease should be eliminated as a possible cause of CAH. Although most patients with Wilson's disease are under 30 years of age, occasional patients are encountered who are older. In 95% of patients with Wilson's disease, the ceruloplasmin level is <20 mg%. Those with levels of 20–30 mg% may demonstrate stimulation by the hepatic inflammatory process, since ceruloplasmin is an acute-phase reactant.[5] If the ceruloplasmin level is low and quantitative studies of hepatic copper are unavailable or nondiagnostic, the next step is a 24-hr urine collection for copper at baseline and after a single dose of 250 mg d-penicillamine. Normal subjects excrete a mean of 30 μg/24 hr with an upper limit of 60 μg/24 hr, while almost all symptomatic patients excrete in excess of 100 μg/24 hr.[6] A four- to eightfold increase in urinary copper is attained in patients with Wilson's disease following a test dose of d-penicillamine. All patients with neurologic symptoms and 95% of patients with hepatic involvement have Kayser–Fleischer rings that should be looked for with a slit lamp by an ophthalmologist.[5]

Hemochromatosis

Iron accumulation in the liver does not directly cause a histologic picture that can be confused with CAH; rather, it is associated with increased fibrous septa that progress to a cirrhosis over many years. It is not associated with piecemeal necrosis, but it continues to be unclear how an advanced cirrhosis does develop in this condition. However, hemochromatosis may occur in the setting of chronic hepatitis, either coexistent because hemochromatosis is the most common genetic defect among Caucasians (associated with an increased incidence of HLA-A3 and B-14) or is secondary to some forms of liver disease, especially notable in alcoholic liver disease and in cirrhosis after portocaval shunt.

Although serum ferritin is elevated in almost all patients with hemochromatosis and can be elevated in very early disease before significant iron accumulation, I have encountered a few patients with increased iron saturation in the absence of significant elevation of serum ferritin; several families have been reported with this pattern. Thus, tests for both serum ferritin and serum iron and iron-binding capacity seem worthwhile. The definitive diagnosis is made by quantitation of iron content on liver biopsy, which will be in excess of 1 g/100 g dry weight. When suspected in advance, liver biopsy should be performed with a reusable needle cleaned with an iron chelator prior to sterilization or with a disposable needle. When excess iron is unexpectedly found on liver biopsy, methods are now available to measure the amount of hepatic iron in fixed tissue. When doubt remains, one should advise a course of phlebotomy and determine whether the patient tolerates this without developing an anemia. The patient does not have hemochromatosis if anemia develops after removal of 2–4 units of blood. This technique will differentiate patients with CAH and iron accumulation from patients with CAH and coexistent hemochromatosis.[7]

α_1-Antitrypsin Deficiency

α_1-Antitrypsin deficiency may cause a syndrome with clinical features indistinguishable from other forms of CAH. Although early reports emphasized preexisting pulmonary disease, patients are now being identified with advanced liver disease and normal pulmonary function. α_1-Antitrypsin is synthesized solely by the liver and represents 90% of the circulating α_1-globulins. A reduction of α_1-globulin was the basis for the initial screening test for the deficiency. A more specific assay for α_1-antitrypsin is now available, but it does not identify some patients with heterozygous defects. Each of these defects has been associated with cirrhosis in case reports. It is unknown whether these defects are coincidental or causative. However, obtaining a protein inhibitor phenotype is the most sensitive way of identifying the possibility that α_1-antitrypsin deficiency may be contributing to CAH. Careful staining of the liver biopsy with periodic acid-Schiff, determining that intrahepatocytic positive granules identified are diastase resistant, is necessary for histologic diagnosis. These lysosomal vacuoles may be missed on casual review of biopsies because they have similar staining properties to normal cytoplasm on the hematoxylin-eosin stain.[8]

Immunologic CAH

Anti-smooth muscle antibody has been identified as a characteristic feature of immunologic CAH and is positive in 52% of cases.[9] Some patients with primary biliary cirrhosis may also have positive antibodies, so it cannot be used to differentiate these two conditions. Patients with systemic lupus erythematosus (SLE) lack this antibody; if positive, it serves as a distinguishing feature when the clinical syndrome resembles SLE and the antinuclear antibody (ANA) is positive. The finding of antibody to double-stranded DNA by the *Crithidia luciliae* immunofluorescence assay or by means of an assay using *Escherichia coli* double-stranded DNA is highly specific for SLE.[10] Rarely, patients have both SLE and CAH, but these can be identified by biopsies of the liver and other organs, such as the kidney. Patients with SLE may have biopsy findings consistent with CPH, but CAH is not part of the spectrum of SLE liver involvement, and the liver vasculature is usually spared from the vasculitis. In the original series of patients with SLE, patients with immunologic CAH were included because of confusion over the meaning of a positive LE cell test.[11] It was formerly thought that anti-smooth muscle antibody was a nonspecific antibody, but recent studies have demonstrated that it is specifically directed against the actin present in the hepatocyte microfilament system.[12] These antibodies have been identified in acute and chronic viral hepatitis in low titers but are virtually diagnostic of immunologic CAH when present in high titers of greater than 1 : 320.

Primary Biliary Cirrhosis

Primary biliary cirrhosis presents diagnostic difficulties in separation from patients with immunologic CAH who have prominent cholestatic features. In addition, the antimicrosomal antibody, which is positive in 96% of patients with primary biliary cirrhosis, is positive in a small proportion of patients with CAH, hence is not a distinguishing feature. The immunologic and histologic boundaries between CAH and primary biliary cirrhosis are blurred in about 15% of patients with these conditions. The final separating test for diagnostic purposes is a therapeutic trial of corticosteroids and azathioprine. By definition, patients with CAH respond to treatment, while those with primary biliary cirrhosis do not.[13] Although this involves somewhat circular reasoning, it does provide the best available method of separation and is a practical means of proceeding with management. Piecemeal necrosis is a feature of primary biliary cirrhosis that occurs in response to patchy bile duct obstruction by inflammation and obliteration. The cirrhosis that develops more closely resembles secondary biliary cirrhosis, which develops behind a bile duct stricture, than it is related to CAH.

Primary Sclerosing Cholangitis

Because of its close association with inflammatory bowel disease, primary sclerosing cholangitis is seldom difficult to separate from CAH. The biopsy picture is now well-known and does not include piecemeal necrosis. Moreover, the cholangiogram obtained by endoscopic retrograde cholangiopancreatography is diagnostic. However, a few patients have a normal cholangiogram and have a variant of primary sclerosing cholangitis termed intrahepatic small duct sclerosing cholangitis.[14] Since the primary sclerosing cholangitis process is patchy, the diagnostic lesions may be missed on liver biopsy, leaving the diagnosis cholestasis of unknown etiology. Since piecemeal necrosis is not a part of primary sclerosing cholangitis, and since the anti-smooth muscle and antimitochondrial antibodies are not present, a diagnosis of CAH is not entertained. However, a few patients with ulcerative colitis have true CAH, noted especially with fivefold elevations of aminotransferases.[14]

REFERENCES

1. Weiss JS, Gautam A, Lauff JJ, et al: The clinical importance of a protein-bound fraction of serum bilirubin in patients with hyperbilirubinemia. *N Engl J Med* **309**:147–150, 1983.
2. Black M, Billing BH: Hepatic bilirubin UDP-glucuronyl transferase activity in liver disease and Gilbert's syndrome. *N Engl J Med* **280**:1266–1271, 1969.
3. Greenfield SM, Soloway RD, Carithers RL Jr, et al: Evaluation of post-prandial serum bile acid response as a test of liver function. *Dig Dis Sci* **31**:785–791, 1986.
4. Koretz RL, Stone O, Gitnick GL: The long-term course of non A, non B post-transfusion hepatitis. *Gastroenterology* **79**:893–898, 1980.
5. Sternlieb I, Scheinberg IH: Wilson's disease, in Wright R, Alberti KGMM, Karran S, Millward-Sadler GH (eds): *Liver and Biliary Disease*. WB Saunders, Philadelphia, 1979, pp. 774–787.
6. Cartwright GE, Lodges RE, Gubler CJ, et al: Studies on copper metabolism. XIII. Hepatolenticular degeneration. *J Clin Invest* **33**:1487–1501, 1954.
7. Powell LW: Hemochromatosis and related iron storage diseases, in Wright R, Alberti KGMM, Karran S, Millward-Sadler GH (eds): *Liver and Biliary Disease*. WB Saunders, Philadelphia, 1979, pp. 788–804.
8. Triger DR, Millward-Sadler GH: Alpha-1-antitrypsin deficiency and liver disease, in Wright RS, Alberti KGMM, Karran S, Millward-Sadler GH (eds): *Liver and Biliary Disease*. WB Saunders, Philadelphia, 1979, pp. 805–821.
9. Czaja AJ, Davis GL, Ludwig J, et al: Autoimmune features as determinants of prognosis in steroid-treated chronic active hepatitis of uncertain etiology. *Gastroenterology* **85**:713–717, 1983.
10. Gurian LE, Rogoff TM, Ware AJ, et al: The immunologic diagnosis of chronic active "autoimmune" hepatitis: Distinction from systemic lupus erythematosus. *Hepatology* **5**:397–402, 1985.
11. Harvey AM, Shulman LE, Tumulty PA, et al: Systemic lupus erythematosus: Review of the literature and clinical analysis of 138 cases. *Medicine (Baltimore)* **33**:291–437, 1954.
12. Lidman K, Biberfeld G, Fagraeus A, et al: Anti-actin specificity of human smooth muscle antibodies in chronic active hepatitis. *Clin Exp Immunol* **24**:266–272, 1976.

13. Geubel AP, Baggenstoss AH, Summerskill WHJ: Responses to treatment can differentiate chronic active liver disease with cholangiolitic features from the primary biliary cirrhosis syndrome. *Gastroenterology* **71**:444–449, 1976.
14. Linder KD, Wiesner RH, LaRusso NF, Dickson ER: Chronic active hepatitis: Overlap with primary biliary cirrhosis and primary sclerosing cholangitis, in Czaja AJ, Dickson ER (eds): *Chronic Active Hepatitis: The Mayo Clinic Experience.* Dekker, New York, 1986, pp. 171–188.

Chronic Active Hepatitis
Management

ROGER D. SOLOWAY

INTRODUCTION AND PERSPECTIVE

When the first reports of resolution of severe chronic active hepatitis (CAH) in response to prednisone with or without imuran were published 17 years ago,[1-3] enthusiasm was high because this described the first medical regimens that gastroenterologists could employ to alter the course of liver disease in a large group of patients. Before this, only supportive therapy was available except for the removal of alcohol in patients with alcoholic liver disease and the use of *d*-penicillamine in the treatment of Wilson's disease.[4] However, as with most advances in therapy, time has tempered enthusiasm, and experience has further defined and restricted the proportion of patients in whom treatment with prednisone and imuran are appropriate. The initiation of treatment for this condition was important from several respects: (1) the results demonstrated that the natural history of chronic liver disease could be altered, and (2) success stimulated research interest in this area.

I am a therapeutic enthusiast, but I have gradually become more conservative over time as more information has become available. My enthusiasm has been in contrast to the stance of most investigators and clinicians involved in the treatment of CAH who have been reluctant to treat until studies support that decision. My aggressiveness stems from a long-standing belief that a significant number of patients progress to cirrhosis, in the absence of symptoms; the clinician must make an aggressive attempt to prevent this process. This approach requires the use of liver biopsy, even in patients with either asymptomatic dis-

ROGER D. SOLOWAY • Department of Medicine, University of Texas Medical Branch, Galveston, Texas 77550-2778.

ease or mild biochemical abnormalities, or both, once the 6-month criterion for duration of biochemical abnormality has been met. An initial liver biopsy provides the baseline against which subsequent liver biopsies can be evaluated objectively for progression. This is true even with the knowledge that serial biopsies have been found to be accurate for the degree of chronic active hepatitis but provide low accuracy for the presence or extent of cirrhosis.[5,6] Because of the inaccuracy of detection of cirrhosis, I recommend laparoscopic examination, in selected patients, in determining the site for percutaneous needle biopsy as well as the extent of cirrhosis. Once the extent of disease has been determined, the course of follow-up and management for the patient can be outlined and the prognosis established with greater objectivity.

This chapter reviews the current indications, limitations, and consequences of treatment for various forms of CAH and suggests areas in which advances might be made. Finally, areas are pointed out in which treatment questions remain and some ways in which these questions might be addressed.

CHRONIC PERSISTENT HEPATITIS

Once the diagnosis of chronic persistent hepatitis (CPH) has been established by liver biopsy, the patient can be reassured that the condition is compatible with no change in life expectancy and can be monitored periodically by blood studies. Such patients should have normal liver blood studies except for transaminase[7]; if periodic monitoring (once each year) demonstrates abnormalities, especially a decrease in albumin, a repeat liver biopsy should be considered. I have also monitored my patients with periodic fasting and postprandial levels of serum bile acids[8] and with the indocyanine dye excretion test,[9] as a more sensitive means of assessing changes in liver function, and have observed changes in these tests before observing changes in traditional liver blood studies.

Occasionally, patients with CPH will complain of severe incapacitating. fatigue. The characteristic story is that they feel reasonably well on arising but rapidly tire with effort. Some patients have found that resting for several hours enables them to continue their duties for the remainder of the day. Some patients may sleep 10–12 hr each day. This pattern of fatigue distinguishes it from depression or malingering. This type of fatigue is characteristic of liver disease but is unpredictable in its occurrence from patient to patient, and its occurrence is not correlated with the severity of the condition. However, in individual cases, recurrence of fatigue may signal the recrudescence of hepatitis. Since most forms of hepatitis have a waxing and waning history, recurrence of this symptom may be a helpful signal. In the setting of incapacitating chronic fatigue, when temporizing measures have failed, I have empirically used prednisone 5–10 mg/day for periods of 3–6 months with relief of the fatigue in some patients. Such treatment must be initiated with the plan to discontinue it, if there has been no subjective response during that period.

AUTOIMMUNE CHRONIC ACTIVE HEPATITIS

Periportal Hepatitis (Mild Chronic Active Hepatitis)

Although patients with mild CAH were initially included in the first trials of treatment,[2] long-term results brought into question whether these patients need treatment at all or whether the natural history of this part of the spectrum of CAH more resembles that of chronic persistent hepatitis.[10] Although I initially treated these patients, as the natural history of this portion of the CAH spectrum has become known, I have felt comfortable in close observation of these patients with periodic monitoring biopsies. If several biopsies show no progression, I have advised that no treatment should be initiated and further biopsies need not be undertaken unless there is some change in one of the monitoring blood studies apart from the aminotransferases, which may fluctuate. Thus, the management of nonprogressive periportal hepatitis is identical to that of CPH and treatment is only initiated in those uncommon cases in which fatigue is incapacitating. I initiate treatment in this condition when serial biopsies demonstrate progressive disease, even in the absence of symptoms. In such patients, the concern is the silent progression to cirrhosis. I have considered it better to treat if in doubt about progression. Such patients are most likely to respond to therapy quickly,[11] making the length of treatment short and maintaining remission with azathioprine,[12] for good long-term management.

Moderate and Severe Chronic Active Hepatitis (Periportal Hepatitis with Bridging or Multilobular Necrosis)

For patients with these histologic lesions and significant biochemical activity indicated by a 10-fold rise in aminotransferase or a fivefold rise in aminotransferase coupled with a twofold rise in gammaglobulin, the original arbitrary therapeutic suggestions of prednisone or imuran, or both,[2] still are recommended.[13]

Prednisone

The recommended regimen for patients below age 40, or for whom childbearing is still a possibility, is prednisone 60 mg/day tapered to 20 mg after 1 month and maintained until histologic remission is achieved.[2] For patients above age 40, or in whom prednisone alone has not been successful, a regimen of prednisone 30 mg/day tapered to 10 mg after 1 month and maintained together with azathioprine 50 mg/day[13] is recommended because of its decreased toxicity. In my uncontrolled experience in patients with diabetes mellitus or psychiatric manifestations attributable to steroids, prednisone 5–10 mg/day has been well tolerated and, in combination with azathioprine, has been effective treatment for CAH. Others have used low-dose steroids without the initial loading dose with success in a group of patients with variable severity.[1] Alternate-day prednisone was used in one study with a success rate better than that of the control group but significantly less than the group taking prednisone and azathioprine.[14] However, the method for testing the alternate-day program, abrupt discontinuation with raising the dose in relationship to symptoms, was counter to those studies that demonstrate a beneficial effect of this program in other diseases. The recommended regimen is to maintain the previous dose, doubling the dose on the alternate day, and then gradually tapering and eliminating the lower dose followed by a tapering of the remaining increased alternate-day dose. This program proceeds on the unproved theory that it may be effective in maintaining suppression while not inducing remission. This remains a reasonable alternative since steroid side effects are unlikely to arise during the first 3 months of treatment.

Azathioprine

In doses of 50–100 mg/day, azathioprine is tolerated without the usual side effects of leukopenia or thrombocytopenia. These side effects may be difficult to assess when hypersplenism is present, but the initial blood counts and the development of splenomegaly and signs of portal hypertension may help clarify the situation. If necessary, the dose can be reduced and the response of white blood cells and platelets monitored.

Treatment Failures

When disease is progressive and unresponsive to standard regimens, most patients will respond to 60 mg prednisone coupled with 150 mg azathioprine until a biochemical response is achieved.[15] In the Mayo group, 20% of patients were in this category. Institution of this regimen reduced mortality in this subgroup from 75% to less than 20%.[15] Such patients may never be able to achieve a histologic remission and may require such doses for years.[15] In this situation, pulse doses of prednisone, administered every several weeks, may also bring the disease under control, when other measures have failed. I have treated a young girl with aminotransferase levels of more than 1200 for 18 months despite continued treatment with 60 mg prednisone with pulse doses of 250 mg prednisone every 2 weeks with reduction of her aminotransferase to the 150–200 U range.

The course of pulse doses had to be stopped because of the development of significant anxiety and fatigue. With the advent of liver transplantation, such therapy with its side effects and hazards of infection must be balanced against the risks of transplantation. The physician caring for such patients must make the decision for transplantation when the risks of further treatment outweigh the risks of transplantation. This is an individual decision that is difficult to make but, if the patient is becoming more fatigued or losing muscle mass or the complications of advanced liver disease such as ascites or encephalopathy progress, the decision to opt for transplantation should be made.

Maintenance of Histologic Remission

It is now well-known that once remission is attained, stopping azathioprine and tapering prednisone over a 6-week period results in a 50% relapse rate within 6 months.[10,13] Patients were then destined to a series of treatment cycles with increased risk for steroid toxicity due to cumulative steroid exposure. Recently, a new approach was reported from the United Kingdom that greatly reduced the relapse rate. The prednisone was gradually tapered and the azathioprine was maintained for years thereafter.[12] My personal experience supports this method, and it should now be considered the procedure of choice for tapering medication. I have also had success with gradual institution over months of alternate-day prednisone in this same situation. The advantage of these regimens is that the disease remains suppressed while steroid side effects are minimized or eliminated. These observations suggest that the original Mayo Clinic protocol for the cessation of treatment was too short and that drugs and regimens that may not induce remission are capable of maintaining it once it has been achieved.

CAH with Less Biochemical Severity

No controlled study has addressed the question of whether those patients with disease of less biochemical activity require the same type or intensity of treatment. Since the Mayo Clinic studies continued to require disease of the original significant activity for admission, their results cannot address this question. In the absence of data, individual conclusions made by treating physicians must suffice. Since I have concluded that the pattern on biopsy is the basis for estimation of severity, I treat such patients with a regimen identical to that suggested for CAH with greater biochemical activity. The decision for or against treatment needs to be made frequently by the gastroenterologist because studies[16] have indicated that 95% of patients with CAH, even in large university referral centers, either do not fulfill the criteria for biochemical activity required by the Mayo Clinic studies or are clearly viral in origin. A recent uncontrolled report indicates that the course of CAH without cirrhosis was benign, even if untreated, while CAH with cirrhosis was a condition necessitating treatment.[17] The accompanying editorial[18] indicated that studies had demonstrated differing results.

Drug- or Alcohol-Induced CAH

It is has been known for decades that removal of alcohol leads to a prompt improvement in most cases of alcoholic liver disease. A few patients with non-alcoholic CAH have Mallory's hyaline, confusing interpretation, and there has been a report of alcoholic liver disease presenting as CAH.[19] Using the same approach, it is been suggested and now widely adopted that prompt discontinuation of drugs causing CAH causes a rapid symptomatic, biochemical, and histologic improvement without other therapy.[20] This unique response is both therapeutic and diagnostic.

Wilson's Disease

Wilson's disease may present with a clinical picture indistinguishable from immunologic CAH. It is very important to identify this condition so that patients can be treated with specific therapy, d-penicillamine.[4] Immunosuppressive treatment is not effective in this condition.

α_1-Antitrypsin Deficiency

It is clear that the homozygous condition may result in cirrhosis for which there is no known treatment. If a heterozygous protein inhibitor (π-type) phenotype is present with some PAS-positive diastase-resistant granules present on liver biopsy, the relationship to a concomitant CAH is unclear. Such patients should undergo a trial of treatment if they meet the criteria outlined above for autoimmune CAH.[21] Patients with progressive disease unresponsive to treatment are candidates for liver transplantation.

Primary Biliary Cirrhosis

The distinction between CAH and primary biliary cirrhosis cannot be decided on clinical, biochemical, immunological or histological grounds in about 15% of patients with CAH, since a proportion of patients with CAH present with predominant cholestatic features. In this setting, a therapeutic trial of standard treatment for CAH is the abitrary method used to separate the two conditions. Patients with CAH respond to treatment while patients with primary biliary cirrhosis are unresponsive.[22] If such a treatment trial is undertaken, one must decide beforehand to discontinue it if there is no response in 6 months, since the most likely candidates for steroid toxicity are women above age 40 with a chronic elevation of serum bilirubin and a decreased level of albumin.[23]

Hepatitis B Chronic Active Hepatitis

Only about 10% of patients with hepatitis B develop CAH but, when present, it is more severe and progressive than Non-A, Non-B CAH. In a series from Rotterdam,[24] only 5% of patients with HB_sAg-positive CAH met the Mayo Clinic treatment criteria.[2] When examined in retrospect, 22 patients with hepatitis B CAH had been entered into the Mayo Clinic studies. Although corticosteroids have been shown to enhance short-term survival and induce remission in CAH in general, these end points were less frequently achieved in patients with hepatitis B. Histologic remission was 15% versus 68% in HB_sAg-negative CAH, while treatment failure was 54% versus 16% in HB_sAg-negative CAH.[25] This increased rate of failure occurred when doses of prednisone were reduced to conventional levels (10–20 mg/day) and responded to increased prednisone dosage.[25] During treatment lasting as long as 8 years, no effect of treatment on the level of HBV replication, as measured by the levels of HB_cAg, was detected. However, there was a lower than expected seroconversion rate from HB_eAg to anti-HB_e.[25] It has been shown that patients treated with steroids have an increased proportion of hepatocytes infected with HBV when liver biopsies are examined.[26] At present there is no enthusiasm for long-term corticosteroids in these patients due to the negative results of 3 separate series.[27-29] Norton Greenberger[29] recently stated that "most gastroenterologists believe that steroids are not indicated in the routine management" of hepatitis B CAH. I do not believe that the role of prednisone has been fully defined. There may be subpopulations of patients with hepatitis B that may be suitable candidates for steroid treatment alone or with azathioprine.

Steroids remain an option in clinical trials in combination with antiviral agents. They are being employed in short courses in an effort to activate the disease following acute steroid withdrawal so that treatment with antiviral agents such as interferon may become more effective.[30] Steroids may be useful alone when used in a short course (10 weeks) and then withdrawn rapidly.[30,31] Patients with mild disease appear to have little problem with this program, even if enzymes peak following withdrawal.[30] However, this procedure is hazardous in patients with advanced disease who may severely decompensate transiently[31] or who may occasionally die. In one study, 14 of 16 patients (87.5%) became persistently negative for HBV DNA, and 10 patients who were positive for HB_eAg became negative. Five of these patients became anti-HB_e positive. In controls, only 3 of 15 became negative for HBV DNA and none seroconverted their HB_eAg status during a 1-year follow-up.[31]

When HB_eAg converts to anti-HB_e, cirrhosis has been believed to have been developed, and hepatitis becomes quiescent. This is not true in all such patients. In one series from Italy,[26] 24% of patients with anti-HB_e had circulating HBV DNA. CAH was present in 19 of 20 patients, and 4 of 6 patients with cirrhosis had "active" cirrhosis. These patients assemble HB_cAg in the hepatocyte cytoplasm rather than in the nucleus.

A series of studies have examined the effects of interferons from various sources alone or in combination with arabinose monophosphate (ara MP), and the results have been marginally in favor of a beneficial effect, but side effects have been significant. However, decreased doses of interferon may be as effective and have less toxicity. These doses are currently being employed in ongoing studies. Patients with progressive HB_sAg CAH should be referred to centers conducting treatment trials, so that the most efficacious program can be determined as quickly as possible.

Patients with HB_sAg have come to transplantation, if they are negative for HIV, the immunodeficiency virus. Unfortunately, since HBV may be present in areas other than the liver, the new graft is frequently eventually infected with the virus despite administration of HBV vaccine.

Hepatitis D Chronic Active Hepatitis

Studies indicate that this incomplete RNA virus, which depends on the presence of hepatitis B for its expression, since excess HB_sAg forms its outer coat, is not a new virus. Retrospective studies of banked sera have indicated that it has been present for at least 20–25 years in the United States.[32] However, its influence on the course of hepatitis B in the United States is incompletely known. No results of treatment of CAH patients with both the hepatitis B and D viruses have been published.

Non-A, Non-B (NANB) Chronic Active Hepatitis

This type of hepatitis is defined as following an episode of acute hepatitis that in turn followed an episode of transfusion by the appropriate interval. As many as 50% of patients with acute NANB hepatitis may develop CAH following acute hepatitis, which may progress to cirrhosis.[33,34] This condition has progressed slowly in most cases. However, in cases in which progressive disease has been documented by serial biopsy, empirical treatment with steroids or steroids and azathioprine have been instituted and have produced a low rate of success. Recently, hope has been renewed for specific treatment for this condition, following the report[35] that 10 male patients with NANB CAH with elevations of aminotransferase for a mean of 6 years had responded to subcutaneous injections of recombinant human α-interferon. Within 1–4 weeks, sustained decreases occurred in eight patients. Two patients showed a rise in aminotransferase after treatment was discontinued and had a second biochemical remission after treatment was reinstituted. Three patients who underwent liver biopsy demonstrated a marked decrease in necrosis and inflammation. Most patients were free of side effects when the dose was decreased to 1 million units three times weekly. This rapid improvement is in contrast to the slow response in hepatitis B CAH and suggests to Hoofnagle et al.[35] that the disease process in NANB is due to direct cell injury in contrast to HB CAH, which is thought to be mediated through immune mechanisms.

Nonspecific Chronic Active Hepatitis

The nomenclature of CAH is becoming increasingly complex as we gain more knowledge, but it is important to separate the known from the unknown. This is not served well by lumping all patients who do not have specific viral or immunological markers into a NANB category, encompassing both viral and nonviral etiologies. This type of categorization impedes definition of both the natural history and response to treatment. I believe that in cases in which markers may have cleared with the development of a less active phase of the disease or that have never had markers present, in whom no clear-cut history of previous viral or posttransfusion hepatitis is present, the designation should be nonspecific hepatitis so that no etiology is implied. The plan of treatment for this group is unclear, but a number of these patients have already been given therapy in treatment trials.[13–15,22] When severe disease is present, such patients appear to respond to therapy similarly to patients with immunologic CAH.[36,37] Studies have not been performed in patients with mild to moderate disease. However, the recommendations made above for immunologic CAH would appear to be the practical approach, until data become available, i.e., treat patients with progressive disease and those with bridging or multilobular necrosis, since their chance of progression to cirrhosis is significant.

MANAGEMENT WITHOUT BIOPSY

Rarely, patients are first seen whose clotting studies are too prolonged to allow percutaneous liver biopsy. It was determined early in the course of the Mayo Clinic studies that such patients be treated for CAH, provided markers for viral hepatitis were not present. Although the response rate was low because of the advanced nature of their disease, such patients always had CAH when biopsied later after improvement or evaluation at autopsy.[38]

REFERENCES

1. Cook GC, Mulligan, Sherlock S: Controlled prospective trial of corticosteroid therapy in active chronic hepatitis. *QJ Med* **158**:159–185, 1971.
2. Soloway RD, Summerskill WHJ, Baggenstoss AH, et al: Clinical, biochemical, and histological remission of severe chronic active liver disease: A controlled study of treatments and early prognosis. *Gastroenterology* **63**:820–833, 1972.
3. Murray-Lyon IM, Stern RB, Williams R: Controlled trial of prednisone and azathioprine in active chronic hepatitis. *Lancet* **1**:735–737, 1973.
4. Sternlieb I, Scheinberg IH: Wilson's disease, in Wright R, Alberti KGMM, Karran S, Millward-Sadler GH (eds): *Liver and Biliary Disease*. WB Saunders, Philadelphia, 1979, pp. 774–787.
5. Scheuer PJ: Liver biopsy in the diagnosis of cirrhosis. *Gut* **11**:275–278, 1970.
6. Soloway RD, Baggenstoss AH, Schoenfield LJ, Summerskill WHJ: Observer error and sampling variability tested in evaluation of hepatitis and cirrhosis by liver biopsy. *Am J Dig Dis* **16**:1082–1086, 1971.
7. Becker MD, Scheuer PJ, Baptista A, Sherlock S: Prognosis of chronic persistent hepatitis. *Lancet* **1**:53–57, 1971.
8. Greenfield SM, Soloway RD, Carithers RL Jr, et al: Evaluation of post prandial serum bile acid response as a test of liver function. *Dig Dis Sci* **31**:785–791, 1986.
9. Leevy CM, Smith F, Longueville J, et al: Indocyanine green clearance as a test of hepatic function. *JAMA* **200**:236–240, 1967.
10. Czaja AJ, Ammon HV, Summerskill WHJ: Clinical features and prognosis of severe chronic active liver disease (CALD) after corticosteroid-induced remission. *Gastroenterology* **78**:518–523, 1980.
11. Czaja AJ, Ammon HV, Summerskill WHJ: Clinical features and prognosis of severe chronic active liver disease (CALD) after corticosteroid-induced remission. *Gastroenterology* **78**:518–523, 1980.
12. Stellon AJ, Hegarty JE, Portmann B, Williams R: Randomised controlled trial of azathioprine withdrawal in autoimmune chronic active hepatitis. *Lancet* **1**:668–670, 1985.
13. Ammon HV: Assessment of treatment regimens, in Czaja AJ, Dickson ER (eds): *Chronic Active Hepatitis: The Mayo Clinic Experience*. Dekker, New York, 1986, pp. 33–46.
14. Summerskill WHJ, Korman MG, Ammon HV, Baggenstoss AH: Prednisone for chronic active liver disease: Dose titration, standard dose, and combination with azathioprine. *Gut* **16**:876–883, 1975.
15. Schalm SW, Ammon HV, Summerskill WHJ: Failure of customary treatment in chronic active liver disease: Causes and management. *Ann Clin Res* **8**:221–227, 1976.
16. Koretz RL, Lewin KF, Higgins J, et al: Chronic active hepatitis: Who meets treatment criteria? *Dig Dis Sci* **25**:695–699, 1980.
17. Graham W, Cooksley E, Bradbear RA, et al: The prognosis of chronic active hepatitis without cirrhosis in relation to bridging necrosis. *Hepatology* **6**:345–348, 1986.
18. Combes B: The initial morphologic lesion in chronic hepatitis: Important or unimportant. (Editorial.) *Hepatology* **6**:518–522, 1986.
19. Galambos JT: Natural history of alcoholic hepatitis. III. Histological changes. *Gastroenterology* **63**:1026–1035, 1972.
20. Maddrey WC, Boitnott JK: Drug-induced chronic liver disease. *Gastroenterology* **72**:1348–1353, 1977.
21. Ludwig J: Morphology of chronic active hepatitis: Differential diagnosis and therapeutic implications, in Czaja AJ, Dickson ER (eds): *Chronic Active Hepatitis: The Mayo Clinic Experience*. Dekker, New York, 1986, pp. 83–104.
22. Geubel AP, Baggenstoss AH, Summerskill WHJ: Responses to treatment can differentiate

chronic active liver disease with cholangiolitic features from the primary biliary cirrhosis syndrome. *Gastroenterology* **71**:444–449, 1976.

23. Uribe M, Go VLW: Prednisone pharmacokinetics and toxicity in chronic active liver disease and health, in Czaja AJ, Dickson ER (eds): *Chronic Active Hepatitis: The Mayo Clinic Experience.* Dekker, New York, 1986, pp. 47–69.

24. Schalm SW, Blankenstein M, Heijtink RA: Mortality and morbidity of chronic hepatitis B infection. *Neth J Med* **26**:205, 1983, (abst).

25. Schalm SW, Davis GL, Shiels MT: Chronic active hepatitis type B, in Czaja AJ, Dickson ER (eds): *Chronic Active Hepatitis: The Mayo Clinic Experience.* Dekker, New York, 1986, pp. 47–69.

26. Giusti G, Ruggiero G, Galanti B, et al: Treatment of chronic active hepatitis: A retrospective review of 130 patients. *Hepatogastroenterology* **28**:245–249, 1981.

27. Tsuji T, Naito K, Tokuyama K, et al: Follow-up two years after corticosteroid therapy for chronic active hepatitis type B. *Hepatogastroenterology* **27**:85–90, 1980.

28. European Association for the Study of Liver Diseases: A multicenter randomized clinical trial of low-dose steroid treatment in chronic active HBsAg position liver disease. *Gastroenterology* **86**:1317, 1984 (abst).

29. Greenberger NJ: Editorial comment, in Greenberger NJ, Moody FG (eds): *The Year Book of Digestive Diseases 1987.* Year Book Medical, Chicago, 1987, pp. 273.

30. Perrillo RP, Regenstern FG: Corticosteroid therapy for chronic active hepatitis B: Is a little too much? *Hepatology* **6**:1416–1418, 1986.

31. Nair PV, Tong MJ, Stevenson D, et al: A pilot study on the effects of prednisone withdrawal on serum hepatitis B virus DNA and HB$_e$Ag in chronic active hepatitis B. *Hepatology* **6**:1319–1324, 1986.

32. De Cock KM, Govindarajan IS, Chin KP, Redeker AG: Delta hepatitis in the Los Angeles area: A report of 126 cases. *Ann Intern Med* **105**:108–114, 1986.

33. Koretz RL, Suffin SC, Gitnick GL: Post-transfusion chronic liver disease. *Gastroenterology* **71**:797–803, 1976.

34. Koretz RL, Stone O, Mousa M, Gitnick GL: Non-A, non-B post-transfusion hepatitis—A decade later. *Gastroenterology* **88**:1251–1254, 1985.

35. Hoofnagle JH, Mullen KD, Jones DB, et al: Treatment of chronic non-A, non-B hepatitis with recombinant human alpha interferon: A preliminary report. *N Engl J Med* **315**:1575–1578, 1986.

36. Soloway RD, Summerskill WHJ, Baggenstoss AH, Schoenfield LJ: "Lupoid" hepatitis, a nonentity in the spectrum of chronic active liver disease. *Gastroenterology* **63**:458–465, 1972.

37. Czaja AJ, Davis GL, Ludwig J, et al: Autoimmune features as determinants of prognosis in steroid-treated chronic active hepatitis of uncertain etiology. *Gastroenterology* **85**:713–717, 1983.

38. Soloway RD, Summerskill WHJ, Baggenstoss AH, et al: Clinical, biochemical and histological remission of severe chronic active liver disease: A controlled study of treatments and early prognosis. *Gastroenterology* **63**:1820–1833, 1972.

Chronic Active Hepatitis
Prognosis

ROGER D. SOLOWAY

INTRODUCTION

The outline of this chapter will follow the format on the chapter on treatment so that sections can be easily compared. Therefore, I will try to avoid duplication of information and will proceed on the assumption that the reader will refer to the treatment chapter if questions concerning terminology arise. This chapter will contain only a limited number of references since only a portion of the natural history of many of these conditions is known and the natural history continues to evolve. Much of what is said here is based on personal experience and the biases which derive from it.

CHRONIC PERSISTENT HEPATITIS

Chronic Portal and Lobular Hepatitis

The chapter on treatment described the approach to the histologic sub-categories of chronic persistent hepatitis (CPH), but the end result is that the prognosis is the same. Almost all patients have a benign prognosis, and the condition will either persist for years or perhaps for the patient's unaltered life span. The reason that we do not know whether this condition can persist for a patient's entire life is that blood has not been banked for long enough to determine this. The observation that hepatitis B CPH has persisted for more than 14

ROGER D. SOLOWAY • Department of Medicine, University of Texas Medical Branch, Galveston, Texas 77550-2778.

years on the basis of a review of stored sera,[1] suggests that the disease can continue indefinitely without shortening life expectancy. Reports of CPH becoming uncommonly progressive are alluded to in the literature.[2,3]

Patients with nonviral disease may have a condition compatible with a normal life expectancy. This may not be true for patients in whom CPH is due to viruses, since there may be some incidence of hepatocellular carcinoma.[4] We do not have sufficient evidence to estimate the frequency of this occurrence, since there appears to be a 30- to 40-year latency in the development of hepatocellular carcinoma following chronic acute hepatitis (CAH) and cirrhosis in populations in whom there is a 100% perinatal infection rate.[5,6] A large group of patients with CPH type B acquired later in life have not been followed in the United States for a sufficiently long enough period to make this decision. There appears to be a difference in the natural history of chronic hepatitis B virus (HBV) disease acquired during the neonatal period and that contracted in adult life.

Inactive Periportal Hepatitis

If possible, CPH following inactivation of CAH, must be identified histologically and separated from CPH without any such antecedent disease, since CAH in remission (inactive CAH) may have as much as a 50% chance of relapse after discontinuation of treatment.[7,8] We do not know whether disease that undergoes a spontaneous remission has a similar rate of relapse. From studies of the natural history of severe CAH, about 20% of patients develop a spontaneous remission.[9] Such patients may have histologic tell-tale signs of past CAH such as the presence of inactive scars of bridging or multilobular necrosis or an expanded portal tract indicating previous periportal hepatitis (CAH). Now that alternative forms of discontinuing therapy have been introduced,[10] the prognosis of this lesion developing after successful treatment may change and patients may have a more benign course with fewer relapses.

CHRONIC ACTIVE HEPATITIS

Periportal Hepatitis

Mild CAH

As information concerning the natural history of CAH has evolved, it has become clear that the prognosis of CAH without bridging or multilobular necrosis (so-called mild CAH) may be more benign than CAH with these lesions. However, recent studies[11,12] and the accompanying editorial[13] indicate that controversy concerning the prognosis of this lesion still exists. Most physicians believe that patients with periportal hepatitis are very likely to have non-progressive disease, but some studies suggest that a proportion of these patients may progress to cirrhosis.[3] Moreover, identification of those patients who will progress is uncertain based on the initial biopsy.[11–13] For the present, a reasonable course is to undertake two or three biopsies over a period of years to assess whether the disease is progressing. If the severity of the hepatitis is unchanged, such patients may be followed by their biochemical course. If doubt remains, further biopsies may be taken or a laparoscopy may be performed to look for cirrhosis or to determine whether there is an area of the liver to biopsy that is likely to show greater involvement. The prognosis of patients with this lesion may vary from excellent (because the disease will not progress) to guarded (because progressive disease is developing that will eventuate in cirrhosis).

Periportal Hepatitis with Bridging and/or Multilobular Necrosis Moderate to Severe CAH

Disease of this severity presents a spectrum of increased risks for the development of cirrhosis dependent on its etiology and on as yet poorly defined host factors.

Resolving Viral Hepatitis. If the liver biopsy has been taken during the course of a slowly resolving acute viral hepatitis, the elements of the histologic picture that in a chronic setting would be considered poor prognostic features are likely to resolve completely, leaving the patient with postnecrotic scarring where lobular collapse has occurred. In these cases, the overall hepatic architecture is largely intact, and cirrhosis will probably not develop. Even if mild cirrhosis develops, the process usually will not result in the development of portal hypertension.

Drug Hepatitis. Characteristically, if the hepatitis is attributable to medications or alcohol, removal of the agent almost always arrests the process and complete healing occurs. If the process has continued undetected for an extended period, cirrhosis can develop, but this is quite rare. Since the particular drug is the enciting agent, its removal means that the process can be completely arrested. This is unique, because the causative agent cannot be removed in a similar manner for either viral or immunologic disease. There are case reports of continuing progressive disease despite withdrawal of the agent, such as alcohol.[14] However, no absolute proof can be provided to show that the drug that was removed was the primary cause of the process or simply a contributing factor. This is because there is no certain way to know that a given drug has caused a hepatitis except if a complete and rapid cure occurs within weeks after drug withdrawal.

Viral Hepatitis. The prognosis for CAH due to viral disease varies with the causative agent. Once CAH of moderate or greater severity develops during the course of chronic hepatitis B, the course is more rapid and more clinically severe than in CAH due to the Non-A, Non-B viruses. Fortunately, this course develops on only 10% of patients with hepatitis B,[15,16] while it develops in 50% of patients with Non-A, Non-B hepatitis.[17-19] Untreated, the natural history of these diseases is that infection with the HBV leads to death from terminal liver failure or from the complications of cirrhosis more rapidly than with Non-A, Non-B disease. The long-term effects of antiviral treatments for these conditions is unclear because the trials are only in their earliest stages and we must await follow-up studies, as occurred with the Mayo Clinic studies for immunologic CAH,[12] to determine the actual prognosis. We must also assess the effect of new treatment regimens before, during, and after liver transplantation to determine whether this modality can be applied successfully to advanced viral disease, since early experience has indicated that patients may develop graft infections,[20] as the virus may reside in sites other than the liver.[21,22]

Chronic active hepatitis due to the combination of hepatitis B and D viruses is, in general, more aggressive than with hepatitis B alone[23] (see Chapter 7). However, as this disease has been identified and followed, since testing has become generally available, it is clear that an aggressive course is not always followed.[24,25] What factors account for the different courses in patients infected with the same virus is unknown, but they probably reside in differences in host characteristics on which the viruses depend.

Immunologic Chronic Active Hepatitis. Since a number of treatment programs have been successful in achieving clinical, biochemical, and histologic resolution of immunologic CAH, the prognosis is dependent on the initial features of the hepatitis,[11,12] the presence of cirrhosis,[12] and the success of the treatment program for a given patient. Since treatment programs have now been modified after remission has been accomplished,[10] it may be possible to have a sustained and even permanent remission without developing significant drug toxicity. Most of the reports to date differentiate between the presence and absence of cirrhosis on the initial biopsy. Clearly, the presence of cirrhosis decreases the treatment response rate, increases the time to achieve a remission, and increases the rate of relapse.[8] However, once histologic remission has been achieved, newer regimens should be able to maintain patients without relapse. It is not yet known whether elimination of piecemeal necrosis will prevent continued progression of the cirrhotic process or whether it continues unabated once initiated. However, in some of the late follow-ups in the Mayo Clinic series,[12] progression to cirrhosis occurred in patients who had undergone histologic remission, accompanied in most cases by a biochemical flare. Perhaps if such flares can be prevented, most progression can be prevented. Since 4% of most autopsy series are composed of patients with undetected, so-called latent cirrhosis, not clinically apparent and not contributing to the patient's death, it is possible for the process to arrest at any point. Whether this is the exception or the rule awaits continued long-term follow-up. Intermediate-term follow-up evaluation of patients who have been successfully treated suggests that fewer patients develop the long-term complications of cirrhosis than with untreated disease or in patients with alcoholic cirrhosis. It is not clear whether this is a result of the natural course of this disease or of intervention with treatment. It must be remembered that 20% of controls underwent spontaneous resolution of severe CAH,[9] and some of these patients may have had cirrhosis.

Patients who fail treatment run the risk of steroid toxicity and are therefore excellent candidates for liver transplantation at an early stage in their disease before signs of steroid toxicity occur. This needs to be carefully assessed by physicians involved in a transplantation program; such patients should be followed in conjunction with programs early in their course so that familiarity with the patient over time will permit a reasoned decision concerning transplantation to be made at the appropriate time.

Chronic Active Hepatitis with Cholestatic Features. The prognosis of such patients depends entirely on their response to treatment for CAH.[26] If the patient responds, the prognosis is similar to that of CAH patients without cholestasis. If they do not respond, the prognosis resembles that for primary biliary cirrhosis. Since a number of treatment programs for this condition have now been proposed, we must await the long-term results of these programs to determine whether the natural history of primary biliary cirrhosis will be altered.

Wilson's Disease. Treated before the process reaches the cirrhotic stage, Wilson's disease is completely curable and compatible with a normal life expectancy, provided *d*-penicillamine is taken for the rest of the patient's life.[27] Once cirrhosis has developed, the prognosis is variable and cannot be predicted. However, treatment should not be pursued beyond that which is undertaken for immunologic CAH. That is, the patient should be considered for transplantation when the risk of continued treatment exceeds the risks of the operation. This needs to be an individualized decision made by experienced gastroenterologists and surgeons who have participated in longitudinal follow-up of the patient.

α_1-*Antitrypsin Deficiency.* There is no treatment program directed at α_1-antitrypsin deficiency; therefore, the only resort when the condition is advancing is transplantation. However, it has been suggested that the deficiency has made patients susceptible to other forms of chronic hepatitis.[28] These other forms of CAH should be ruled out and treated, if appropriate, with short courses of medication to see if a remission can be induced. This is especially so when the mixed phenotype condition is present and only a few cells exhibit the periodic acid-Schiff (PAS)-positive, diastase-resistant vacuoles,[29] since it is not known what role this mild degree of deficiency plays in the CAH process: initiating or facilitating.

Nonspecific Hepatitis. It is impossible to predict the prognosis of non-specific hepatitis if, because of lack of markers, one cannot be sure that group of patients is ill secondary to one or many etiologies. For practical purposes, patients should be designated as resembling either immunologic or viral CAH and treated accordingly with steroids and azathioprine or interferon. The same rules apply to the patient in whom cirrhosis has intervened. It is our hope that future studies will delineate the causes of CAH in this group of patients so that a more specific approach can be taken for their management.

CIRRHOSIS

All cirrhosis is not equal. Although studies have indicated that cirrhosis is associated with a poorer prognosis in every aspect that has been measured, the severity of the prognosis must vary with the extent of the cirrhosis. Since it has been difficult to grade individual patients accurately as to severity of cirrhosis, we do not have applicable results. Future studies should indicate whether both minimal and advanced disease is associated with a diminished prognosis. Quantitative hepatic function testing may indicate how extensive the cirrhotic process must be before prognosis is altered. Only then can accurate individual predictions be undertaken. Future studies should also address the question of whether fibrosis, leading to portal hypertension and further development of the cirrhotic process continues after treatment induces a complete remission of piecemeal necrosis. If ongoing fibrosis can be measured, we need to differentiate between the effects of development of fibrous septa and sinusoidal fibrosis.

Much progress has been made in the categorization and definition of the natural history of chronic liver disease, making the institution of treatments more appropriate for the individual patient. However, the lack of a definitive message in so many areas in this chapter should indicate that additional data and newer diagnostic methods need to be obtained.

REFERENCES

1. Becker MD, Baptista A, Scheuer PJ, Sherlock S: Prognosis of chronic persistent hepatitis. *Lancet* 1:53–57, 1970.
2. Ludwig J, Czaja AJ, Wolf AM: Prognosis of lobular hepatitis in patients with unresolved viral or chronic hepatitis. *Gastroenterology* 79:1034, 1980 (abst).

3. Dietrichson O: Chronic persistent hepatitis. A clinical, serological and prognostic study. *Scand J Gastroenterol* **10**:249–255, 1975.

4. Liau Y-F, Tai D-I, Chu C-M, et al: Early detection of hepatocellular carcinoma in patients with chronic type B hepatitis. A prospective study. *Gastroenterology* **90**:263–267, 1986.

5. Beasley RP, Hwang L-Y: Hepatocellular carcinoma and hepatitis B virus. *Semin Liver Dis* **4**:113–121, 1984.

6. Kew MC, Marcus R, Geddes EW: Some characteristics of Mocabican Sangaans with primary hepatocellular cancer. *S Afr Med J* **51**:306–309, 1977.

7. Czaja AJ, Ammon HV, Summerskill WHJ: Clinical features and prognosis of severe chronic active liver disease (CALD) after corticosteroid-induced remission. *Gastroenterology* **78**:518–523, 1980.

8. Ammon HV: Assessment of treatment regimens, in Czaja AJ, Dickson ER (eds): *Chronic Active Hepatitis: The Mayo Clinic Experience.* Dekker, New York, 1986, pp. 33–46.

9. Soloway RD, Summerskill WHJ, Baggenstoss AH, et al: Clinical, biochemical, and histological remission of severe chronic active liver disease: A controlled study of treatments and early prognosis. *Gastroenterology* **63**:820–833, 1972.

10. Stellon AJ, Hegarty JE, Portmann B, Williams R: Randomised controlled trial of azathioprine withdrawal in autoimmune chronic active hepatitis. *Lancet* **1**:668–670, 1985.

11. Graham W, Cooksley E, Bradbear RA, et al: The prognosis of chronic active hepatitis without cirrhosis in relation to bridging necrosis. *Hepatology* **6**:345–348, 1986.

12. Davis GL, Czaja AJ, Ludwig J: Development and prognosis of histologic cirrhosis in corticosteroid-treated hepatitis B surface antigen-negative chronic active hepatitis. *Gastroenterology* **87**:1222–1227, 1984.

13. Combes B: The initial morphologic lesion in chronic hepatitis: Important or unimportant. (Editorial.) *Hepatology* **6**:518–522, 1986.

14. Galambos JT: Natural history of alcoholic hepatitis. III. Histological changes. *Gastroenterology* **63**:1026–1035, 1972.

15. Nielson JO, Dietrichson O, Juhl E: Incidence and meaning of the "e" determinant among hepatitis-B-antigen positive patients with acute and chronic liver diseases. *Lancet* **2**:913–915, 1974.

16. Redeker AG: Viral hepatitis: Clinical aspects. *Am J Med Sci* **270**:9–16, 1975.

17. Dienstag JL, Alter JH: Non-A, non-B hepatitis: Evolving epidemiologic and clinical perspective. *Semin Liver Dis* **6**:67–95, 1986.

18. Koretz RL, Suffin SC, Gitnick GL: Post-transfusion chronic liver disease. *Gastroenterology* **71**:797–803, 1976.

19. Koretz RL, Stone O, Mousa M, Gitnick GL: Non-A, non-B post-transfusion hepatitis—A decade later. *Gastroenterology* **88**:1251–1254, 1985.

20. Dusheiko G, Song E, Bowyer S, et al: Natural history of hepatitis B virus infection in renal transplant recipeints—a 15 year follow-up. *Hepatology* **3**:330–336, 1983.

21. Lauchart W, Muller R, Pichlmayr R: Immune prophylaxis of hepatitis B virus reinfection in recipients of human liver allografts. *Transplant Proc* **19**:2387–2389, 1987.

22. Rossi G, Gridelli B, Colledan M, et al: Results of 24 orthotopic liver transplants in Milan. *Transplant Proc* **19**:3832–3834, 1987.

23. Rizzetto M: The delta agent. *Hepatology* **3**:729–737, 1983.

24. Shiels MT, Czaja AJ, Taswell HF, et al: Frequency and significance of delta antibody in acute and chronic hepatitis B: A United States experience. *Gastroenterology* **89**:1230–1234, 1985.

25. De Cock KM, Govindarajan S, Chin KP, Redeker AG: Delta hepatitis in the Los Angeles area: A report of 126 cases. *Ann Intern Med* **105**:108–114, 1986.

26. Geubel AP, Baggenstoss AH, Summerskill WHJ: Responses to treatment can differentiate chronic active liver disease with cholangiolitic features from the primary biliary cirrhosis syndrome. *Gastroenterology* **71**:444–449, 1976.

27. Sternlieb I, Scheinberg IH: Wilson's disease, in Wright R, Alberti KGMM, Karran S, Millward-Sadler GH (eds): *Liver and Biliary Disease*. WB Saunders, Philadelphia, 1979, pp. 774–787.
28. Hodges JR, Millward-Sadler GH, Barbatis C, et al: Heterozygous MZ alpha-1-antitrypsin deficiency in adults with chronic active hepatitis and cryptogenic cirrhosis. *N Engl J Med* **304**:557–560, 1981.
29. Ludwig J: Morphology of chronic active hepatitis: Differential diagnosis and therapeutic implications, in Czaja AJ, Dickson ER (eds): *Chronic Active Hepatitis: The Mayo Clinic Experience*. Dekker, New York, 1986, pp. 83–104.

Index